W9-CCK-573

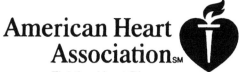

American Heart Associationsm

Fighting Heart Disease and Stroke

Monograph Series

OBESITY:
IMPACT ON CARDIOVASCULAR DISEASE

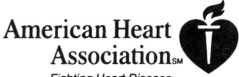

American Heart Association℠

Fighting Heart Disease and Stroke

Monograph Series

OBESITY:
IMPACT ON CARDIOVASCULAR DISEASE

Edited by

Gerald F. Fletcher, MD
Professor of Medicine, Mayo Medical School, Cardiovascular
Division, Mayo Clinic Jacksonville, Jacksonville, Florida

Scott M. Grundy, MD, PhD
Professor of Internal Medicine and Biochemistry Director and Chairman,
Departments of Clinical Nutrition and Internal Medicine,
The Center for Human Nutrition, University of Texas
Southwestern Medical Center at Dallas, Dallas, Texas

Laura L. Hayman, PhD, RN, FAAN
Carl W. and Margaret Davis Walter Professor, Frances Payne Bolton
School of Nursing, Case Western Reserve University,
Cleveland, Ohio

FUTURA

Futura Publishing
Company, Inc.
Armonk, NY

Library of Congress Cataloging-in-Publication Data

Obesity: impact on cardiovascular disease/edited by Gerald
  Fletcher, Scott Grundy, Laura Hayman.
      p.   cm.
    Includes bibliographical references and index.
    ISBN 0-87993-418-2 (hard cover: alk. paper)
    1. Obesity—Complications.   2. Obesity in children—Complications.
  3. Cardiovascular system—Diseases—Risk factors.   4. Cardiovascular
  system—Diseases—Etiology.   5. Obesity—Epidimiology.
  I. Fletcher, Gerald F., 1935– . II. Grundy, Scott M.
  III. Hayman, Laura Lucia.
    [DNLM: 1. Obesity—complications.   2. Cardiovascular Diseases—
  etiology.   3. Exercise Therapy.   WD 210 01214 1999]
  RA645.023024   1999
  616.1'071—dc21
  DNLM/DLC
  for Library of Congress   99-34125
                                                                   CIP

Copyright © 1999
Futura Publishing Company, Inc.

Published by
Futura Publishing Company, Inc.
135 Bedford Road
Armonk, New York 10504

LC #: 98-17362
ISBN #: 0-87993-418-2

Every effort has been made to ensure that the information in this book
is as up to date and accurate as possible at the time of publication.
However, due to the constant developments in medicine, neither the
author, nor the editor, nor the publisher can accept any legal or any
other responsibility for any errors or omissions that may occur.

Printed in the United States of America on acid-free paper.

Contributors

Judith M. Ashley, PhD, RD,   Associate Professor and Associate Director, Nutrition Education and Research Program, University of Nevada School of Medicine, Reno, Nevada

Gerard P. Aurigemma, MD,   Division of Cardiology, University of Massachusetts Medical Center, Worcester, Massachusetts

Michael W. Brands, PhD,   Associate Professor, Department of Physiology and Biophysics and Center for Excellence in Cardiovascular –Renal Research, University of Mississippi Medical Center, Jackson, Mississippi

George A. Bray, MD,   Professor and Executive Director, Pennington Biomedical Research Center, Louisiana State University, Baton Rouge, Louisiana

Lora E. Burke, PhD, MPH, RN,   Postdoctoral Fellow in Cardiovascular Behavioral Medicine, Department of Psychiatry, School of Medicine, University of Pittsburgh, Pittsburgh, Pennsylvania

Trudy L. Burns, PhD,   Professor, Divisions of Biostatistics and Epidemiology, Department of Preventive Medicine and Environmental Health, University of Iowa, Iowa City, Iowa

Stephen R. Daniels, MD, PhD,   Professor, Division of Cardiology, Department of Pediatrics and Environmental Health, University of Cincinnati College of Medicine, Cincinnati, Ohio

Robert H. Eckel, MD   Professor, Department of Medicine and Physiology, Division of Endocrinology, Metabolism, and Diabetes, University of Colorado Health Sciences Center, Denver, Colorado

Gerald F. Fletcher, MD   Professor of Medicine, Mayo Medical School, Cardiovascular Division, Mayo Clinic Jacksonville, Jacksonville, Florida

John P. Foreyt, PhD,   Professor, Department of Medicine, Baylor College of Medicine, Houston, Texas

Scott M. Grundy, MD, PhD,   Professor of Internal Medicine and Biochemistry Director and Chairman, Departments of Clinical Nutrition and Internal Medicine, The Center for Human Nutrition, University of Texas Southwestern Medical Center at Dallas, Dallas, Texas

John E. Hall, PhD,   Professor and Chairman, Department of Physiology and Biophysics and Center for Excellence in Cardiovascular–Renal Research, University of Mississippi Medical Center, Jackson, Mississippi

Laura L. Hayman, PhD, RN, FAAN,   Carl W. and Margaret Davis Walter Professor, Frances Payne Bolton School of Nursing, Case Western Reserve University, Cleveland, Ohio

Jeffrey Henegar, PhD,   Instructor, Department of Physiology and Biophysics and Center for Excellence in Cardiovascular–Renal Research, University of Mississippi Medical Center, Jackson, Mississippi

James O. Hill, PhD,   Center for Human Nutrition, University of Colorado Health Sciences Center, Denver, Colorado

Barbara V. Howard, PhD,   President, MedStar Research Institute, Washington, DC

Daniel W. Jones, MD,   Professor, Department of Physiology and Biophysics and Center for Excellence in Cardiovascular–Renal Research, University of Mississippi Medical Center, Jackson, Mississippi

Marguerite R. Kinney, RN, DNSc, FAAN,   Professor Emerita, School of Nursing, University of Alabama School of Nursing, Birmingham, Alabama

Ronald M. Krauss, MD   Senior Scientist and Head, Department of Molecular Medicine, Lawrence Berkeley National Laboratory, University of California, Berkeley, Berkeley, California

Adamandia D. Kriketos, PhD,   Center for Human Nutrition, University of Colorado Health Sciences Center, Denver, Colorado

Lewis H. Kuller, MD, DrPH,   Professor and Chair Department of Epidemiology, University Professor of Public Health, University of Pittsburgh, Graduate School of Public Health, Pittsburgh, Pennsylvania

Kathy McManus, MS, RD,   Manager, Clinical Nutrition, Brigham and Women's Hospital, Boston, Massachusetts

Katherine M. Newton, PhD,   Assistant Scientific Investigator, Center for Health Studies, Group Health Cooperative of Puget Sound, Seattle, Washington

Eva Obarzanek, PhD, RD, MPH,   Research Nutritionist, Division of Epidemiology and Clinical Applications, National Heart, Lung, and Blood Institute, Bethesda, Maryland

W. S. Carlos Poston, PhD,   Assistant Professor, Department of Medicine, Baylor College of Medicine, Houston, Texas

Eugene W. Shek, PhD,   Research Associate, Department of Physiology and Biophysics and Center for Excellence in Cardiovascular–Renal Research, University of Mississippi Medical Center, Jackson, Mississippi

Sachiko T. St. Jeor, PhD, RD,   Professor and Director, Nutrition Education and Research Program, University of Nevada School of Medicine, Reno, Nevada

Marcia L. Stefanick, PhD,   Associate Professor of Medicine, Stanford Center for Research in Disease Prevention, Stanford University, Palo Alto, California

Mary Ellen Sweeney, MD,   Assistant Professor of Medicine, Emory University School of Medicine and Director of the Hypertension and Lipid Metabolism Clinics, Veterans Administration Medical Center, Department of Medicine, Decatur, Georgia

Acknowledgement

To the leadership of the Council on Cardiovascular Nursing for their vision, tenacity, and support which led to the origination and successful culmination of the American Heart Association Scientific conference, "Obesity: Impact on Cardiovascular Disease".

Preface

In 1977 the Nutrition Committee of the American Heart Association (AHA) issued a statement for healthcare professionals on obesity and heart disease. This statement was developed as part of the American Heart Association's effort to place more emphasis on obesity as a contributing factor to heart disease. The statement recognized that obesity is a predisposing factor for several major cardiovascular risk factors including high blood pressure, disorders of cholesterol and lipid metabolism, and diabetes. It also noted that obesity is becoming increasingly prevalent not only in the United States but worldwide. Even milder forms of overweight can lead to the development of cardiovascular risk factors in susceptible individuals. Risk generally rises with the progressive accumulation of body fat, and many Americans have become markedly obese; these persons are at particularly high risk, especially for diabetes. For these reasons, the American Heart Association specifically has recognized overweight and obesity as risk factors and will devote increased resources to address the problem in the United States.

To support this emphasis on obesity, several councils and committees of the AHA (Council on Cardiovascular Nursing; Council on Arteriosclerosis, Thrombosis, and Vascular Biology; Council on Cardiovascular Disease in the Young; Council on Clinical Cardiology, Epidemiology and Prevention; Council on High Blood Pressure Research; The Nutrition Committee; and Prevention Coordinating Committee) in 1998 sponsored a conference on the impact of obesity on cardiovascular disease. The current volume is authored by the participants of this conference. The purpose of the conference was to evaluate current research data pertaining to the causation and cardiovascular sequela of obesity. The conference was designed to cover a broad range of topics in the obesity field. The topics addressed in the conference are mentioned briefly.

There is an increasing interest in the role of genetics in the causation of obesity, and this issue was put into perspective relative to the known environmental factors affecting body weight. Of increasing concern is the alarming increase in the prevalence of obesity in childhood and adolescence. At the same time, it is recognized that much of obesity in the adult population is the result of weight gain during young adulthood. Thus the focus of causation of obesity is being shifted to earlier ages with more emphasis on genetics and early developmental influences. At the same time, changes in eating and exercise habits in our society undoubtedly play a major role in the rise in obesity prevalence. These changes in habits require a continuing evaluation of the balance between energy intake and energy expenditure in the etiology of obesity, along with genetic and environmental factors that affect each.

The presence of obesity is associated with multiple metabolic alterations. These can lead to changes in cardiac function, essential hypertension, abnormalities in lipoprotein metabolism, insulin resistance, and glucose intolerance. Recent advances have provided new information on the biochemical mechanisms underlying the adverse metabolic effects of obesity; a better understanding of these mechanisms offers new targets for therapy to reduce the metabolic complications. Although pharmacologic interventions hold promise for both reducing obesity and mitigating the complications of being overweight, behavorial interventions remain the mainstay of therapy. The adverse impact of obesity on all segments of the economy also is being recognized increasingly. The many complications of obesity have a major impact on economics in the managed care setting.

All of these issues along with others were presented as discussed by the speakers and participants in this conference. The current volume to follow provides a detailed summary of the presentation and compiles a useful resource for many of the major issues related to the impact of obesity on cardiovascular disease.

Scott M. Grundy, MD, PhD

References

1. Eckel RH, for the Nutrition Committee. Obesity and heart disease. A statement for healthcare professionals from the Nutrition Committee, American Heart Association. *Circulation* 1997;96:3248–3250.

Contents

PART 1
Epidemiology of Obesity

PART 2
Pathophysiology of Obesity

PART 3
Assessment, Interventions, Treatment, and Outcomes

Epidemiology of Obesity

Chapter 1

The Epidemiology of Obesity in Adults in Relationship to Cardiovascular Disease

Lewis H. Kuller, MD, DrPH

Distribution of Measures of Obesity

Obesity is by definition an increase in body fat.[1] In men, the average amount of body fat is approximately 15%–20%, and in women 25%–30%. The percentage of body fat increases with age in both men and women.[1] Few studies have evaluated the relationship between the percentage of body fat and either cardiovascular risk factors or risk of disease, because of prior difficulties of the measurement of the total body fat or percent body fat in population studies.[2] The definitions of obesity and its relationship to disease therefore have been dependent primarily on measurements of weight, height, or relatively simple estimates of anthropometric characteristics such as waist circumference, skinfolds, and bioelectric impedance.[3]

In 1985 a National Institutes of Health (NIH) conference reviewed the use of body mass index (BMI) (weight in kilograms divided by height in meters squared) for classification of obesity.[4] Overweight was defined as a BMI of >27.8 for men and 27.3 for women. A 1985 Food and Agricultural Organization (FAO), World Health Organization (WHO) expert committee defined obesity as a BMI >30 for men and >28.6 for women.[5] In 1995 a WHO committee modified the cut points and classified obesity into three categories: grade 1, overweight, 25.0–29.9 kg/m^2; grade 2, overweight, 30–39.9 kg/m^2; and grade 3, morbid obesity, >40 kg/m^{-2}. Several modifications of this classification recently have been proposed (Table 1).[4,6]

From: Fletcher GF, Grundy SM, Hayman LL (eds). *Obesity: Impact on Cardiovascular Disease*. Armonk, NY: Futura Publishing Co., Inc.; © 1999.

Table 1

Classification of Obesity and Age-Adjusted Prevalence for NHANES III

	BMI	Prevalence (%) age 20–74
Preobese	25.0–29.9	32.0
Class I obesity	30.0–34.9	14.4
Class II obesity	35.0–39.9	5.2
Class III obesity	≥40	2.9

Reproduced with permission from Reference 4.

There is a high correlation between measurements of obesity and the percentage of body fat. Men at each level of obesity will have a lower percent body fat than women.[1] The percentage of body fat in relationship to the BMI will increase in older ages, even if there is no substantial weight gain.[1] In the Healthy Women's Study in Pittsburgh we evaluated various measures of obesity among postmenopausal women. There is a very high correlation (0.8) between BMI, body weight, and the percent body fat as measured by dual X-ray absorptiometry (DEXA). However, at each level of BMI there is substantial variation in the percentage of body fat (Figure 1). The percent of body fat by BMI category also will vary by age.[1]

The distribution of obesity based on the new NIH criteria recently was reported from the Third National Health and Nutrition Examina-

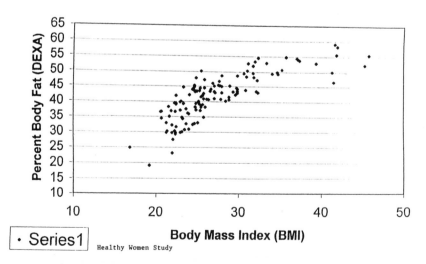

Figure 1. Relationship between percent body fat and body mass index (BMI) at the eighth post; $r = 0.81$, $P = 0.00$.

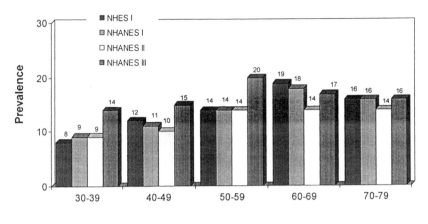

Figure 2. The prevalence of grade I obesity (BMI 30.0–34.9) in women grouped according to age with results from various US studies 1980–1994. Reproduced with permission from Reference 4.

tion Survey (NHANES III) (1988–1994) and compared with previous US national surveys (Figures 2-5).[4] The age-adjusted prevalence of overweight (BMI 25.0–29.9) is approximately 40% in men and 24% in women, and has not changed substantially since 1960–1962. The prevalence of grade I obesity (BMI 30.0–34.9) has increased in men from the

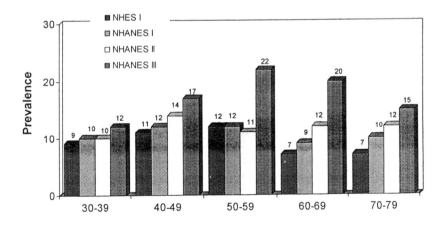

Figure 3. The prevalence of class I obesity in men grouped according to age with results from various US studies 1980–1994. Reproduced with permission from Reference 4.

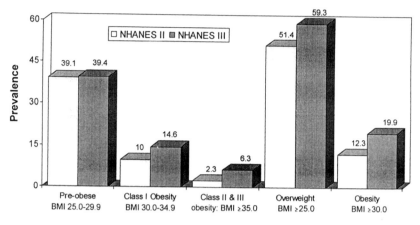

All Race-Ethnic Group Men

Figure 4. The change in age-adjusted prevalence in obesity and overweight subjects between National Health and Nutritional Examination Survey (NHANES II) (1976–1980) and NHANES III (1988–1994) for men aged 20–74 years in all race and ethnic groups. Reproduced with permission from Reference 4.

years 1960–1962 to 1988–1994 from approximately 9% to 15% and in women from approximately 10% to 14%. The prevalence of grade II obesity (BMI of 35.0–39.9) over the same comparison of years has increased in men from 1.3% to 3.6% and in women from 3.3% to 6.8%, and for grade III (BMI > 40.0) in men from 0.3% to 1.8% and in women from 1.3% to 3.9%. There has been a substantial increase in the prevalence of obesity, BMI > 30 in older men, that is, 55+, and in younger women. The increase in obesity for younger men, that is, <40, has been relatively modest, except for small increases in those with extreme obesity. The change in overweight obesity between NHANES II (1976–1980) and NHANES III (1988–1994) has been greatest for the classes II and III obesity (Figures 4 and 5). These new findings, if substantiated by further analysis, do not support the widely held view that there is an overall increase in obesity in the US population across all age, race, and sex groups. The increase may be limited to specific age groups and especially to those at the tail ends of the weight distribution (Figures 4 and 5) between 1976–1980 and 1988–1994, NHANES II and III.

This higher prevalence of obesity among older men suggests two possibilities both related to a cohort effect. The following is the most likely explanation: (1) smoking cessation, which began in the 1960s and 1970s, in men would be associated with an increase in obesity caused by weight gain following smoking cessation and (2) an improvement in longevity, secondary to the reduction in cigarette smoking. There

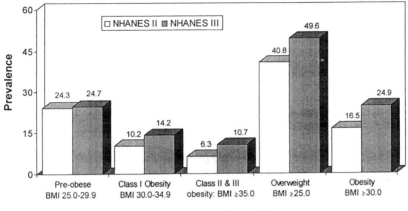

All Race-Ethnic Group Women

Figure 5. The change in age-adjusted prevalence in obesity and overweight subjects between NHANES II (1976–1980) and NHANES III (1988–1994) for women aged 20–74 years from all race and ethnic groups. Reproduced with permission from Reference 4.

has been a very substantial decline in coronary heart disease (CHD) mortality, even in older men. This is attributed to the substantial decline in cigarette smoking in men. This would result in a growing population of older obese men. The high prevalence of cigarette smoking began at a later chronological time in women than men. The greater weight gain among younger women also may be in part related to smoking cessation. In women there also has been an effort to increase weight gain during pregnancy.[7]

The higher weights and weight gains associated with smoking cessation have been noted in other populations besides the United States. A recent publication from the Monitoring of Trends and Determinants in Cardiovascular Diseases (MONICA) Project of the WHO showed that in about every population for both men and women aged 35–64, there was an approximate 2–3 unit lower BMI in smokers as compared with nonsmokers and a substantial increase in the BMI associated with smoking cessation.[8] Smoking cessation may have played an important role but alone does not account for all of the trends in overweight and obesity in the United States.

The percentages of all grades of obesity are substantially higher in black and Mexican American women than for non-Hispanic white women. For men, the prevalence of measures of obesity and overweight are similar in whites, blacks, and Mexican Americans. The higher prevalence of obesity among black and Mexican American women is much more striking at younger ages, under the age of 60. For white women, the prevalence of obesity increases with age, approximately up to age 80, while for blacks and Mexican Americans the prevalence of obesity tends to peak at approximately age 50–59. For men also the prevalence of obesity tends to peak at approximately age 50–59.[4]

The prevalence of obesity and increase in obesity over time usually is substantially greater in lower socioeconomic status (SES) and less educated women. A much weaker association of SES is reported for men.[9,10]

In the past it has been believed, and perhaps rightfully so, that decreased physical activity and increased consumption of caloric dense foods were primary determinants of this epidemic of obesity.[11–13] There has been a decrease in the percentage of fat calories in the diet. An increase in total caloric intake with little change in the total grams of fat in the diet has been observed. Also, there may have been a modest increase in leisure time physical activity in the United States.[14]

The continued controversy as to whether fat calories are more important than carbohydrate calories is not going to be resolved by more observational studies using poor instruments to quantify total calories, fat calories, and carbohydrates.[11] There is a strong association between total fat calories and caloric intake. The intake of more caloric dense foods probably is a contributor to obesity. This argument about fat and carbohydrate calories is of little relevance in the United States. There are probably very few obese individuals who consume a low-fat, high-carbohydrate diet.[15–17]

Obesity and Health

The relationship between obesity and cardiovascular risk factors and cardiovascular disease (CVD) has been documented by numerous studies.[18,19] The following are the major issues that remain unresolved: (1) whether there is a threshold level of obesity and increase in prevalence of cardiovascular risk factors, (2) whether the increase in risk factors primarily is a function of weight gain over time or the extent of overweight/obesity at a specific age, and (3) whether weight gain between different ages has similar effects on cardiovascular risk factors? Weight gain is associated with increased cardiovascular risk factors. Are the changes in risk factors with weight gain a function of increased caloric intake, decreased energy expenditure, or changes in specific types of calories and nutrients, namely fat, saturated fat, salt intake, or dietary cholesterol? Is the relationship between measures of obesity and risk of CVD linear, or is there a threshold effect? Is there a relationship between the distribution of body fat and risk of CVD, independent of the level of obesity? Is the association of measures of obesity and distribution of body fatness and subsequent risk of CVD age dependent? What are the possible pathophysiological processes that relate obesity and distribution of body fat to the risk of CVD?

There is solid evidence that weight loss is associated with a decrease in cardiovascular risk factors [such as blood pressure, low-density lipoprotein cholesterol (LDLC), and blood glucose levels]. Evidence that weight reduction is associated with a decrease in morbidity and mortality caused by CVD is weaker, and the magnitude of the effect is still unknown.[20–22]

Blood Pressure

There are numerous studies that have documented the association of measures of obesity and cardiovascular risk factors. The strongest and probably most consistent relationships are with blood pressure levels and diabetes mellitus.[23–26] Weight gain and measures of obesity are important determinants of blood pressure levels.[27] The association appears to be continuous across the measures of BMI or waist circumference from relatively low levels (a BMI of approximately 22–23 or even lower). The association of weight and weight gain and blood pressure levels is consistent across most populations. Weight loss, independent of a decrease in salt intake, is associated with a decrease in blood pressure.[28,29]

In the Dormont High School Follow-up Study, there was a very substantial increase in weight between ages 17 and 47, 50.5 pounds in men and 28.3 pounds for women.[30] There was a strong association of systolic blood pressure (SBP) at age 47 and both baseline weight and weight change from age 17. Increases in SBP also were related strongly to weight change. Blood pressure levels track from childhood through adolescents as does weight.

In the Intersalt Study, the relationship between BMI and both SBP and diastolic blood pressure (DBP) was evaluated in 52 centers around the world for both men and women. The population varied by levels of blood pressure, obesity, and sodium intake and other dietary and psychosocial variables. In 51 of the 52 centers in men and in 46 of the 52 centers in women, there was a positive association between BMI and SPB, significant in 29 for men and 30 for women. The pooled regression coefficient for increase in SBP a one-unit increase in BMI was approximately 0.92 for men and 0.72 for women. A one-BMI unit increase is associated with an approximate 1-mm greater SBP.[31]

The variation in change in blood pressure and increase or decrease in relation to weight change is substantial within a population. This likely is caused by other factors such as specific nutrients and genetic host susceptibility. The response of the blood pressure to a controlled weight gain or weight loss may be a very good method for the evaluation of genetic or host susceptibility, especially if the change in blood pressure per unit change in weight is consistent within individuals.

Studies in Nigeria, a population in transition, provide another important opportunity to evaluate the effects of weight change on blood pressure in an African population with similar genetic heritage to the US black population. A study by Bunker et al.[32] of senior and junior government employees in Benin City, Nigeria showed that BMI was higher for the senior as compared with the junior employees, related to both a diet higher in calories and fat, and decreased physical activity as compared with junior grade employees. The blood pressure and cholesterol levels were both higher in the senior employees as compared with the junior employees. There was a strong relationship between BMI and higher blood pressure levels. There appeared to be a threshold of a BMI of approximately 21–23 and higher blood pressure levels. The waist circumference was not very different than for US blacks even though the BMI was substantially lower. There was a strong association of greater waist circumference and higher blood pressure levels from approximately 80 cm. In spite of the lower BMI and relatively low-fat diet, there was a very high prevalence of hypertension, with levels beginning to approach that of the US black population, especially among older senior service employees in Nigeria. The increased prevalence of obesity among African populations is likely to contribute to a major epidemic of hypertensive disease and complications such as heart disease and stroke in the future in these populations.

In the Coronary Artery Risk Development in Young Adults (CARDIA) Study,[18–30] and in the Atherosclerosis Risk in the Community (ARIC),[33–52] the prevalence of hypertension, hyperlipidemia, and diabetes among black men and women were related to the degree of obesity as measured by the sum of skin folds.[26] In CARDIA, the percentage of body fat and waist-to-hip ratio were related strongly to cardiovascular risk factors.[53–56] There were no substantial differences in the association of measures of body fatness and blood pressure by race or sex. Over a 7-year follow-up in CARDIA, BMI increased in all four race and sex groups, greater in blacks than in whites, especially in black women. Waist circumference also increased substantially in all four race and sex groups, similar in black and white men, and greater in black women as compared with white women.

In the Nurses Health Study,[27] both BMI at age 18 and current BMI were related strongly to the risk of subsequent hypertension. In the nurse's study, the risk appeared to be linear from a BMI of approximately 20 upward. This would be consistent with the previous studies in Nigeria. Weight gain since age 18 was associated with a substantial increase in the risk of hypertension. The effects of weight change were greater for younger women <45 as compared with women >55 years of age. Weight loss was associated with a decrease in blood pressure, primarily among women with an initial BMI of >22 at age 18.

The risk of disease associated with blood pressure levels is continuous from relatively low levels of blood pressure. Thus, approaches to the prevention of weight gain could have a major impact on lowering the distribution of blood pressure in the population and decrease in vascular disease, including both CHD and stroke.

Among individuals with elevated blood pressure, obesity appears to increase the risk of CHD. However, there is some suggestion that nonobese hypertension may be associated more closely with specific hypertension pathology such as retinopathy, intracerebral hemorrhage, and renal failure. In the Hypertension Detection and Follow-up Program, lower BMI was associated with higher total mortality and the efficacy of treatment comparing special care versus referred care was greater for participants with lower body weight (Figure 6).[23]

The Trials of Hypertension Prevention (TOHP) is one of the few studies that directly evaluated weight loss, independent of a decrease in salt intake, and changes in systolic and SBP, in a randomized clinical trial of nonhypertensives, that is, SBP <90. There was an approximate 4.4-kg weight loss at 6 months in the intervention group and an

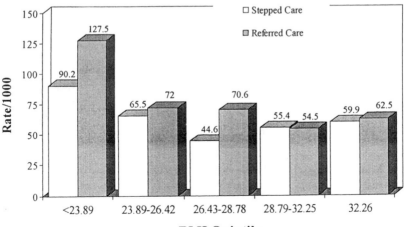

Figure 6. Baseline BMI and 5-year mortality rate, adjusted for age, sex, and race of all participants. Reproduced with permission from Reference 23.

approximate 6-mm decrease in blood pressure, as compared with little weight loss in the control group, and a 2.2-mm decrease in blood pressure, probably caused by regression to the mean. The results would suggest about a 1-mm decrease in SBP per 1-kg reduction in body weight. These findings are similar to the estimates from the Intersalt Study. The decrease in blood pressure with weight loss was similar in magnitude to that of salt reduction. Interestingly, the combination of salt reduction and weight loss did not have any greater effect on reducing blood pressure, than weight loss alone, or salt reduction alone. It was extremely difficult to maintain long-term weight loss after 36 months of follow-up, there was only a 0.2-kg decrease in weight in the intervention group and a 1.8-kg increase in the control group or an approximate 2-kg or 4-lb difference between the groups. The results of TOHP strongly support at least the short-term effects of weight loss, independent of reducing salt on blood pressure levels.[28,29]

The Treatment of Mild Hypertension Study (TOMH) Study showed that nonpharmacologic therapies (including weight loss and exercise) were not nearly as effective as nonpharmacologic therapies combined with drug therapy to reduce blood pressure among hypertensive patients.[57] This study should have laid to rest the argument that nonpharmacologic therapy of hypertension, alone, is an effective alternative therapy to drug therapy. Unfortunately, there remains interest in the treatment of hypertension with nonpharmacologic therapies alone. The reduction of CVD in relation to blood pressure level is a function of the decrease in blood pressure. It seems unwarranted to focus on a small reduction in blood pressure associated with weight reduction among hypertensives as opposed to a much larger decrease in blood pressure associated with drug therapy. On the other hand, the combination of nonpharmacologic therapy (such as weight reduction and exercise) plus drug therapy to lower blood pressure probably is more efficacious than pharmaceutical blood pressure therapy alone.

The Trials of Nonpharmacologic Intervention in the Elderly (TONE) Study[58] was a randomized control trial of nonpharmaceutical intervention in the elderly. There were 585 overweight individuals with SBPs lower than 145 mm and SBP less than 85 while on drug therapy in the study. Participants were assigned to either a weight loss program, salt reduction, or a control group. The average reduction in weight for the participants assigned to weight loss was approximately 3.8 kg at the 9-, 18-, and 30-month follow-up versus a 0.9-kg reduction for those not assigned to weight loss. The main end point was remaining free of cardiovascular events or developing high blood pressure after being taken off antihypertensive drug therapy during follow-up. At 30 months, 39.2% of those in the weight loss versus 26.2% of those in the placebo were event free (ratio 0.70). These results were similar to those for sodium reduction, versus no sodium reduction.

The recently reported Dietary Approaches to Stop Hypertension (DASH) Study[59] has shown that, at least in the short-term, reduction of total fat intake, even without weight reduction, decreases blood pressure levels. These results must be verified such as in the Women's Health Initiative (WHI). If the findings are consistent (ie, that lower fat intake reduces blood pressure independent of weight change), then it might suggest that at least some of the associations between increasing weight and blood pressure are related primarily to higher fat intakes. However, the previous studies in the literature do not suggest a major effect on blood pressure of reducing fat calories on decreasing blood pressure without weight loss.

Lipids

There is a positive association between BMI and blood LDLC and triglyceride (TG) levels, and an inverse association with high-density lipoprotein cholesterol (HDLC).[60–62] Weight gain is associated with an increase in total LDLC and with a decrease in HDLC. However, the association of BMI and blood cholesterol levels is not consistent across populations. There are populations with very high prevalence of obesity and weight gain (especially early in life) and relatively low LDLC levels. Within these populations there still may be an association of cholesterol level and BMI. The low-cholesterol levels in these populations are related primarily to their reduced total cholesterol and saturated fat intake as compared with US populations.

The percentage of specific saturated fat and dietary cholesterol are the most important determinants of LDLC levels. It is probable that obesity is an important determinant of higher LDLC only in populations that consume diets relatively high in saturated fat and cholesterol. In such populations weight gain is associated strongly with increased LDLC and weight lowering to decrease LDLC levels.

In the Healthy Women Study (HWS) we demonstrated that there was about a pound per year increase in weight among peri- to postmenopausal women and that weight gain was related very strongly to increase in LDLC. The increase in weight was associated with a rise in LDLC for women both taking and not taking hormone replacement therapy (HRT).[63]

The relationship of waist circumference or increased visceral fat, independent of BMI, is associated much less consistently with high LDLC. Waist circumference is associated strongly with higher TGs and lower HDLC. In the HWS the amount of visceral fat was estimated by computerized tomography (CT). The relationship of increased visceral fat was related much more strongly to HDLC, TGs, blood pressure, and insulin than to LDLC levels. BMI and weight gain, on the other hand, were related strongly to LDLC.

Lipid-lowering drugs are extremely effective in reducing LDLC and risk of CHD and stroke. Reduction of LDLC with drug therapy among obese individuals with HDLC levels may be far more advantageous than attempting a substantial weight reduction and diet alone to lower LDLC and risk of CVD.[33] The combination of nonpharmacologic therapies, low-saturated fat and -cholesterol diet, weight reduction and exercise, and pharmacologic therapies may be the best approach.

Glucose, Insulin

Higher BMI and especially increased truncal or abdominal fat clearly is an important determinant of blood glucose levels, insulin resistance, and the development of diabetes.[33–35] Among diabetics, the association of BMI with increase in mortality is not consistent across populations. In western countries with a high prevalence of atherosclerosis, BMI clearly is a risk factor, for increased CVD mortality among diabetics. However, in other populations the association is much weaker. It is unclear whether levels of blood glucose are a continuous risk factor for CVD or whether the association primarily was at higher levels of blood glucose or diabetes.[37,38] Obesity and genetic characteristics are the major determinants of diabetes in the population. Prevention of weight gain probably will play a major role in reducing the prevalence of diabetes in the population.

In CARDIA there was a consistent linear association between weight gain and changes in serum insulin levels.[56] The results were similar for all race and sex groups. The mean change in fasting glucose also was related directly to weight gain, similar in the four race and sex groups. The increase in glucose levels was related directly to an increase in fasting insulin levels. The changes in fasting insulin levels and weight were related very closely to decreased physical activity. In multivariate models, changes in BMI and in waist circumference were related strongly to changes in serum insulin and glucose levels in all four race and sex groups.

The current Diabetes Prevention Trial will, hopefully, provide important answers with regard to, at least, the potential for prevention of diabetes. Other planned clinical trials finally may provide information about the most successful ways of lowering blood glucose and reducing clinical CVD.

Risk of Cardiovascular Disease

Measures of obesity and weight gain clearly are related to the risk of CVD, including CHD, stroke, and total mortality in most populations.[39-46] This association is stronger at younger than older ages. A critical question is whether obesity is an independent cardiovascular risk factor or whether the association of obesity or body fat distribution and CVD primarily is operating through the effects of obesity or weight gain on elevated blood pressure, cholesterol, diabetes, etc. (ie, cardiovascular risk factors).

There is still considerable controversy as to whether there is a weight threshold associated with increased total mortality. Troiano et al[18] have reviewed the relationship between obesity and mortality (Figure 7). The association of mortality and body weight was included in a metaanalysis of 19 prospective studies of approximately 600 000 white men and women over a 15–30 year follow-up. All cause mortality was lowest at a BMI in the range of 23–28 kg/m². The association was suggested to be independent of smoking and concurrent illness.

New studies have been able to evaluate the relationship between measures of obesity, other risk factors, and atherosclerosis either at postmortem examination and noninvasive methods of measuring atherosclerosis. In the Cooperative Multicenter Study, Pathobiological Determinants of Atherosclerosis in Youth (PDAY), 1532 young persons, 15–34 years of age, who died of external causes and were autopsied at a medical examiner's laboratory, had quantitative studies of atherosclerosis of the aorta and right coronary arteries.[47] The thickness of the panniculus adiposus and BMI was used to measure the degree

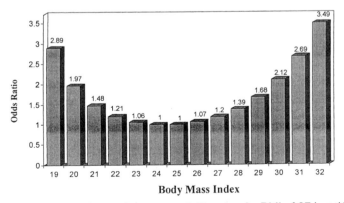

Figure 7.   Differences from minimum mortality rate of a BMI of 27 in a 10-year follow-up and a BMI of 24 with 30-year follow-up. Reproduced with permission from Reference 18.

of adiposity. The thickness of the panniculus and BMI was associated with more extensive fatty streaks and also with higher prevalence of raised lesions in the right coronary artery. The effects persisted after adjustment for lipoprotein profiles and history of cigarette smoking. The glycohemoglobin level exceeding 8% also was associated with more extensive lesions in the right coronary artery. Interestingly, neither the level of BMI nor the thickness of the panniculus were associated with the prevalence of raised lesions in either the thoracic or abdominal aorta.

In the Muscatine Study, electron beam CT was used to evaluate coronary artery calcification in 474 women and 386 men ages 29–43. Coronary artery calcification was present in 33% of the men and 15% of the women. In multiple logistic regression analysis for the prevalence of coronary artery calcification the highest decile of BMI, odds ratio of 3 (1.8–5.2) for men and women was a key predictor. Men and women who had high BMI or SBP in the highest tertile had a 42% prevalence of coronary artery calcification, as compared with 8% for those who had a BMI and SBPs in the lowest tertile. Other predictors of coronary artery calcification include a lower HDLC and higher LDLC.[48]

In the ARIC Study, ages 45–64, the mean BMI was higher in cases with severe carotid atherosclerosis as measured by B-mode ultrasound.[49] The BMI at age 45–64 was substantially higher in black women than in white women but did not differ between black and white men. The associations of change in body weight from age 25 to middle age, established as ages 45–64, was evaluated in ARIC.[62] Between the ages of 25 and 64, there was a reported 12-kg increase in weight in white women, 20.8 kg in black women, 9.7 kg in white men, and 10.1 in black men. Weight change was associated with higher carotid intimal medial thickness in black and white men and white women but not in black women. The differences in intimal medial thickness are associated with a 10-kg increase in weight change and was 0.016 mm in white men at the age of 25 and between the ages of 45 and 64.

The waist-to-hip ratio was studied in relationship to the extent of carotid intimal medial thickness in all four race and sex groups in ARIC. Both BMI and waist-to-hip ratio were significantly related to carotid intimal medial thickness, after adjustment for other risk factors. Diabetes and fasting insulin, but not hyperglycemia, also were related strongly to carotid intimal medial thickness. Carotid intimal medial thickness was a strong predictor of risk of clinical CHD over time, especially among women.[51]

In the Cardiovascular Health Study, age 65+, the prevalence of obesity was 44% at age 65–69, 40% at age 70–74, 31% at age 75–79, and

22% at age 80+; 42% in women and 31% in men.[52,64] Both BMI and waist circumference were related directly to TG levels and inversely to HDLC but not to LDLC levels. The prevalence of obesity was related to hypertension in both men and women. There was a significant association of measures of disability and higher BMI. Higher current weight was related to higher prevalence of fair or poor health and mobility difficulties, especially among women. Body weight was correlated directly with higher left ventricular mass on echocardiography, ventricular septal thickness, and left ventricular posterior wall thickness.

Reported weight at age 50 and current weight were related directly to prevalent CHD among women aged 65+. For men weight at age 50 but not current weight was related to prevalent CHD. Weight gain since age 50 was associated with higher SBP, higher blood cholesterol level, lower HDLC, higher insulin glucose, and a history of diabetes.

The BMI was related directly to a composite index of subclinical CVD in both white and black women and in white men.[65] The waist-to-hip ratio also was related to the prevalence of subclinical disease except in black men. BMI was related directly to carotid intimal medial thickness in both blacks and whites, men and women. The association was stronger in men than in women.

In multivariate analysis, the BMI was a significant predictor of subclinical disease (relative risk 1.067; 1.028 to 1.108) in white men but not in women or black men after adjustment for the other risk factors, such as SBP, LDLC, glucose, smoking, and white blood count.

In the Cardiovascular Health Study, 646 or 12% of the cohort died within 5 years. Weight or measures of BMI or waist circumference were not significant predictors of total or CHD mortality over time after including measures of subclinical disease. Total mortality was associated inversely with increasing age, male sex, low BMI, and high SBP. In multivariate analysis, low weight was associated significantly with increased mortality. The death rate was 46.6/1000 for those in the lowest weight quintile, as compared with 22.5 in the highest quintile (Figure 8).[52]

Furthermore, detailed analysis included only participants with stable or increasing weight since age 50. The mortality rate was highest for women with BMIs <20, while for men there was no longer any association of weight and mortality. High BMI at age 50 was associated with higher total mortality at age 65+ in CHS. The highest mortality was for women who had high BMI at age 50 and low at age 65+. A >10% loss of weight from age 50 to baseline, aged 65+, was associated with higher subsequent mortality in the nonsmoking participants[52]

Subjects with Stable or Increased Weight Since Age 50

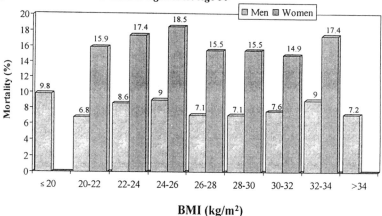

Figure 8. Five-year mortality rate in nonsmoking older adults categorized by baseline BMI and gender as reported by The Cardiovascular Health Study (1996). Reproduced with permission from Reference 52.

In both the ARIC and the CHS, the effect of measures of obesity, BMI, and waist was blunted and modest as a risk factor for CVD after including measures of other risk factors and subclinical CVD. However, hypertension and diabetes were very important determinants of CVD and both risk factors are related strongly to weight gain and obesity.

Not all populations demonstrate an association of obesity and mortality or CVD. The studies by Hodge et al[38] in the Pacific Islands have found no evidence that obesity is associated with an increased risk of mortality over a 10-year follow-up. The prevalence of obesity and diabetes is very high in these populations. There is a substantial increase in risk factors such as LDLC and TGs associated with acculturation in particularly with increases in saturated fat and cholesterol in the diet.

The Strong Heart Study is evaluating cardiovascular risk factors among American Indians. There is a high prevalence of obesity, especially early age of onset of obesity.[65-67] The prevalence of major electrocardiogram (ECG) abnormalities was low in these populations. It was lowest among the Arizona Indian populations that have the highest prevalence of obesity and diabetes. There was little evidence of a relationship between obesity and total mortality in these populations. Definite myocardial infarction (MI) or CHD was related strongly to a history of diabetes, 4.6 prevalence ratio in women and 1.8 in men. In logistic regression analysis, age, diabetes, sex, and cigarette smoking but not BMI or waist circumference were associated with a higher prevalence of CHD. Recent reports suggest that the cardiovascular mortality among Native Americans may be approximately that of US white populations.[68]

Body Fat Distribution

The distribution of body fat probably plays a very important role in the risk of CVD.[69] In the recent past, measurements of skin folds or the ratio of waist to hip or more recently just waist measurement, were shown to be a strong predictor of cardiovascular risk factors such as elevated blood pressure, insulin, TGs, low HDLC, and risks of CVD.[70,71] A waist measurement >94 cm for men and 80 cm in women was defined as at risk and >102 cm in men and 88 cm in women at very high risk of CVD. These waist measures are considered to be a surrogate marker for the amount of intra-abdominal or visceral fat.[72] The development of better methods of measuring intra-abdominal fat have provided new approaches to evaluating the distribution of body, total fat, and risk of CVD.

The waist circumference is a good estimate of visceral fat or intra-abdominal fat across the population, that is, individuals with greater waist circumference will almost certainly have greater intra-abdominal fat. This is intuitively logical, because fatter people obviously will weigh more, have greater body fat, and greater fat in most fat depots. However, there is very substantial variation in the amount of visceral or intra-abdominal fat as measured by CT at any specific level of waist circumference. The waist circumference is measuring both intra-abdominal fat and subcutaneous fat in the abdominal region. The amount of visceral or intra-abdominal fat also increases with age in both men and women and especially among postmenopausal women. Weight gain during adult years may be associated with an increase in visceral or intra-abdominal fat. Men have substantially more visceral or intra-abdominal fat than women.[73] Black women have been reported to have lesser amounts of visceral fat given the same BMI.[74] However, the amount of intra-abdominal fat increases in women postmenopausal and is higher in women who have had artificial menopause.[73]

There are, unfortunately, very few studies that have enough information to be able to separate the various components of obesity, both the amount of fatness as well as the distribution of body fat and risk of CVD. The new and better methods of measuring both body fatness and body fat distribution, as well as atherosclerosis, will provide better information with regard to the distribution of fatness measures and, at the least, subclinical atherosclerosis and risk of CVD.

Bjorntorp[73] has proposed that abdominal fat is a major risk factor for CVD and non–insulin-dependent diabetes, and stroke in both men and women. The increased visceral obesity primarily was caused by an endocrine abnormality with elevated sensitivity of the hypothalamic pituitary adrenal axis to increased secretion of a corticotropin-releasing hormone (CRH; ACTH), and increased cortisol secretion, and in women increasing adrenal androgens. Growth hormone releasing hormone (GHRH) and gonadotropin releasing hormone (GRH) are reduced resulting in lower GH) and sex-steroid hormone secretion. Therefore, cortisol and insulin cause an increase in the accumulation of visceral fat and testosterone and GH decrease visceral fat. Estrogen enhances the storage of lipid in the gluteal femoral area.

An increased waist circumference is related strongly to many of the measures of metabolic syndrome X, including insulin levels, higher TG levels, lower HDLC, especially HDL_{2c}, increased plasminogen activator inhibitor-1 (PAI-1), small dense LDLC particles, and higher levels of acute phase proteins, such as C-reactive protein (CRP). Differences in CHD incidence between men and women probably is explained in part but not completely by differences in intra-abdominal fat or waist circumference.[74–79]

The amount of visceral fat is related strongly to measures of inflammation and clotting. The high levels of CRP are related directly to obesity and especially increased intra-abdominal fat, as have been noted in several studies including the HWS and the Cardiovascular Health Studies. Epidemiological studies have documented that markers of inflammation are related directly to the risk of heart attack.[80,81]

Other investigators have questioned the importance of intra-abdominal fat as a measure of risk.[82] The amount of intra-abdominal fat represents a relatively small percentage of total body fat. At least one group of investigators have suggested that measures of total truncal fat, rather than visceral fat, may be a more important predictor of at least insulin resistance.

The measures of fatness are correlated so highly that use of statistical methods to adjust for different distributions of body composition are unlikely to be useful. It would perhaps be preferable to study specific groups of individuals with unique distributions of body fat. For example, we have been studying women who have polycystic ovary. They have an early age increase in the amount of intra-abdominal fat. They have high-androgen levels and low-peak estradiol levels. They have many of the characteristics of so-called metabolic syndrome X at a relatively young age. They have higher LDLC levels than matched controls, especially at younger ages, probably because of the low-peak estrogen levels and increasing body weight. By definition, they should have more extensive atherosclerosis and perhaps higher risks of heart attack, especially at younger ages. Preliminary data have suggested that they do have a higher prevalence of carotid intimal medial thickness and perhaps plaques in the carotid arteries. On the other hand, some studies have suggested that they do not have an increased risk of CHD.[83]

Fujimota has proposed that in some non-Caucasian populations such as in the Japanese, there is an increased susceptibility to central or visceral obesity and the associated metabolic syndrome X.[84,85] Lifestyle changes may play an important role in the development of this syndrome, along with the genetic susceptibility. Prospective studies in Japanese American men have shown visceral fat to be a better predictor of the development of Non–insulin-dependent diabetes mellitus (NIDDM) as compared with the BMI or skin fold measurements. In women, both generalized obesity and visceral fat were associated with risk of NIDDM. There was a significant association of both glucose intolerance and CHD with increased intra-abdominal fat in Japanese–Americans.

The extent of obesity is related directly to the level of estrone and estradiol among postmenopausal women because of the aromatization of androstenedione to estrone in fat tissue. This association accounts, in part, for the lower use of HRT (ie, less symptomatology among obese women), the positive association of postmenopausal obesity and breast cancer, and the negative association of obesity with osteoporosis and hip fracture. The higher BMI among postmenopausal women and the associated higher estrogen levels could, in part, blunt the effects of obesity on the risk of CVD among older women.[86–90] Visceral or intra-abdominal fat, on the other hand, is a small percentage of the total fat and, therefore, the increase in visceral fat or even truncal fat may contribute to CVD, while that of total fat or BMI would be blunted by the higher levels of endogenous estrogen.

There are very few studies in women that have evaluated the effects of weight loss on cardiovascular risk factors, symptomatology, hormone levels, and bone mineral density. We were able to test partially this association in the Women's Healthy Lifestyle Project (WHLP), a trial to prevent weight gain and increase LDLC during the peri- to the postmenopause. The intervention included increasing exercise, low-saturated fat, a low-caloric intake, and decrease in cholesterol in the diet. The intervention group had a substantial weight loss and a significant decrease in LDLC, TGs, and blood pressure. However, there was, a greater loss of bone in the intervention group. The loss of bone was related directly to weight change. Also, there was an increase in bone reabsorption markers suggesting that there was some increase in bone loss. This bone loss was unrelated to the BMI at baseline or the bone density. It was only partially blunted by increase in physical activity and was not related to calcium intake. These results clearly document the need to evaluate the different possible physiological changes that can occur in relation to weight loss. Current follow-up of the WHLP cohort will determine whether the small changes in bone, especially trabecular bone, persist over time.

Prevention of weight gain in women, especially from the peri- to the postmenopause, is likely to decrease the rise in LDLC, blood pressure and blood glucose from the peri- to postmenopause, the development of atherosclerotic disease, clinical CHD, and other vascular diseases when these women are in their 50s, 60s, and 70s but may increase risk of osteoporosis and fracture. In the Study of Osteoporotic Fractures (SOF) among older women, 65+, both the low BMI and the weight loss since age 50 were strong predictors of the risk of hip fracture (Figure 9).[91] The reason for the weight loss or low BMI could not be determined accurately in the study. The association of osteoporosis and weight also has been documented recently in the Rotterdam Aging Study.[92] Body weight and weight loss also are related directly to bone mineral density in men and also are likely to risk a fracture. At a minimum in older individuals, weight reduction should be monitored carefully by measures of bone mineral density and, probably, by bone reabsorption markers. A major effort should be made to determine the best approaches to the prevention of bone loss and, possibly, muscle loss and Sarcopenia among both men and women in voluntary weight reduction therapies. We do not know the effects of weight loss in older individuals on disease risk. Clinical trials to evaluate multiple end points (including breast and prostate cancer, osteoporosis, CVD, Sar-

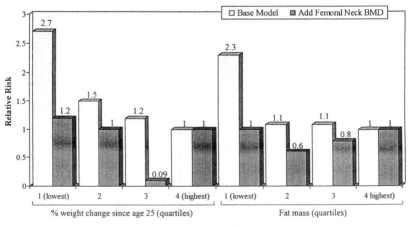

Figure 9. Multivariate association between anthropometric measures of body size and hip fracture. Reproduced with permission from Reference 97.

copenia, and dementia) among older individuals should have a high priority.[93-95]

Discussion

There has been an increase in the prevalence of obesity in the United States and other countries. The increase apparently occurred among older men and younger women. Weight gain is a major determinant of increase in LDLC, TGs, blood pressure, glucose, insulin, and the development of diabetes.[96] Prevention of weight gain, therefore, should have the highest priority and is more likely to be successful than attempting nonpharmacologic weight reduction interventions among individuals who have already gained substantial amounts of weight and have elevated cardiovascular risk factors or clinical CVD. Studies of prevention of weight gain, especially the association of increased energy expenditure, and changes in the consumption of calorically dense foods should have higher priority. Pharmaceutical therapies probably will be needed for treatment of obesity, especially class II and III, and reduction of cardiovascular risk factors.

Few, if any, of the clinical epidemiological studies really have been able to determine whether obesity is an independent risk factor or whether the effects of obesity are moderated by the effects of weight gain and obesity, traditional cardiovascular risk factors (such as LDLC, blood pressure, and TGs) and, perhaps, the effects of obesity on factors related to inflammation, thrombosis, and fibrinolysis.

To be meaningful, studies of obesity and risk of CVD and CHD need to include objective measures of cardiovascular risk factors. It is clear that "adjustment" for these risk factors does reduce the relationship between obesity and risk of CVD. Without such measures of risk factors, the studies of the relationship between obesity and risk of CVD probably are of limited utility. The Null hypothesis, until proven otherwise, is that obesity, except probably at extremes, is not an independent risk factor for CVD but, rather, is an important determinant of cardiovascular risk factors and, hence, obesity indirectly is an important determinant of CVD. However, weight gain may be an independent risk factor especially for development of atherosclerosis.

The hypotheses relating the amount of visceral fat to sex-steroid hormones, cortisone, insulin, inflammation, thrombosis, fibrinolysis, and behavioral changes should be important in the development of CVD. Major efforts to evaluate the interrelationship of fat distribution and hormones, inflammation, behavior, growth factors, and CVD using new techniques [such as CT and magnetic resonance imaging (MRI)] need to be done. The continued emphasis on using BMI, alone, or weight will provide little new information for epidemiological, clinical, or genetic studies.

The interrelationship of obesity and CVD is, clearly, age-race-sex dependent. Age-adjusted studies of BMI, etc. and CVD are uninterpretable and should be avoided. The distribution of measures of weight, BMI, body fat, and visceral fat are continuous in the population. The risk of disease also is linear to at least fairly low BMI, that is, 22 or less. The arbitrary class of overweight or obesity is not based on good epidemiology or pathophysiology. The arbitrary criteria generates misinterpretation of genetic and epidemiology studies (ie, the "search for genes for obesity"). The primary focus should be on prevention of weight gain, study of body fat distribution and disease, and genetic-environmental interactions.

References

1. Gallagher D, Visser M, Sepulveda D, et al. How useful is body mass index for comparison of body fatness across age, sex, and ethnic groups? *Am J Epidemiol* 1996;143:228–239.
2. Luke A, Durazo-Arvizu R, Rotimi C, et al. Relation between body mass index and body fat in black population samples from Nigeria, Jamaica, and the United States. *Am J Epidemiol* 1997;145:620–628.
3. Abernathy RP, Black DR. Healthy body weights: An alternative perspective. *Am J Clin Nutr* 1996;63:448S–451S.
4. Flegal KM, Carroll MD, Kuczmarski RJ, et al. Overweight and obesity in the United States: Prevalence and trends, 1960–1994. *Int J Obes Relat Metab Disord* 1998;22:39–47.
5. Sichieri R, Everhart JE, Hubbard VS. Relative weight classifications in the assessment of underweight and overweight in the United States. *Int J Obes Relat Metab Disord* 1992;16:303–312.
6. WHO Expert Committee on Physical Status. *The Use and Interpretation of Anthropometry. Physical status: The Use and Interpretation of Anthropometry.* 854th ed. Geneva, 1995.
7. Franz MJ, Horton ES Sr, Bantle JP, et al. Nutrition principles for the management of diabetes and related complications. *Diabetes Care* 1994;17:490–518.
8. Molarius A, Seidell JC, Kuulasmaa K, et al. Smoking and relative body weight: An international perspective from the WHO MONICA Project. *J Epidemiol Community Health* 1997;51:252–260.
9. NCHS/CDC NHANES III, Phase I. 1998–1991.
10. Kuczmarski RJ, Flegal KM, Campbell SM, et al. Increasing prevalence of overweight among US adults. The National Health and Nutrition Examination Surveys, 1960 to 1991. *JAMA* 1994;272:205–211.
11. Ravussin E, Swinburn BA. Pathophysiology of obesity. *Lancet* 1992;340:404–408.
12. Prentice AM. Obesity: The inevitable penalty of civilisation? *Br Med Bull* 1997;53:229–237.
13. Prentice AM, Jebb SA. Obesity in Britain: Gluttony or sloth? *BMJ* 1995;311:437–439.

14. Ernst ND, Sempos CT, Briefel RR, et al. Consistency between US dietary fat intake and serum total cholesterol concentrations: The National Health and Nutrition Examination Surveys. *Am J Clin Nutr* 1997;66:965S–972S.
15. Rolls BJ, Castellanos VH, Halford JC, et al. Volume of food consumed affects satiety in men. *Am J Clin Nutr* 1998;67:1170–1177.
16. Bell EA, Castellanos VH, Pelkman CL, et al. Energy density of foods affects energy intake in normal-weight women. *Am J Clin Nutr* 1998;67:412–420.
17. Braam LA, Ocke MC, Bueno-de-Mesquita HB, et al. Determinants of obesity-related underreporting of energy intake. *Am J Epidemiol* 1998;147: 1081–1086.
18. Troiano RP, Frongillo EA Jr, Sobal J, et al. The relationship between body weight and mortality: A quantitative analysis of combined information from existing studies. *Int J Obes Relat Metab Disord* 1996;20:63–75.
19. Manson JE, Stampfer MJ, Hennekens CH, et al. Body weight and longevity. A reassessment. *JAMA* 1987;257:353–358.
20. Bray GA. Obesity: A time bomb to be defused. *Lancet* 1998;352:160–161.
21. Schwartz MW, Brunzell JD. Regulation of body adiposity and the problem of obesity. *Arterioscler Thromb Vasc Biol* 1997;17:233–238.
22. Garn SM. Fractionating healthy weight. *Am J Clin Nutr* 1996;63:412S–414S.
23. Stamler J. Epidemiologic findings on body mass and blood pressure in adults. *Ann Epidemiol* 1991;1:347–362.
24. Landsberg L, Troisi R, Parker D, et al. Obesity, blood pressure, and the sympathetic nervous system. *Ann Epidemiol* 1991;1:295–303.
25. Frohlich ED. Obesity and hypertension. Hemodynamic aspects. *Ann Epidemiol* 1991;1:287–293.
26. Folsom AR, Burke GL, Byers CL, et al. Implications of obesity for cardiovascular disease in blacks: The CARDIA and ARIC Studies. *Am J Clin Nutr* 1991;53:1604S–1611S.
27. Huang Z, Willett WC, Manson JE, et al. Body weight, weight change, and risk for hypertension in women. *Ann Intern Med* 1998;128:81–88.
28. Anonymous. Effects of weight loss and sodium reduction intervention on blood pressure and hypertension incidence in overweight people with high-normal blood pressure. The Trials of Hypertension Prevention, phase II. The Trials of Hypertension Prevention Collaborative Research Group [see Comments]. *Arch Intern Med* 1997;157:657–667.
29. Whelton PK, Kumanyika SK, Cook NR, et al. Efficacy of nonpharmacologic interventions in adults with high-normal blood pressure: Results from phase 1 of the Trials of Hypertension Prevention. Trials of Hypertension Prevention Collaborative Research Group. *Am J Clin Nutr* 1997;65:652S–660S.
30. Yong LC, Kuller LH. Tracking of blood pressure from adolescence to middle age: The Dormont High School Study. *Prev Med* 1994;23:418–426.
31. Dyer AR, Elliott P. The INTERSALT study: Relations of body mass index to blood pressure. INTERSALT Co-operative Research Group. *J Hum Hypertens* 1989;3:299–308.
32. Bunker CH, Ukoli FA, Matthews KA, et al. Weight threshold and blood pressure in a lean black population. *Hypertension* 1995;26:616–623.
33. Stamler J, Briefel RR, Milas C, et al. Relation of changes in dietary lipids and weight, trial years 1–6, to changes in blood lipids in the special intervention and usual care groups in the Multiple Risk Factor Intervention Trial. *Am J Clin Nutr* 1997;65:272S–288S.

34. Abate N. Insulin resistance and obesity. The role of fat distribution pattern. *Diabetes Care* 1996;19:292–294.
35. Yamashita S, Nakamura T, Shimomura I, et al. Insulin resistance and body fat distribution. *Diabetes Care* 1996;19:287–291.
36. Chan JM, Rimm EB, Colditz GA, et al. Obesity, fat distribution, and weight gain as risk factors for clinical diabetes in men. *Diabetes Care* 1994;17:961–969.
37. Chaturvedi N, Fuller JH. Mortality risk by body weight and weight change in people with NIDDM. The WHO Multinational Study of Vascular Disease in Diabetes. *Diabetes Care* 1995;18:766–774.
38. Hodge AM, Dowse GK, Collins VR, et al. Mortality in Micronesian Nauruans and Melanesian and Indian Fijians is not associated with obesity. *Am J Epidemiol* 1996;143:442–455.
39. Eckel RH. Obesity and heart disease: A statement for healthcare professionals from the Nutrition Committee, American Heart Association. *Circulation* 1997;96:3248–3250.
40. Spataro JA, Dyer AR, Stamler J, et al. Measures of adiposity and coronary heart disease mortality in the Chicago Western Electric Company Study. *J Clin Epidemiol* 1996;49:849–857.
41. Kahn HS, Austin H, Williamson DF, et al. Simple anthropometric indices associated with ischemic heart disease. *J Clin Epidemiol* 1996;49:1017–1024.
42. Hubert HB, Feinleib M, McNamara PM, et al. Obesity as an independent risk factor for cardiovascular disease: A 26-year follow-up of participants in the Framingham Heart Study. *Circulation* 1983;67:968–977.
43. Seidell JC, Verschuren WM, van Leer EM, et al. Overweight, underweight, and mortality. A prospective study of 48 287 men and women. *Arch Intern Med* 1996;156:958–963.
44. Rexrode KM, Hennekens CH, Willett WC, et al. A prospective study of body mass index, weight change, and risk of stroke in women. *JAMA* 1997;277:1539–1545.
45. Lee IM, Manson JE, Hennekens CH, et al. Body weight and mortality. A 27-year follow-up of middle-aged men. *JAMA* 1993;270:2823–2828.
46. Jousilahti P, Tuomilehto J, Vartiainen E, et al. Body weight, cardiovascular risk factors, and coronary mortality. 15-year follow-up of middle-aged men and women in eastern Finland. *Circulation* 1996;93:1372–1379.
47. McGill HC Jr, McMahan CA, Malcom GT, et al. Relation of glycohemoglobin and adiposity to atherosclerosis in youth. Pathobiological Determinants of Atherosclerosis in Youth (PDAY) Research Group. *Arterioscler Thromb Vasc Biol* 1995;15:431–440.
48. Burns TL, Mahoney LT, Stanford W, et al. Lifetime risk factor load predicts coronary artery calcification in young adult ment and women: The Muscatine Study. Presented at the 38th Annual Conference on Cardiovascular Disease Epidemiology and Prevention; Santa Fe, NM: American Heart Association; 1998.
49. Heiss G, Sharrett AR, Barnes R, et al. Carotid atherosclerosis measured by B-mode ultrasound in populations: Associations with cardiovascular risk factors in the ARIC study. *Am J Epidemiol* 1991;134:250–256.
50. Stevens J, Tyroler HA, Cai J, et al. Body weight change and carotid artery wall thickness. The Atherosclerosis Risk in Communities (ARIC) Study. *Am J Epidemiol* 1998;147:563–573.
51. Chambless LE, Heiss G, Folsom AR, et al. Association of coronary heart disease incidence with carotid arterial wall thickness and major risk fac-

tors: The Atherosclerosis Risk in Communities (ARIC) Study, 1987–1993. *Am J Epidemiol* 1997;146:483–494.

52. Diehr P, Bild DE, Harris TB, et al. Body mass index and mortality in nonsmoking older adults: The Cardiovascular Health Study. *Am J Public Health* 1998;88:623–629.

53. Folsom AR, Jacobs DR Jr, Wagenknecht LE, et al. Increase in fasting insulin and glucose over seven years with increasing weight and inactivity of young adults. The CARDIA Study Coronary Artery Risk Development in Young Adults. *Am J Epidemiol* 1996;144:235–246.

54. Burke GL, Bild DE, Hilner JE, et al. Differences in weight gain in relation to race, gender, age and education in young adults: The CARDIA Study. Coronary Artery Risk Development in Young Adults. *Ethn Health* 1996;1: 327–335.

55. Slattery ML, McDonald A, Bild DE, et al. Associations of body fat and its distribution with dietary intake, physical activity, alcohol, and smoking in blacks and whites. *Am J Clin Nutr* 1992;55:943–949.

56. Folsom AR, Burke GL, Ballew C, et al. Relation of body fatness and its distribution to cardiovascular risk factors in young blacks and whites. The role of insulin. *Am J Epidemiol* 1989;130:911–924.

57. Neaton JD, Grimm RH Jr, Prineas RJ, et al. Treatment of Mild Hypertension Study. Final results. Treatment of Mild Hypertension Study Research Group. *JAMA* 1993;270:713–724.

58. Whelton PK, Applegate WB, Ettinger WH, et al. Efficacy of weight loss and reduced sodium intake in the Trials of Nonpharmacologic Interventions in the Elderly (TONE). *Circulation* 1996;1996:I178. Abstract.

59. Whelton PK, Appel LJ, Espeland MA, et al. Sodium reduction and weight loss in the treatment of hypertension in older persons: A Randomized Controlled Trial of Nonpharmacologic Interventions in the Elderly (TONE). TONE Collaborative Research Group. *JAMA* 1998;279:839–846.

60. Kuller LH, Meilahn E, Bunker C, et al. Development of risk factors for cardiovascular disease among women from adolescence to older ages. *Am J Med Sci* 1995;310:S91–S100.

61. Denke MA, Sempos CT, Grundy SM. Excess body weight. An underrecognized contributor to high blood cholesterol levels in white American men. *Arch Intern Med* 1993;153:1093–1103.

62. Denke MA, Sempos CT, Grundy SM. Excess body weight. An underrecognized contributor to dyslipidemia in white American women. *Arch Intern Med* 1994;154:401–410.

63. Kuller LH, Heilahn EN, Lassila H, et al. Cardiovascular risk factors during first five years postmenopause in nonhormone replacement therapy users. In: Forte TM, ed. *Hormonal, Metabolic, and Cellular Influences on Cardiovascular Disease in Women.* Armonk, NY: Future Publishing Company, Inc; 1997:273–287.

64. Harris TB, Savage PJ, Tell GS, et al. Carrying the burden of cardiovascular risk in old age: Associations of weight and weight change with prevalent cardiovascular disease, risk factors, and health status in the Cardiovascular Health Study. *Am J Clin Nutr* 1997;66:837–844.

65. Oopik AJ, Dorogy M, Devereux RB, et al. Major electrocardiographic abnormalities among American Indians aged 45 to 74 years (the Strong Heart Study). *Am J Cardiol* 1996;78:1400–1405.

66. Welty TK, Lee ET, Yeh J, et al. Cardiovascular disease risk factors among American Indians. The Strong Heart Study. *Am J Epidemiol* 1995;142:269–287.
67. Kuller L, Fisher L, McClelland R, et al. Differences in prevalence of and risk factors for subclinical vascular disease among black and white participants in the Cardiovascular Health Study. *Arterioscler Thromb Vasc Biol* 1998;18:283–293.
68. Lee ET, Cowan LD, Welty TK, et al. All-cause mortality and cardiovascular disease mortality in three American Indian populations, aged 45–74 years, 1984–1988. The Strong Heart Study. *Am J Epidemiol* 1998;147:995–1008.
69. Arner P. Not all fat is alike. *Lancet* 1998;351:1301–1302.
70. Bouchard C, Bray GA, Hubbard VS. Basic and clinical aspects of regional fat distribution. *Am J Clin Nutr* 1990;52:946–950.
71. Han TS, van Leer EM, Seidell JC, et al. Waist circumference action levels in the identification of cardiovascular risk factors: Prevalence study in a random sample. *BMJ* 1995;311:1401–1405.
72. Carey DG. Abdominal obesity. *Curr Opin Lipidol* 1998;9:35–40.
73. Bjorntorp P. The regulation of adipose tissue distribution in humans. *Int J Obes* 1996:291–302.
74. Kleerekoper M, Nelson DA, Peterson EL, et al. Body composition and gonadal steroids in older white and black women. *J Clin Endocrinol Metab* 1994;79:775–779.
75. Larsson B, Svardsudd K, Welin L, et al. Abdominal adipose tissue distribution, obesity, and risk of cardiovascular disease and death: 13 year follow up of participants in the study of men born in 1913. *Br Med J (Clin Res Ed)* 1984;288:1401–1404.
76. Lean ME, Han TS, Seidell JC. Impairment of health and quality of life in people with large waist circumference. *Lancet* 1998;351:853–856.
77. Albu JB, Murphy L, Frager DH, et al. Visceral fat and race-dependent health risks in obese nondiabetic premenopausal women. *Diabetes* 1997;46:456–462.
78. Meilahn EN, Cauley JA, Tracy RP, et al. Association of sex hormones and adiposity with plasma levels of fibrinogen and PAI-1 in postmenopausal women. *Am J Epidemiol* 1996;143:159–166.
79. Goodman-Gruen D, Barrett-Connor E. Sex differences in measures of body fat and body distribution in the elderly. *Am J Epidemiol* 1996;143:898–906.
80. Tracy RP, Psaty BM, Macy E, et al. Lifetime smoking exposure affects the association of C-reactive protein with cardiovascular disease risk factors and subclinical disease in healthy elderly subjects. *Arterioscler Thromb Vasc Biol* 1997;17:2167–2176.
81. Ridker PM, Morrow DA, Anderson JL. C-reactive protein predicts cardiovascular risk. American Heart Association 70th Scientific Sessions. Orlando, FL, 1997. Abstract.
82. Abate N, Garg A, Peshock RM, et al. Relationships of generalized and regional adiposity to insulin sensitivity in men. *J Clin Invest* 1995;96:88–98.
83. Talbott E, Guzick D, Clerici A, et al. Coronary heart disease risk factors in women with polycystic ovary syndrome. *Arterioscler Thromb Vasc Biol* 1995;15:821–826.
84. Fujimoto WY, Bergstrom RW, Boyko EJ, et al. Susceptibility to development of central adiposity among populations. *Obes Res* 1995;3:179S–186S.

85. Edwards KL, Burchfiel CM, Sharp DS, et al. Factors of the insulin resistance syndrome in nondiabetic and diabetic elderly Japanese-American men. *Am J Epidemiol* 1998;147:441–447.
86. Kuller LH, Gutai JP, Meilahn E, et al. Relationship of endogenous sex steroid hormones to lipids and apoproteins in postmenopausal women. *Arteriosclerosis* 1990;10:1058–1066.
87. Hankinson SE, Willett WC, Manson JE, et al. Alcohol, height, and adiposity in relation to estrogen and prolactin levels in postmenopausal women. *J Natl Cancer Inst* 1995;87:1297–1302.
88. Kuller LH, Cauley JA, Lucas L, et al. Sex steroid hormones, bone mineral density, and risk of breast cancer. *Environ Health Perspect* 1997;105:593–599.
89. Cauley JA, Lucas FL, Kuller LH, et al. Bone mineral density and risk of breast cancer in older women: The study of osteoporotic fractures. Study of Osteoporotic Fractures Research Group. *JAMA* 1996;276:1404–1408.
90. Cauley JA, Gutai JP, Kuller LH, et al. Black-white differences in serum sex hormones and bone mineral density. *Am J Epidemiol* 1994;139:1035–1046.
91. Ensrud KE, Cauley J, Lipschutz R, et al. Weight change and fractures in older women. Study of Osteoporotic Fractures Research Group. *Arch Intern Med* 1997;157:857–863.
92. Burger H, de Laet CE, van Daele PL, et al. Risk factors for increased bone loss in an elderly population: The Rotterdam Study. *Am J Epidemiol* 1998;147:871–879.
93. Stevens J, Cai J, Pamuk ER, et al. The effect of age on the association between body-mass index and mortality. *N Engl J Med* 1998;338:1–7.
94. Singh PN, Lindsted KD. Body mass and 26-year risk of mortality from specific diseases among women who never smoked. *Epidemiology* 1998;9:246–254.
95. Fried LP, Kronmal RA, Newman AB, et al. Risk factors for 5-year mortality in older adults: The Cardiovascular Health Study. *JAMA* 1998;279:585–592.
96. Eckel RH, Krauss RM. American Heart Association call to action: Obesity as a major risk factor for coronary heart disease. *AHA Nutrition Committee Circulation* 1998;97:2099–2100.
97. Ensrud KE, Lipschutz RC, Cauley JA, et al. *Am J Med* 1997;103:274–280.

Chapter 2

Obesity in Children, Adolescents, and Families

Eva Obarzanek, PhD, RD, MPH

Introduction

Obesity in children is a public health problem for the United States; its prevalence is high, it tracks over time as do other cardiovascular disease (CVD) risk factors, and it is associated with other CVD risk factors such as elevated blood pressure and dyslipidemia. In addition, obesity and other CVD risk factors aggregate in families, suggesting children will develop the increased risk present in their adult relatives. This report reviews the health risks of obesity during childhood, focusing on cardiovascular risk.

A Medline search on articles relating to obesity in childhood, ages 1–19, using key words including obesity, childhood, adolescence, hypercholesterolemia, risk factors, CVD, genetics, family history, mortality, and morbidity, was performed to search for articles from 1970 to 1998. In addition, relevant articles found in reference lists were used. Articles were obtained on tracking of weight and other CVD risk factors including blood lipids and blood pressure, obesity and its associations with other CVD risk factors, familial associations of obesity and risk factors relationships, and adult morbidity and mortality relations to childhood obesity.

To summarize the numerous tracking correlations, simple averages were calculated across studies. If male and female correlations were given separately they were averaged as well, because their proportion in the sample population tended to be similar, and there was no consistent trend for higher correlations in one sex versus another. Similarly, race-specific correlations also were included in the simple

From: Fletcher GF, Grundy SM, Hayman LL (eds). *Obesity: Impact on Cardiovascular Disease*. Armonk, NY: Futura Publishing Co., Inc.; © 1999.

averages, because there were not enough separate race-specific correlations to examine race separately. The racial groups most often reported separately were white and black. Thus, the averages reflect both sexes and all racial groups, primarily white and black.

Definition of Obesity in Children

Unlike adults where levels of body mass index (BMI, kg/m^2) could be related to specific health outcomes such as mortality[1,2] and disease,[3,4] no studies examining such relationships exist for children. Despite attempts to associate levels of body fatness with increased prevalence of other CVD risk factors in children,[5] no large-scale studies have been reported to provide the data necessary for consensus on a health-related definition of obesity in children. Generally, it is agreed that BMI, although correlated with fatness, is related to body fat in children less consistently than in adults, because it reflects components of lean body mass and bone, as well as fat, where the proportions of each may shift at various rates at different ages during childhood.[6]

Also, there is no consensus as to which reference population to use to identify a percentile cut point to define obesity in children. Reference populations used include those from the 1963–1970 Health Examination Surveys II and III,[7] the first National Health and Nutrition Examination Survey, (NHANES I) 1971–1974,[8,9] the NHANES II 1976–1980 ,[10] and a combination of the first and second NHANES surveys.[11]

To identify overweight children in treatment guidelines for clinicians, an expert committee identified the age-specific 95th percentile of BMI as an appropriate cut point.[12] The term overweight was used rather than obesity to acknowledge that BMI does not measure body fat. The age-specific 85th percentile of BMI also was recognized as an "at-risk" child, likely to become overweight. Thus, for public health purposes, it is useful to examine the 85th percentile of BMI to estimate population prevalences of children at risk of obesity.[7,13] It is likely that at younger ages, the 85th percentile of BMI overstates the prevalence of obesity; but as adolescents approach adult ages, it is likely that the 85th percentile begins to resemble the degree of fatness found in adults at the 85th percentile.

Obesity Prevalence and Trends in Children

Data from NHANES III, using as the reference population the 1963–1970 Health Examination Surveys, indicate that 21% to 23% of children age 6–17 are overweight, based on the definition of ≥85th

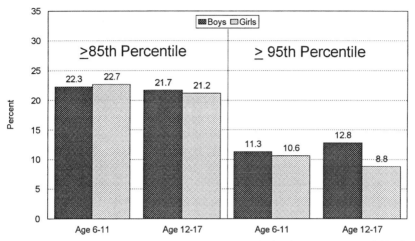

Figure 1. Prevalence of overweight and obesity in National Health and Nutrition Examination Survey (NHANES) III. Adapted with permission from Reference 7.

percentile of BMI, and 9% to 13% of children age 6–17 are obese, based on the definition of ≥95th percentile[7] (Figure 1). Furthermore, the prevalence of overweight is not distributed equally across sex and racial/ethnic groups (Figure 2). In younger children and in adolescents the prevalence of overweight tends to be lowest for whites, particularly girls. Black girls have the highest prevalence of overweight

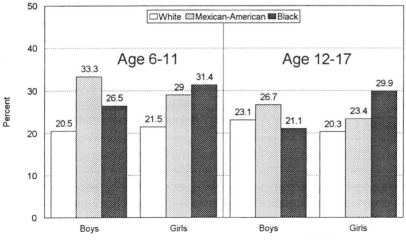

Figure 2. Prevalence of overweight (≥85th percentile) in NHANES III. According to race/sex subgroups. Adapted with permission from Reference 7.

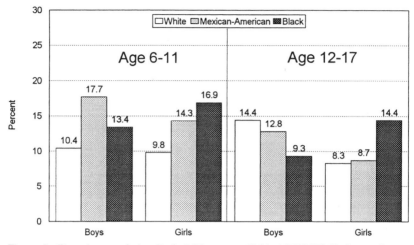

Figure 3. Prevalence of obesity (≥95th percentile) in NHANES III. According to race/sex subgroups. Adapted with permission from Reference 7.

among girls in both age groups. Mexican American boys have the highest prevalence of overweight among boys in the 6–11 year age group, whereas white boys have the highest prevalence among boys in the adolescent 12–17 year age group. These race-sex patterns are similar for the 95th percentile (Figure 3).

The NHANES III has brought to public attention not only the high prevalence of overweight and obesity in American children, but even more unsettling, the increasing secular trend, which is especially evident since the previous survey in 1976–1980.[7] The prevalence of overweight (≥85th percentile) increased similarly in younger and older children of both sexes, from 15% in the earliest 1963–1970 surveys to 22%–23% in the latest survey, a 50% increase.[7] In boys and girls age 6–11 the prevalence of obesity (≥95th percentile) shows a doubling from the earliest surveys to the latest survey, from 5% to 11%. In the 12–17 year age group, the prevalence of obesity (≥95th percentile) more than doubled in boys, from 5% to 13%, and increased 1.7-fold in girls, from 5% to 9%.[7]

Tracking of Weight and Cardiovascular Disease Risk Factors

If weight and CVD risk factors during childhood were independent of weight and CVD risk factors in adulthood, then childhood levels may not increase CVD risk. However, there is abundant evidence that weight and CVD risk factors track to varying degrees from childhood to adulthood. Tracking of weight and other risk factors typically has been measured by the following methods: correlations between weight and risk factors at one age with weight and risk factors at another, examination of the maintenance of a child's percentile ranking in weight and risk factor from childhood to older ages, and relative risk ratios that calculate the likelihood of becoming overweight as an adult if overweight as a child.

Tracking of Weight and Body Mass Index

Twenty-two studies reported 187 tracking correlations with varying measures (including weight, BMI, weight for height, and skin folds), varying lengths of follow-up, and varying initial ages for the first measurement.[14-35] Tracking usually is higher with measures of weight or with weight and height compared with skin fold measures. Figure 4 illustrates how the correlation coefficients change according to the age at the first measurement and the number of years of follow-up between the two measurements. Initial ages reflect the preschool (age 1–4), prepubertal (age 5–8), pubertal (age 9–14), and older adolescent (age 15–20) ages. No matter what the initial age is, the correlation coefficients decrease as the follow-up period increases. For very short term follow-up periods of 1–3 years, the correlation coefficients are little affected by the initial age of the first measurement, ranging from

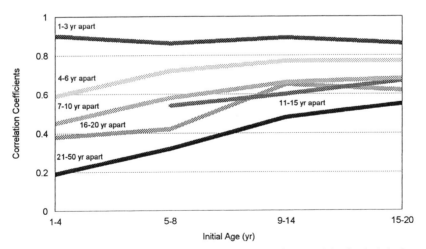

Figure 4. Tracking of weight, body mass index (BMI), or weight-for-height for various follow-up periods: mean correlation coefficients. $N = 187$ correlation coefficients from 22 studies.

Table 1

Tracking of Weight, BMI, or Weight for Height:
Mean Correlation Coefficients

Overall				Initial age (years)				
No. of years apart	N^*	1–4	N^*	5–8	N^*	9–14	N^*	15–20
1–3	1	0.90	11	0.86	17	0.89	1	0.86
4–6	4	0.59	14	0.72	25	0.77	5	0.77
7–10	3	0.45	11	0.58	13	0.66	3	0.68
11–15	0	—	9	0.54	13	0.60	5	0.67
16–20	4	0.38	6	0.42	8	0.65	7	0.62
21–50	4	0.19	8	0.32	13	0.48	2	0.55

					Initial age (years)							
		1–4			5–8			9–14			15–20	
By sex	$N^†$	M	F	$N^†$	M	F	$N^†$	M	F	$N^†$	M	F
1–3	0	—	—	7	0.81	0.86	9	0.89	0.89	0	—	—
4–6	7	0.40	0.60	11	0.68	0.73	18	0.78	0.80	4	0.79	0.74
7–10	2	0.24	0.51	7	0.60	0.63	7	0.68	0.62	2	0.68	0.71
11–15	0	—	—	9	0.53	0.54	12	0.64	0.60	5	0.70	0.65
16–20	4	0.38	0.37	5	0.43	0.43	7	0.71	0.59	7	0.57	0.66
21–50	4	0.17	0.21	8	0.34	0.31	13	0.48	0.47	2	0.56	0.53

* Number of correlation coefficients obtained from 22 studies.
† Number of correlation coefficients obtained from 16 studies.

0.86 to 0.90 across all the ages. At all longer follow-up periods, tracking is lowest for very young children age 4 years and under. For the very longest follow-up period of 21–50 years the correlation coefficients continue to increase across the entire range of initial age, reaching 0.55 when the initial age is the oldest. Although some individual studies reported a trend for somewhat higher tracking in one sex versus another (which sometimes depended on age),[15,22,30] when all the studies providing separate correlations by sex were averaged together no consistent sex differences were observed (Table 1).[14–17,19,21,22,24,27–31,33–35]

There were insufficient numbers of studies comparing tracking correlations by race.

Several studies examined rankings of various upper percentiles, ranging from the top tertile to the top 5th percentile, covering a follow-up period of 3 years to over 20 years, with initial age ranging from 1–4 years to 16 years or more.[14,17,18,20,22,29,32,34,35] They all showed greater than expected occurrence of high percentile BMI or weight for height than if there were no tracking, ranging from 12 percentage points greater than expected[34] to as much as 60 percentage points greater than expected.[32] As for tracking of correlation coefficients, the persistence of percentile ranking is more likely to occur at older initial ages and with shorter intervals between measurements. It has been noted that the greater maintenance of percentile rankings occurs particularly at the higher levels of overweight. Thus, children at the 95th or higher percentiles tend to maintain their percentile ranking more than children at the 75th to 90th percentiles.[22,29]

In a review article, Serdula et al[36] calculated the probability of being overweight at follow-up if overweight as a child from data of several published studies. The relative risk of being overweight at follow-up was 2.0 to 6.5 in individuals who were overweight initially compared with children who were not overweight initially. The relative risk increased as the initial age increased and decreased as the interval between measurements increased. Since that review was published other studies provided information on relative risk, showing similar relative risk of 4.3[37] or even higher relative risks of 10.3 to 28.3.[38]

Taken together, these studies show that obesity in adulthood is not independent of obesity in childhood. The correlation coefficients are moderately high, high percentile rankings are maintained over time, and relative risks are well above 1. Nevertheless, not all obese children will become obese adults. Studies have observed from 26% to as high as 75% of obese children remained obese as an adult.[36–38] It may therefore be difficult to identify with precision the individual obese child who will become an obese adult. Of obese young adults in their 20s to early 30s, only approximately one-quarter were obese children.[28,29] Nevertheless, the evidence is very strong that in general obese children are likely to become obese adults.

Tracking of Cardiovascular Disease Risk Factors

Other CVD risk factors also track from childhood to adulthood, although to a lesser extent than does weight.[14,16,18,20,24,31–33,39–61] Because there are fewer correlation coefficients reported for other CVD risk factors than there are for weight, patterns are more difficult to discern. The most consistent pattern with all the risk factors is that the correlation coefficients decrease with increasing intervals between measurements. The pattern of lower tracking correlation coefficients when initial ages are younger and when the intervals between measurements are greater was less consistent than was observed for weight. Table 2 shows the average of all correlation coefficients together across all initial ages and all follow-up periods. The correlation

Table 2

Mean Tracking Correlations of CVD Risk Factors

	N*	Mean	Range	N*	Boys	Girls
TC	102	0.60	0.35–0.78	78	.61	0.58
LDL-C	71	0.60	0.38–0.82	48	.56	0.52
HDL-C	72	0.40	−0.09–0.75	50	.39	0.37
TG	71	0.37	0.14–0.71	53	.39	0.37
SBP	131	0.43	0.19–0.73	91	.39	0.40
DBP	127	0.30	−0.12–0.57	91	.28	0.28

* N = number of correlation coefficients from 11–19 studies.

coefficients are highest for total cholesterol (TC) and low-density lipoprotein cholesterol (LDL-C) at r = 0.60, moderate for triglycerides (TG), high-density lipoprotein cholesterol (HDL-C), and systolic blood pressure (SBP), ranging from 0.37 to 0.43, and somewhat lower for diastolic blood pressure (DBP), at r = 0.30. DBP is more difficult to measure in children than SBP, and studies varied in whether they used the fourth or fifth Korotkoff sounds for DBP. There was little difference between boys and girls in the magnitude of these tracking correlations. Tracking also is evident from linear regression analyses relating follow-up values to baseline values. The most consistent greatest predictor of follow-up levels of a risk factor is the baseline level of that risk factor.[37,49]

The lower magnitude of CVD risk factor correlation coefficients compared with those for weight may be attributed in part to differences in measurement precision and day-to-day within-person variability. Body weight and BMI can be measured with good precision and low-measurement error, while lipids and blood pressure have higher measurement error. Tracking correlations increased considerably from 0.45 to 0.69 for 3-year tracking in SBP[62] and from 0.57 to 0.78 from initial visit to the next follow-up if the total number of cholesterol measurements increased from two to five or more.[43] With the multiple measures, these risk factor tracking coefficients approach those seen in adults and those seen for weight in children.

Relationship between Obesity and Cardiovascular Disease Risk Factors

Obesity has been associated with CVD risk factors in children. Studies from the Bogalusa Heart Study, Muscatine, National Heart, Lung, and Blood Institute Growth and Health Study (NGHS), as well as other pediatric populations, have shown that weight, BMI, and/or skin folds are correlated with CVD risk factors. Averaging the cross-sectional correlation coefficients reported across sex and age, the mean correlation coefficients in children over the age of 3 range from −0.18 to 0.37 for the various risk factors (Table 3).[18,26,44,45,51,63–80] These associations have been found in boys and girls, whites, blacks, Asians, and Hispanics.[45,74,76,80] As with tracking correlations, correlations between weight and risk factors are smaller at younger preadolescent ages, particularly for blood lipids, than at older ages. Moderate correlations of 0.3 to 0.4 with SBP are already evident by age 6–9[69] and 9–10.[74] Correlations between weight and cholesterol have been found to be weaker in blacks than whites in some studies,[76,79] but this has not been observed consistently at all ages and in both sexes.[45,74]

In addition to cross-sectional studies, longitudinal studies have observed correlations between childhood levels of or change in BMI or skin folds and adult levels of CVD risk factors, ranging from −0.06 to 0.4 (Table 4).[26,44,69] Those with the larger gains in weight, BMI, or triceps skin folds had greater increases in risk factor levels (or decreases for HDL-C) compared with children who have not gained weight or were in the lowest tertile of weight or weight gain (Table 5).[16,44,81] Finally, in linear regression models of follow-up levels of CVD risk factors, baseline levels of BMI and change in BMI were the next most predictive factors, after baseline level of the risk factor, for predicting follow-up levels.[37]

Some studies have observed race differences in the magnitude of the change in CVD risk factors with increasing obesity in children. Thus, although there is an association between CVD risk factors and obesity in both blacks and whites, the extent of change in a risk factor has been observed to be less in blacks than in whites for lipids[44,79] and for blood pressure.[39] More research investigating this possible differential relationship between the races should be conducted.

Table 3

Mean Correlations Between Obesity and CVD Risk Factors

	*N**	Mean	Range
TC	25	0.07	−0.06–0.20
LDL-C	15	0.11	−0.02–0.24
HDL-C	15	−0.18	−0.03––0.35
TG	12	0.20	0.02–0.29
SBP	26	0.37	0.15–0.60
DBP	26	0.26	0.02–0.49

* *N* = number of correlation coefficients from 6–10 studies.

Table 4

Correlations Between Childhood Obesity and Adult Level of Risk Factors

Study	Description	Correlation coefficients
Freedman, 1985, N = 1598, age 5–12 years {46}	Change in triceps vs. change in risk factor (5-yr follow-up)	0.21 (TC) 0.28 (LDL-C) −0.06 (HDL-C) 0.17 (TG)
Myers, 1995, N = 1457, age 5–14 years {82}	Childhood ponderal index vs. adult risk factor (15.7-yr follow-up)	0.12 (TC) 0.09 (SBP)
Higgins, 1983, N = 2101, age 6–17 years {128}	Childhood BMI vs. adult risk factor (15-yr follow-up)	0.24–.34 (SBP) 0.19–.33 (DBP)

In general, although the magnitude of the cross-sectional correlations between obesity and risk factors are modest, the longitudinal observations provide additional evidence that obesity is associated causally with risk factors in children.

Clustering of Risk Factors in Overweight Children

Webber[80] observed that being in the upper quartile of a BMI $(kg/m^{2.77})$ tended to occur together or cluster with elevated levels of

Table 5

Change in CVD Risk Factors with Weight or Skin Folds Change

Study	Weight or skin folds change	Risk factor change
Dwyer, 1998, N = 5106, age 9 years {45}	Gained weight vs. never gained weight (3-yr follow-up)	+4.9% TC −5.3% HDL-C +2.4% SBP
Freedman, 1985, N = 1598, age 5–12 years {46}	Highest vs. lowest tertile change in triceps (5-yr follow-up)	+7.8% TC +11.2% LDL-C −2.9% HDL-C +19.3% TG
Clarke, 1986, N = 2925, age 6–15 years {41}	Increased from lowest four quintiles to highest quintile vs. remained in the lowest quintile of BMI (10-yr follow-up)	+19.2 percentiles SBP +9.9 percentiles DBP

cholesterol and blood pressure in school children. Twice as many children as expected were in the top quartile for all three risk factors. Children age 6–12 with multiple risk factors had 1.2 to 1.6 higher BMI units and 2.6 to 3.6 mm higher subscapular skin folds than those without multiple risk factors.[82] Other observations showed that overweight children and young adults (age 5–24) in the upper tertile of subscapular skin folds had 2 to 4 times greater occurrence than expected of three risk factors, including LDL-C + very LDL-C (VLDL-C)–to–HDL-C ratio, SBP, and insulin, while children in the lowest tertile of subscapular skin folds have approximately only 0.3 to 0.7 the expected occurrence of these three risk factors.[83] The prevalence of having a cluster of risk factors, defined by a multiple risk factor index score above the 75th percentile, was highest (approximately 37%) in 5–17 year olds who were at the top tertile of ponderal index and was lowest (approximately 14%) in those in the lowest tertile of ponderal index.[40] Furthermore, change in ponderal index (kg/m^3) over 8 years was related to the prevalence of being above the 75th percentile of the multiple risk factor index score. Thus, about 37% of those who were in the highest tertile of gain in ponderal index were above the 75th percentile of the multiple risk factor index score compared with only approximately 16% for those who were in the lowest tertile of gain in ponderal index. In addition, this clustering of risk factors was likely to follow the adolescents into adulthood. The tracking correlation over 8 years of this multiple risk index score was higher $(r = 0.64)$ than the tracking correlations of each individual risk factor of SBP $(r = 0.54)$, TC–to–HDL-C ratio $(r = 0.57)$, and insulin level $(r = 0.34)$.[40]

Srinivasan[37] observed that adults overweight since their adolescence 12 years earlier were 3.0 to 5.8 times as likely to have at least two other risk factors as lean adults who had been lean adolescents. Myers et al.[26] reported that the percentage of adults with a cluster of risk factors (≥75th percentile in TC, SBP, and ponderal index) increased in relation to the number of risk factors (≥75th percentile) they had during childhood 15 years earlier. Approximately 20% of young adults had a cluster of risk factors if they had three risk factors during childhood compared with approximately 4% who had only one risk factor or 1% with no risk factors during childhood.[26] These data show that heavy children have a higher than expected occurrence of two or more risk factors and that this clustering likely is to be maintained through adulthood. This sequence of events suggests that overweight children with a cluster of risk factors would be at substantial risk of developing coronary heart disease (CHD) in the future.

Fat Patterning and Cardiovascular Disease Risk Factors

In adults evidence has been accumulating that much of the risk of obesity lies in the location of the excess adipose tissue. Central adiposity is related to increased incidence in CVD, stroke, and Type 2 diabetes mellitus.[84] The component of abdominal fat that is likely to be the major factor accounting for this relationship is visceral fat.[84] Although there is no evidence linking central adiposity with disease in children, observations from the Bogalusa Heart Study indicate that the association between obesity and CVD risk factors in over 3500 children and young adults, age 5–24, is attenuated when adjusted for subscapular skin folds, an index of central adiposity.[83,85] Similarly, in NGHS, an investigation on obesity development in 2379 girls age 9 and 10 at baseline, it was observed that within overweight girls, greater central adiposity assessed by a ratio of subscapular and suprailiac skin folds to total skin folds was associated with higher risk factor levels and clustering of high blood pressure and high levels of lipids than overweight girls without central adiposity (Morrison, personal communication, 1998). Caprio et al.[86] reported significant associations in 10 obese adolescent girls between visceral fat, assessed by imaging techniques, and TGs ($r = 0.53$) and HDL-C ($r = -0.54$) but not with LDL-C or blood pressure. However, other reports have found inconsistent or no associations between fat distribution and CVD risk factors independent of overall obesity.[87–91] Because the data are limited and inconsistent in children, and because in general overall adiposity is correlated highly with regional adiposity, overall adiposity is still the best overall measure of risk in children.

Familial Aggregation of Cardiovascular Disease Risk Factors and Obesity

CVD risk factors tend to occur in families, suggesting the influence of shared genetics as well as shared environment. Correlation coefficients of risk factors within family members averaged across several studies, including sib pairs and parent-child pairs, range from 0.14 for SBP to 0.28 for HDL-C (Table 6).[18,63,68,74,92–98]

Children whose family members have a history of disease tend to have higher risk factor levels as well. Children with a family history of coronary artery disease (CAD), including myocardial infarction, had 7–8 mg/dL (5%–7%) higher levels of TC and LDL-C, 1 mg/dL (2%) lower levels of HDL-C, and 2 mg/dL (3%) higher TG than children

Table 6

Correlations Within Families of Risk Factors

N*	Risk factor	Correlation coefficient	Range
36	TC	0.27	0.17–0.40
8	LDL-C	0.26	0.12–0.35
10	HDL-C	0.28	0.04–0.46
8	TG	0.17	0.11–0.25
20	SBP	0.17	−0.03–0.49
20	DBP	0.14	0.09–0.25

* N = number of correlation coefficients from 13 studies.

without a family history of CAD.[99–103] Similarly, children with a family history of hypertension had 2 mm Hg (2%) higher SBP and 1 mm Hg (1.5%) higher DBP than children without a family history of hypertension.[99,100,102] Conversely, two studies observed that parents and grandparents of children at the 95th percentiles of TC had approximately 65 mg/dL (40%) and 20 mg/dL (10%) higher TC levels than parents and grandparents of children at the 5th percentile or less of TC.[104,105] These studies also reported higher mortality and frequency of CAD in the parents and grandparents of children with high-cholesterol levels.[104,105]

It has long been observed that obesity tends to run in families.[106] Children with heavy parents are more likely to be heavy than children without heavy parents. Morrison et al[74] reported a risk ratio of 1.9 and 1.7 for overweight white and black mothers having an overweight daughter compared with nonoverweight mothers. More recently, Whitaker et al[38] observed risk ratios of 2:3 for a child to be obese if they had one obese parent. If the child had two obese parents, the risk ratio ranged from 2 to 15. The range reflects the age of the child, with the higher ratios occurring for younger children age 5 or less. Conversely, relatives of heavy children are 12%–20% heavier than relatives of lean children.[107]

Obesity and CVD risk factors are related between children and their families as well. Children who came from families with a history of hypertension had 4% higher BMI and those who came from families with a history of CAD had 10%–13% higher subscapular skin folds than children with no family history of hypertension or CAD.[99–101] Conversely, Burns et al[107] reported that relatives of heavy children have approximately 4 mg/dL (5%) higher LDL-C, 8 mg/dL (16%) lower HDL-C, 15 mg/dL (15%) higher TG, 11 mm Hg (10%) higher SBP, 4 mm Hg (5%) higher DBP, and 25% higher CVD death rates than relatives of lean children.

Childhood Obesity and Adult Morbidity and Mortality

There are several reports linking obesity in youth with adult morbidity and mortality. In follow-up of up to 37 years of obese 18-year-old military men with BMI $\geq$ 31, Sonne-Holm et al[108] reported relative risk ratio of 1.67 for mortality in obese versus a nonobese control group ($P < 0.02$) and noted most of this mortality occurred during early ages (18–29 years). Mossberg[109] likewise had 40 years of follow-up data on overweight children admitted to a hospital and found that these adults who had been overweight as children had 20% higher prevalence of chronic disease including CVD, hypertension, and diabetes compared with an external nonobese reference population, which was significant with all diseases combined ($P < 0.001$) but not for any individual disease. There also was a 1.7 time greater number of deaths than expected, most of which were caused by CVD, although this was not significant.

In a population-based study, Abraham et al[110] noted that adults who had been overweight (120% or more relative weight) during childhood had higher levels (not significant) of fasting blood sugar, SBP, and DBP in adulthood 40 years later. More recently, after 42 years of follow-up of 13 146 children age 5–18, all-cause mortality was reported to be 1.5 to 1.6 higher in adults who were in the upper quintile of relative weight compared with the lowest quintile of relative weight during childhood.[111] Similarly, a 55-year follow-up of 508 school children initially aged 13–18 reported that adult men who were overweight during childhood had 2.3 times higher mortality from CAD and 1.8 times higher mortality from all causes compared with men who were normal weight during childhood.[112] There was no association with obesity and mortality in women who were overweight as adolescents. However, overweight during adolescence was associated with 1.8 to 2.1 times increased risk of CAD for both men and women and with 8.1 times increased risk of functional impairment (difficulty with activities of daily living) in women compared with their lean counterparts. These studies are the most compelling evidence of deleterious effects of childhood obesity on health later in adulthood.

Etiology of Obesity

The factors related to the cause of obesity are described only briefly below. Greater understanding of the factors related to obesity is pivotal to help design interventions to prevent and treat obesity.

Genetics

Ample evidence exists that weight is in part determined genetically.[106] However, the role of the environment is recognized strongly to be contributory to obesity as well. Although much research currently is underway to determining genes responsible for human obesity, there currently is no practical application for intervention on obesity using information based on an individual's genetic composition.

Socioeconomic Status

A consistent inverse association has been found between socioeconomic status and obesity in adult women, primarily white women[113]; however, the role of race independent of socioeconomic status is less clear.[114] The relationship between socioeconomic status and obesity is less consistent in children. A recent report in a cohort of 9- and 10-year-old girls suggested that household education and income is related inversely to obesity in white girls but this is less clear in black girls.[115]

Diet

Although overall caloric intake as part of energy balance is important, studies generally have not observed a direct relation between energy intake and body weight in childhood.[116] Several studies have reported a direct relationship between percent of calories from fat and body weight in children in cross-sectional analyses.[116–118] Longitudinal investigations will help further clarify the role of energy intake and macronutrient composition in the development of obesity.

Physical Activity

Evidence is accumulating that physical activity is an important factor related inversely to body weight[119] and fat gain.[52] Studies evaluating the type and amount of physical activity that favorably influences weight and weight gain are important to help design interventions to prevent obesity.

Television Viewing

Because the early intriguing reports that television viewing is related directly to obesity[120] and fat gain,[121] the factors accounting for this association have not been determined. Increased snacking, less time spent being physically active, and reduced resting metabolic rate[121,122] are among the explanations offered. Interventions to decrease sedentary activities have been suggested as a promising area for intervention.[123]

Psychosocial

Associations between obesity and numerous psychosocial factors, including self-esteem,[124,125] body image,[126] family influences,[127] and culture,[128] have been examined. Prospective studies will help identify psychosocial factors related to obesity development and may help guide intervention approaches to prevent obesity.

Conclusions

As in adults, obesity in children is associated cross-sectionally and longitudinally with single and multiple CVD risk factors. The presence of substantial tracking of weight and CVD risk factors, familial associations of weight and CVD risk factors, and consistent cross-sectional and longitudinal relationships between obesity and CVD risk factors suggests that obese children likely are to have elevated risk of CVD observed in their adult relatives. The increased probability of elevated CVD risk is supported further by studies showing increased rates of disease and mortality in adults who were obese as children. Taken together, these studies strongly suggest that childhood obesity confers future elevated CVD risk. Given its high and increasing prevalence, obesity is a significant public health problem, and there is a pressing need for public health solutions to prevent obesity in childhood.

References

1. Troiano RP, Frongillo EA Jr, Sobal J, et al. The relationship between body weight and mortality: A quantitative analysis of combined information from existing studies. *Int J Obes Relat Metab Disord* 1996;20:63–75.
2. Manson JE, Willett WC, Stampfer MJ, et al. Body weight and mortality among women. *N Engl J Med* 1995;333:677–685.

3. Willett WC, Manson JE, Stampfer MJ, et al. Weight, weight change, and coronary heart disease in women. Risk within the "normal"' weight range. *JAMA* 1995;273:461–465.
4. Brown CD, Donato KA, Obarzanek E. Body mass index and prevalence of risk factors for cardiovascular disease. *Obess Res* In press.
5. Williams DP, Going SB, Lohman TG, et al. Body fatness and risk for elevated blood pressure, total cholesterol, and serum lipoprotein ratios in children and adolescents. *Am J Public Health* 1992;82:358–363.
6. Obarzanek E. Methodological issues in estimating the prevalence of obesity in childhood. *Ann N Y Acad Sci* 1993;699:278–279.
7. Troiano RP, Flegal KM, Kuczmarski RJ, et al. Overweight prevalence and trends for children and adolescents. The National Health and Nutrition Examination Surveys 1963 to 1991. *Arch Pediatr Adolesc Med* 1995;149: 1085–1091.
8. Must A, Dallal GE, Dietz WH. Reference data for obesity: 85th and 95th percentiles of body mass index (wt/ht2) and triceps skinfold thickness. *Am J Clin Nutr* 1991;53:839–846.
9. Must A, Dallal GE, Dietz WH. Reference data for obesity: 85th and 95th percentiles of body mass index (wt/ht2): A correction. *Am J Clin Nutr* 1991;54:19–23.
10. Muecke L, Simons-Morton B, Huang IW, et al. Is childhood obesity associated with high-fat foods and low physical activity? *J Sch Health* 1992;62:19–23.
11. Campaigne BN, Morrison JA, Schumann BC, et al. Indexes of obesity and comparisons with previous national survey data in 9- and 10-year-old black and white girls: The National Heart, Lung, and Blood Institute Growth and Health Study. *J Pediatr* 1994;124:675–680.
12. Himes JH, Dietz WH. Guidelines for overweight in adolescent preventive services: Recommendations from an expert committee. The Expert Committee on Clinical Guidelines for Overweight in Adolescent Preventive Services. *Am J Clin Nutr* 1994;59:307–316.
13. Troiano RP, Flegal KM. Overweight children and adolescents—description, epidemiology, and demographics. *Pediatrics* 1998;101:497–504.
14. Angelico F, Del Ben M, Barbato A, et al. Eleven-year tracking of established cardiovascular risk factors in Italian school-aged children. *Ann Ig* 1997;9:193–200.
15. Casey VA, Dwyer JT, Coleman KA, et al. Body mass index from childhood to middle age: a 50-y follow-up. *Am J Clin Nutr* 1992;56:14–18.
16. Clarke WR, Schrott HG, Leaverton PE, et al. Tracking of blood lipids and blood pressures in school age children: The Muscatine Study. *Circulation* 1978;58:626–634.
17. Clarke WR, Lauer RM. Does childhood obesity track into adulthood? *Crit Rev Food Sci Nutr* 1993;33:423–430.
18. Clarke WR, Woolson RF, Lauer RM. Changes in ponderosity and blood pressure in childhood: The Muscatine Study. *Am J Epidemiol* 1986;124: 195–206.
19. Freedman DS, Shear CL, Burke GL, et al. Persistence of juvenile-onset obesity over eight years: The Bogalusa Heart Study. *Am J Public Health* 1987;77:588–592.
20. Frerichs RR, Webber LS, Voors AW, et al. Cardiovascular disease risk factor variables in children at two successive years. The Bogalusa Heart Study. *J Chronic Dis* 1979;32:251–262.

21. Garn SM, Pilkington JJ, Lavelle M. Relationship between initial fatness level and long-term fatness change. *Ecol Food Nutr* 1984;14:85–92.

22. Guo SS, Roche AF, Chumlea WC, et al. The predictive value of childhood body mass index values for overweight at age 35 y. *Am J Clin Nutr* 1994;59:810–819.

23. Lissau-Lund-Sorensen I, Sorensen TI. Prospective study of the influence of social factors in childhood on risk of overweight in young adulthood. *Int J Obes Relat Metab Disord* 1992;16:169–175.

24. Michels VV, Bergstralh EJ, Hoverman VR, et al. Tracking and prediction of blood pressure in children. *Mayo Clin Proc* 1987;62:875–881.

25. Miller FJ, Billewicz WZ, Thomson AM. Growth from birth to adult life of 442 Newcastle upon Tyne children. *Br J Prev Soc Med* 1972;26:224–230.

26. Myers L, Coughlin SS, Webber LS, et al. Prediction of adult cardiovascular multifactorial risk status from childhood risk factor levels. The Bogalusa Heart Study. *Am J Epidemiol* 1995;142:918–924.

27. Shapiro LR, Crawford PB, Clark MJ, et al. Obesity prognosis: A longitudinal study of children from the age of 6 months to 9 years. *Am J Public Health* 1984;74:968–972.

28. Stark O, Atkins E, Wolff OH, et al. Longitudinal study of obesity in the National Survey of Health and Development. *Br Med J* 1981;283:13–17.

29. Power C, Lake JK, Cole TJ. Body mass index and height from childhood to adulthood in the 1958 British born cohort. *Am J Clin Nutr* 1997;66:1094–1101.

30. Rolland-Cachera MF, Bellisle F, Sempe M. The prediction in boys and girls of the weight/height index and various skinfold measurements in adults: A two-decade follow-up study. *Int J Obes* 1989;13:305–311.

31. Wattigney WA, Webber LS, Srinivasan SR, et al. The emergence of clinically abnormal levels of cardiovascular disease risk factor variables among young adults: The Bogalusa Heart Study. *Prev Med* 1995;24:617–626.

32. Webber LS, Cresanta JL, Voors AW, et al. Tracking of cardiovascular disease risk factor variables in school-age children. *J Chronic Dis* 1983;36:647–660.

33. Webber LS, Cresanta JL, Croft JB, et al. Transitions of cardiovascular risk from adolescence to young adulthood. The Bogalusa Heart Study, II: Alterations in anthropometric blood pressure and serum lipoprotein variables. *J Chronic Dis* 1986;39:91–103.

34. Weststrate JA, Van Klaveren H, Deurenberg P. Changes in skinfold thicknesses and body mass index in 171 children, initially 1 to 5 years of age: A 5 1/2-year follow-up study. *Int J Obes* 1986;10:313–321.

35. Zack PM, Harlan WR, Leaverton PE, et al. A longitudinal study of body fatness in childhood and adolescence. *J Pediatr* 1979;95:126–130.

36. Serdula MK, Ivery D, Coates RJ, et al. Do obese children become obese adults? A review of the literature. *Prev Med* 1993;22:167–177.

37. Srinivasan SR, Bao W, Wattigney WA, et al. Adolescent overweight is associated with adult overweight and related multiple cardiovascular risk factors: The Bogalusa Heart Study. *Metabolism* 1996;45:235–240.

38. Whitaker RC, Wright JA, Pepe MS, et al. Predicting obesity in young adulthood from childhood and parental obesity. *N Engl J Med* 1997;337:869–873.

39. Bao W, Srinivasan SR, Wattigney WA, et al. Usefulness of childhood low-density lipoprotein cholesterol level in predicting adult dyslipidemia

and other cardiovascular risks. The Bogalusa Heart Study. *Arch Intern Med* 1996;156:1315–1320.

40. Bao W, Srinivasan SR, Wattigney WA, et al. Persistence of multiple cardiovascular risk clustering related to syndrome X from childhood to young adulthood. The Bogalusa Heart Study. *Arch Intern Med* 1994;154: 1842–1847.

41. Bao W, Srinivasan SR, Berenson GS. Tracking of serum apolipoproteins A-I and B in children and young adults: The Bogalusa Heart Study. *J Clin Epidemiol* 1993;46:609–616.

42. Berenson GS, Harsha DW, Webber LS, et al. Contrasts by race and sex of cardiovascular risk factors in children and young adults: The Bogalusa Heart Study. *Cardiovasc Risk Factors* 1992;2:81–95.

43. Freedman DS, Byers T, Sell K, et al. Tracking of serum cholesterol levels in a multiracial sample of preschool children. *Pediatrics* 1992;90:80–86.

44. Freedman DS, Burke GL, Harsha DW, et al. Relationship of changes in obesity to serum lipid and lipoprotein changes in childhood and adolescence. *JAMA* 1985;254:515–520.

45. Hait HI, Lemeshow S, Rosenman KD. A longitudinal study of blood pressure in a national survey of children. *Am J Public Health* 1982;72:1285–1287.

46. Hofman A, Valkenburg HA, Maas J, et al. The natural history of blood pressure in childhood. *Int J Epidemiol* 1985;14:91–96.

47. Kallio MJ, Salmenpera L, Siimes MA, et al. Tracking of serum cholesterol and lipoprotein levels from the first year of life. *Pediatrics* 1993;91:949–954.

48. Laskarzewski P, Morrison JA, deGroot I, et al. Lipid and lipoprotein tracking in 108 children over a four-year period. *Pediatrics* 1979;64:584–591.

49. Lauer RM, Clarke WR. Childhood risk factors for high adult blood pressure: The Muscatine Study. *Pediatrics* 1989;84:633–641.

50. Lauer RM, Lee J, Clarke WR. Factors affecting the relationship between childhood and adult cholesterol levels: The Muscatine Study. *Pediatrics* 1988;82:309–318.

51. Lauer RM, Anderson AR, Beaglehole R, et al. Factors related to tracking of blood pressure in children. U.S. National Center for Health Statistics Health Examination Surveys Cycles II and III. *Hypertension* 1984;6:307–314.

52. Orchard TJ, Donahue RP, Kuller LH, et al. Cholesterol screening in childhood: Does it predict adult hypercholesterolemia? *The Beaver County experience J Pediatr.* 1983;103:687–691.

53. Porkka KV, Viikari JS, Taimela S, et al. Tracking and predictiveness of serum lipid and lipoprotein measurements in childhood: a 12-year follow-up. The Cardiovascular Risk in Young Finns Study. *Am J Epidemiol* 1994;140:1096–1110.

54. Porkka KV, Viikari JS, Akerblom HK. Tracking of serum HDL-cholesterol and other lipids in children and adolescents: The Cardiovascular Risk in Young Finns Study. *Prev Med* 1991;20:713–724.

55. Rosner B, Hennekens CH, Kass EH, et al. Age-specific correlation analysis of longitudinal blood pressure data. *Am J Epidemiol* 1977;106:306–313.

56. Sporik R, Johnstone JH, Cogswell JJ. Longitudinal study of cholesterol values in 68 children from birth to 11 years of age. *Arch Dis Child* 1991;66:134–137.

57. Stuhldreher WL, Orchard TJ, Donahue RP, et al. Cholesterol screening in childhood: Sixteen-year Beaver County Lipid Study Experience. *J Pediatr* 1991;119:551–556.
58. Twisk JW, Kemper HC, Mellenbergh DJ, et al. Factors influencing tracking of cholesterol and high-density lipoprotein: The Amsterdam Growth and Health Study. *Prev Med* 1996;25:355–364.
59. Voors AW, Webber LS, Berenson GS. Time course study of blood pressure in children over a three-year period. Bogalusa Heart Study. *Hypertension* 1980;2:102–108.
60. Webber LS, Srinivasan SR, Wattigney WA, et al. Tracking of serum lipids and lipoproteins from childhood to adulthood. The Bogalusa Heart Study. *Am J Epidemiol* 1991;133:884–899.
61. Zinner SH, Margolius HS, Rosner B, et al. Stability of blood pressure rank and urinary kallikrein concentration in childhood: An eight-year follow-up. *Circulation* 1978;58:908–915.
62. Gillman MW, Rosner B, Evans DA, et al. Use of multiple visits to increase blood pressure tracking correlations in childhood. *Pediatrics* 1991;87:708–711.
63. Connor SL, Connor WE, Henry H, et al. The effects of familial relationships, age, body weight, and diet on blood pressure and the 24 hour urinary excretion of sodium, potassium, and creatinine in men, women, and children of randomly selected families. *Circulation* 1984;70:76–85.
64. Daniels SR, Obarzanek E, Barton BA, et al. Sexual maturation and racial differences in blood pressure in girls: The National Heart, Lung, and Blood Institute Growth and Health Study. *J Pediatr* 1996;129:208–213.
65. Dahlstrom S, Viikari J, Akerblom HK, et al. Atherosclerosis precursors in Finnish children and adolescents. II. Height, weight, body mass index, and skinfolds, and their correlation to metabolic variables. *Acta Paediatr Scand Suppl* 1985;318:65–78.
66. Ellison RC, Sosenko JM, Harper GP, et al. Obesity, sodium intake, and blood pressure in adolescents. *Hypertension* 1980;2:78–82.
67. Gilliam TB, Katch VL, Thorland W, et al. Prevalence of coronary heart disease risk factors in active children, 7 to 12 years of age. *Med Sci Sports* 1977;9:21–25.
68. Gillum RF. Resting pulse rate of children and young adults associated with blood pressure and other cardiovascular risk factors. *Public Health Rep* 1991;106:400–410.
69. Higgins MW, Hinton PC, Keller JB. Weight and obesity as predictors of blood pressure and hypertension. In: Loggie JMH, Horan MJ, Gruskin AB, Hohn AR, Dunbar JB, Havlik RJ, eds. NHLBI Workshop on Juvenile Hypertension. New York, NY: Biomedical Information Corporation, 1983:125–143.
70. Khoury P, Morrison JA, Kelly K, et al. Clustering and interrelationships of coronary heart disease risk factors in schoolchildren, ages 6–19. *Am J Epidemiol* 1980;112:524–538.
71. Kikuchi DA, Srinivasan SR, Harsha DW, et al. Relation of serum lipoprotein lipids and apolipoproteins to obesity in children: The Bogalusa Heart Study. *Prev Med* 1992;21:177–190.
72. Lauer RM, Connor WE, Leaverton PE, et al. Coronary heart disease risk factors in school children: The Muscatine Study. *J Pediatr* 1975;86:697–706.
73. Liebman M, Chopin LF, Carter E, et al. Factors related to blood pressure in a biracial adolescent female population. *Hypertension* 1986;8:843–850.
74. Morrison JA, Payne G, Barton BA, et al. Mother-daughter correlations of obesity and cardiovascular disease risk factors in black and white house-

holds: The NHLBI Growth and Health Study. *Am J Public Health* 1994;84: 1761–1767.
75. Moussa MA, Skaik MB, Selwanes SB, et al. Factors associated with obesity in school children. *Int J Obes Relat Metab Disord* 1994;18:513–515.
76. Resnicow K, Morabia A. The relation between body mass index and plasma total cholesterol in a multiracial sample of US schoolchildren. *Am J Epidemiol* 1990;132:1083–1090.
77. Voors AW, Webber LS, Frerichs RR, et al. Body height and body mass as determinants of basal blood pressure in children—The Bogalusa Heart Study. *Am J Epidemiol* 1977;106:101–108.
78. Srinivasan SR, Ehnholm C, Wattigney WA, et al. Relationship between obesity and serum lipoproteins in children with different apolipoprotein E phenotypes: The Bogalusa Heart Study. *Metabolism* 1994;43:470–475.
79. Wattigney WA, Harsha DW, Srinivasan SR, et al. Increasing impact of obesity on serum lipids and lipoproteins in young adults. The Bogalusa Heart Study. *Arch Intern Med* 1991;151:2017–2022.
80. Webber LS, Voors AW, Srinivasan SR, et al. Occurrence in children of multiple risk factors for coronary artery disease: The Bogalusa Heart Study. *Prev Med* 1979;8:407–418.
81. Dwyer JT, Stone EJ, Yang M, et al. Predictors of overweight and overfat-ness in a multiethnic pediatric population. Child and Adolescent Trial for Cardiovascular Health Collaborative Research Group. *Am J Clin Nutr* 1998;67:602–610.
82. Raitakari OT, Porkka KV, Rasanen L, et al. Clustering and six year cluster-tracking of serum total cholesterol, HDL-cholesterol and diastolic blood pressure in children and young adults. The Cardiovascular Risk in Young Finns Study. *J Clin Epidemiol* 1994;47:1085–1093.
83. Smoak CG, Burke GL, Webber LS, et al. Relation of obesity to clustering of cardiovascular disease risk factors in children and young adults. The Bogalusa Heart Study. *Am J Epidemiol* 1987;125:364–372.
84. Bjorntorp P. Visceral obesity: A civilization syndrome. *Obes Res* 1993;1: 206–222.
85. Shear CL, Freedman DS, Burke GL, et al. Body fat patterning and blood pressure in children and young adults. The Bogalusa Heart Study. *Hypertension* 1987;9:236–244.
86. Caprio S, Hyman LD, McCarthy S, et al. Fat distribution and cardiovascular risk factors in obese adolescent girls: Importance of the intraabdominal fat depot. *Am J Clin Nutr* 1996;64:12–17.
87. Baumgartner RN, Siervogel RM, Chumlea WC, et al. Associations between plasma lipoprotein cholesterols, adiposity and adipose tissue distribution during adolescence. *Int J Obes.* 1989;13:31–41.
88. Becque MD, Hattori K, Katch VL, et al. Relationship of fat patterning to coronary artery disease risk in obese adolescents. *Am J Phys Anthropol* 1986;71:423–429.
89. Gutin B, Basch C, Shea S, et al. Blood pressure, fitness, and fatness in 5- and 6-year-old children. *JAMA* 1990;264:1123–1127.
90. Moussa MA, Skaik MB, Selwanes SB, et al. Contribution of body fat and fat pattern to blood pressure level in school children. *Eur J Clin Nutr* 1994;48:587–590.
91. Stallones L, Mueller WH, Christensen BL. Blood pressure, fatness, and fat patterning among USA adolescents from two ethnic groups. *Hypertension* 1982;4:483–486.

92. Burns TL, Moll PP, Lauer RM. The relation between ponderosity and coronary risk factors in children and their relatives. The Muscatine Ponderosity Family Study. *Am J Epidemiol* 1989;129:973–987.
93. Chen W, Srinivasan SR, Bao W, et al. Sibling aggregation of low- and high-density lipoprotein cholesterol and apolipoproteins B and A-I levels in black and white children: The Bogalusa Heart Study. *Ethn Dis* 1997;7:241–249.
94. Friedlander Y, Bucher KD, Namboodiri KK, et al. Parent-offspring aggregation of plasma lipids in selected populations in North America and Israel. The Lipid Research Clinics Prevalence Study. *Am J Epidemiol* 1987; 126:268–279.
95. Greenberg RA, Green PP, Roggenkamp KJ, et al. The constancy of parent-offspring similarity of total cholesterol throughout childhood and early adult life. The Lipid Research Clinics Program Prevalence Study. *J Chronic Dis* 1984;37:833–838.
96. Lee J, Lauer RM, Clarke WR. Lipoproteins in the progeny of young men with coronary artery disease: Children with increased risk. *Pediatrics* 1986;78:330–337.
97. Shear CL, Frerichs RR, Weinberg R, et al. Childhood sibling aggregation of coronary artery disease risk factor variables in a biracial community. *Am J Epidemiol* 1978;107:522–528.
98. Wilson DK, Klesges LM, Klesges RC, et al. A prospective study of familial aggregation of blood pressure in young children. *J Clin Epidemiol* 1992; 45:959–969.
99. Bao W, Srinivasan SR, Wattigney WA, et al. The relation of parental cardiovascular disease to risk factors in children and young adults. The Bogalusa Heart Study *Circulation* 1995;91:365–371.
100. Blonde CV, Webber LS, Foster TA, et al. Parental history and cardiovascular disease risk factor variables in children. *Prev Med* 1981;10:25–37.
101. Greenlund KJ, Valdez R, Bao W, et al. Verification of parental history of coronary artery disease and associations with adult offspring risk factors in a community sample: The Bogalusa Heart Study. *Am J Med Sci* 1997; 313:220–227.
102. Shear CL, Webber LS, Freedman DS, et al. The relationship between parental history of vascular disease and cardiovascular disease risk factors in children: The Bogalusa Heart Study. *Am J Epidemiol* 1985;122:762–771.
103. Widhalm K, Koch S, Pakosta R, et al. Serum lipids, lipoproteins and apolipoproteins in children with and without familial history of premature coronary heart disease. *J Am Coll Nutr* 1992;11:32S–35S.
104. Moll PP, Sing CF, Weidman WH, et al. Total cholesterol and lipoproteins in school children: Prediction of coronary heart disease in adult relatives. *Circulation* 1983;67:127–134.
105. Schrott HG, Clarke WR, Wiebe DA, et al. Increased coronary mortality in relatives of hypercholesterolemic school children: The Muscatine Study. *Circulation* 1979;59:320–326.
106. Bouchard C. Genetic factors in obesity. *Med Clin North Am.* 1989;73:67–81.
107. Burns TL, Moll PP, Lauer RM. Increased familial cardiovascular mortality in obese schoolchildren: The Muscatine Ponderosity Family Study. *Pediatrics* 1992;89:262–268.
108. Sonne-Holm S, Sorensen TI, Christensen U. Risk of early death in extremely overweight young men. *Br Med J* 1983;287:795–797.
109. Mossberg HO. 40-year follow-up of overweight children. *Lancet* 1989;2: 491–493.

110. Abraham S, Collins G, Nordsieck M. Relationship of childhood weight status to morbidity in adults. *HSMHA Health Rep* 1971;86:273–284.
111. Nieto FJ, Szklo M, Comstock GW. Childhood weight and growth rate as predictors of adult mortality. *Am J Epidemiol* 1992;136:201–213.
112. Must A, Jacques PF, Dallal GE, et al. Long-term morbidity and mortality of overweight adolescents. A follow-up of the Harvard Growth Study of 1922 to 1935 [see comments]. *N Engl J Med* 1992;327:1350–1355.
113. Sobal J, Stunkard AJ. Socioeconomic status and obesity: A review of the literature. *Psychol Bull* 1989;105:260–275.
114. Kaufman JS, Cooper RS, McGee DL. Socioeconomic status and health in blacks and whites: The problem of residual confounding and the resiliency of race. *Epidemiology* 1997;8:621–628.
115. Kimm SY, Obarzanek E, Barton BA, et al. Race, socioeconomic status, and obesity in 9- to 10-year-old girls: The NHLBI Growth and Health Study. *Ann Epidemiol* 1996;6:266–275.
116. Obarzanek E, Schreiber GB, Crawford PB, et al. Energy intake and physical activity in relation to indexes of body fat: The National Heart, Lung, and Blood Institute Growth and Health Study. *Am J Clin Nutr* 1994;60:15–22.
117. Gazzaniga JM, Burns TL. Relationship between diet composition and body fatness, with adjustment for resting energy expenditure and physical activity, in preadolescent children. *Am J Clin Nutr* 1993;58:21–28.
118. Tucker LA, Seljaas GT, Hager RL. Body fat percentage of children varies according to their diet composition. *J Am Diet Assoc* 1997;97:981–986.
119. US. Department of Health and Human Services. *Physical Activity and Health: A Report of the Surgeon General.* Center for Disease Control and Prevention; 1996; National Center for Chronic Disease Prevention and Health Promotion; i.
120. Thomson ME, Cruickshank FM. Survey into the eating and exercise habits of New Zealand pre-adolescents in relation to overweight and obesity. *N Z Med J* 1979;89:7–9.
121. Dietz WH Jr, Gortmaker SL. Do we fatten our children at the television set? Obesity and television viewing in children and adolescents. *Pediatrics* 1985;75:807–812.
122. Klesges RC, Shelton ML, Klesges LM. Effects of television on metabolic rate: Potential implications for childhood obesity. *Pediatrics* 1993;91:281–286.
123. Epstein LH, Valoski AM, Vara LS, et al. Effects of decreasing sedentary behavior and increasing activity on weight change in obese children. *Health Psychol* 1995;14:109–115.
124. French SA, Story M, Perry CL. Self-esteem and obesity in children and adolescents: A literature review. *Obes Res* 1995;3:479–490.
125. Kimm SY, Barton BA, Berhane K, et al. Self-esteem and adiposity in black and white girls: The NHLBI Growth and Health Study. *Ann Epidemiol* 1997;7:550–560.
126. Moore DC. Body image and eating behavior in adolescents. *J Am Coll Nutr* 1993;12:505–510.
127. Brown KM, Schreiber GB, McMahon RP. Maternal influences on body satisfaction in black and white girls aged 9 and 10. The NHLBI Growth and Health Study. *Ann Behav Med* 1995;17:213–220.
128. Kumanyika SK, Morssink C, Agurs T. Models for dietary and weight change in African-American women: Identifying cultural components. *Ethn Dis* 1992;2:166–175.

Chapter 3

Developmental Aspects of Obesity: Genetic Influences

Trudy L. Burns, PhD

Introduction

The American Heart Association recently has reclassified obesity as a major, modifiable risk factor for coronary heart disease.[1] Human obesity is a familial disorder. But family members share dietary factors, cultural factors, lifestyle factors, and genetic factors; so the observation of familial aggregation does not ensure that genetic factors are involved. Variation in human body fat is caused by a complex interaction of genetic, nutritional, metabolic, social, psychological, and energy expenditure variables. Multiple genes are likely to impact on the body's ability to control its weight, and the specific genetic defects are likely to vary from one family to another.

Obesity is classified as a "complex phenotype" because, with few exceptions to date, obesity does not appear to follow a simple Mendelian pattern of inheritance. When the simple correspondence between genotype and phenotype breaks down, etiologic complexities arise. The lack of correspondence occurs when the same genotype can result in different phenotypes (because of the effects of chance, environment, or interactions with other genes) or different genotypes can result in the same phenotype. Conceptually, the genotype defines the boundary conditions or capacity of the system that determines how body weight and body composition respond to the environment, and nongenetic factors determine at what point within these boundaries the system operates. In other words, the genotype determines what can happen and the environment determines what does happen.

From: Fletcher GF, Grundy SM, Hayman LL (eds). *Obesity: Impact on Cardiovascular Disease.* Armonk, NY: Futura Publishing Co., Inc.; © 1999.

Three Sequential Steps in the Scientific Investigation of Genetic Influences

Numerous body size phenotypes, like many other traits of medical relevance, have been the focus of three sequential steps of scientific investigation, in an attempt to better characterize the genetic component of their etiology.[2] The first step in this process is to determine whether there is evidence for familial aggregation. If evidence for familial aggregation is found, the second step is to determine whether this aggregation can be attributed to environmental, cultural, and/or genetic factors. If evidence is found that genetic factors play a role, the third step is to identify the specific genetic mechanism.

The first step, the assessment of familial aggregation, has been addressed repeatedly in numerous investigations using twin studies, separation studies, studies with relative pairs, and nuclear families, which consist of parents and their offspring. When a phenotype shows evidence for familial aggregation, correlations among various pairs of family members can be used to estimate the heritability h^2, that is, the proportion of the total phenotypic variance that is caused by additive genetic effects. In the extreme case, when all of the observed variability in a trait can be attributed to genetic variability, the heritability is equal to 1.

Familial Aggregation—Twin Studies

The classical twin study provides a simple approach that can be used to investigate the contribution of shared genes and/or shared environmental factors to the determination of a body size phenotype. The principle of the twin study design is that monozygotic (MZ) twins share all of their genes in common; dizygotic (DZ) twins on the average share only one-half of their genes in common, like full siblings, while both types of twins share their rearing environment in common. Therefore, if there is no difference in the intraclass correlation coefficients[3] between samples of MZ (r_{MZ}) and DZ (r_{DZ}) twins, the implication is that the factors that determine the phenotype primarily are nongenetic. However, if there is a difference in the intraclass correlation coefficients, with the MZ correlation expected to be higher than the DZ correlation, the implication is that genetic factors do play a role in the determination of the phenotype, that is, that it is heritable. The classical estimate of heritability h^2, based on twin data, is $h^2 = 2(r_{MZ} - r_{DZ})$. This simple estimate of heritability, which assumes additive genetic effects, has a number of shortcomings[4] that can be minimized using more modern model-fitting approaches.[5]

Twin studies have focused on both children[6] and adults,[7,8] as well as twins reared together and twins reared apart.[9–11] Bodurtha et al[6] investigated the familial aggregation of skin fold thicknesses and the body mass index (BMI) in 11-year-old twins from Virginia. Under the best-fitting model of inheritance, the heritabilities for triceps and subscapular skin folds and BMI were 0.75, 0.77, and 0.87, respectively. In 1955, the National Academy of Sciences–National Research Council (NAS-NRC) Twin Registry was initiated, at which time it contained 15 924 male twin pairs born between 1917 and 1927 and ascertained through the Veterans Administration.[7] Stunkard et al[8] investigated the heritability of BMI measured at the time of induction into the service, and 25 years later (self-reported) using 4071 of the pairs. The BMI heritability at the time of induction (average age 20 years) was 0.77, while 25 years later, the BMI heritability was 0.84. The greater heritability at 45 years of age may reflect the effect of self-reporting, but there also was evidence from the analytical results that the assumption of additive genetic effects might not hold at the older age, and this could result in a biased heritability estimate.

Stunkard et al[9] used data from the Swedish Adoption/Twin Study of Aging for an investigation of twins reared together versus twins reared apart (mean age 59 years). MZ twins reared apart showed very similar intraclass correlation coefficients when compared with MZ twins reared together for both male pairs [$r_{MZ} = 0.70$ ($n = 49$) versus 0.74 ($n = 66$)] and female pairs [$r_{MZ} = 0.66$ ($n = 44$) versus 0.66 ($n = 48$)]. DZ twins showed slightly less consistency in the intraclass correlation coefficients for males [$r_{DZ} = 0.15$ ($n = 75$) versus 0.33 ($n = 89$)] and females [$r_{DZ} = 0.25$ ($n = 143$) versus 0.27 ($n = 119$)]. Model-fitting results suggested that for men, 32% of the observed variance in BMI was caused by additive genetic effects, 37% was caused by nonadditive genetic effects, and 31% was caused by nonshared environmental factors. For women, the fitted model suggested that 17% of the observed BMI variance was caused by additive genetic effects, 57% was caused by nonadditive genetic effects, and 26% was caused by nonshared environmental factors. These twin study results suggest that a very high proportion of the body size variability among twin pairs is genetic in origin.

Familial Aggregation—Adoption Studies

The concept of studying twins raised apart was developed in an attempt to allow the separation of shared genetic effects from shared environmental effects. Adoption studies take advantage of the fact that children are separated from their biological parents at birth and adopted by an unrelated family. So, this design also provides the appropriate contrasts to help separate shared genetic effects from shared environmental effects. Resemblance between the adoptee and their adoptive family members is presumed because of shared environmental factors, while resemblance among the adoptive (biological) family members themselves is presumed because of both shared genetic and shared environmental factors. If information on the biological relatives of the adoptee is available, an additional comparison can be made, because resemblance between the adoptee and biological family members is presumed because of shared genetic effects, especially if the adoptee is separated from the biological relatives early in life. In general, adoption studies have found that shared environmental effects may play a minor role in determining familial resemblance of body size measures; however, shared genetic effects play a major role.[12,13]

Familial Aggregation—Family Studies

Sibling and parent-offspring correlations have been estimated in many populations and these estimates typically are between 0.15 and 0.30 for body size measures such as the BMI, individual skin fold thicknesses, the waist-to-hip circumference ratio, and total body fat.[14-16] Assuming an additive genetic model for the determination of these phenotypes, the maximum heritability is estimated to be between 0.30 and 0.60, that is, twice the correlation coefficient between pairs of first-degree relatives. Therefore, numerous investigations, conducted over many years, using several alternative study designs, found ample evidence for the familial aggregation of body size measures to justify taking the second step to try to discriminate among environmental, cultural, and/or genetic factors that may contribute to the observed familial aggregation.

Segregation Analysis

During the 1970s and 1980s statistical methods were developed[17-20] that allowed investigators to address formally this second step. These methods of analysis focus on transmission of the phenotype through generations in a family and thus require that, at a minimum, data are available for parents and their offspring. Complex multigenerational pedigrees can provide even more information regarding segregation patterns if they can be identified and examined. Segregation analysis attempts to delineate the mode of inheritance of a phenotype that shows evidence of familial aggregation by fitting and comparing different etiologic models. These models allow for factors such as polygenic loci, which are multiple genetic loci—each with a small effect on the determination of the phenotype, a single genetic locus with a major effect, as well as various environmental factors, and combinations of genetic and environmental factors.

Inherent in the methodology used to estimate the degree of familial aggregation using correlation coefficients, is the assumption that a single normal distribution adequately describes the quantitative phenotype of interest, and that the genetic component of variance is attributable to the additive effects of polygenic loci. However, the observed distribution of a phenotype also could be a composite of a number of component distributions that might exist because of genetic effects that are associated with much larger phenotypic differences. Several studies have found statistical evidence that there is a substantial nonadditive (major gene) component involved in the determination of BMI, fat mass, abdominal visceral fat, and a relative fat pattern, with the different genotypes at the major locus being associated with different component distributions.[21–27]

The role of genetic and environmental factors in determining variability in BMI has been investigated using complex segregation analysis in several different populations, using a variety of sampling designs and with surprisingly consistent results.[22–24,28] A segregation analysis of BMI by Price et al[22] using 961 randomly ascertained families from the Lipid Research Clinics family studies suggested that polygenic loci accounted for 34% of the variability in BMI. There also was evidence for a significant nonadditive effect caused by segregation at a recessive major locus, and the frequency of homozygotes at the locus was estimated to be 4.4%.

Similar results were obtained by Province et al[23] from a segregation analysis of BMI using 9226 individuals in 3281 unselected nuclear families from Tecumseh, MI. Polygenic loci were estimated to account for 41% of the BMI variability among children and 20% of the variability among adults, and a recessive major locus accounted for another 20% of the variability. Approximately 6% of the individuals in this population was estimated to be homozygous for the recessive major gene.

A family study conducted in Muscatine, IA investigated familial aggregation of BMI in 284 families.[24] Probands were selected from among the 1783 students who participated in the Muscatine biennial school surveys conducted in 1977, 1979, and 1981 based on relative weight patterns. The following four study groups were identified: (1) a random group ($n = 72$), a random sample of students from the entire pool; (2) a lean group ($n = 70$), students in the lowest quintile of relative weight on all three surveys; (3) a gain group ($n = 70$), students who gained at least two quintiles of relative weight over the 4-year period; and (4) a heavy group ($n = 72$), students in the highest quintile of relative weight on all three surveys. The parents, siblings, a related aunt or uncle, and a first cousin also were examined.[24] Complex segregation analysis suggested that 35% of the variability in BMI was caused by segregation at a recessive major locus, 42% was caused by additive polygenic effects at multiple other loci, and 23% was caused by unidentified environmental effects. The model also suggested that 6% of the Muscatine population was homozygous for the high-BMI allele at the major locus, and 37% of the population was heterozygous carriers of the high-BMI allele.

Hasstedt et al[21] investigated a relative fat pattern index [RFPI = subscapular skin fold/(subscapular skin fold + suprailiac skin fold)] in 59 Utah pedigrees ascertained through cases of cardiovascular disease. Complex segregation analysis supported a recessive mode of inheritance of RFPI, with 42% of the variance caused by segregation at the major locus, 10% caused by variability at polygenic loci, and 48% caused by random environmental effects. On the basis of the fitted recessive model, 22% of the individuals in this population were estimated to be homozygous for the gene associated with increased RFPI.

Interestingly, in each of these four populations, the major gene was found to act in a recessive fashion—as do the majority of the rodent major-obesity genes that have been identified.[29] Subsequent to the early segregation analysis publications, a number of more recent investigations have found evidence for major gene effects in the determination of body size measures in other populations.[25–28,30,31] Segregation analysts now are focusing on fitting models to determine whether the major genetic loci identified from univariate analyses of single phenotypes are one in the same locus, by fitting bivariate segregation models that allow for the identification of common sources of phenotypic variation. A bivariate analysis of BMI and fat mass conducted by Borecki et al[31] provided evidence for two pleiotropic recessive loci, together accounting for 64% and 47% of the variance in BMI and fat mass, respectively. Hasstedt et al[32] previously had found evidence for a second recessive major locus effect in the determination of BMI by fitting a two-locus segregation analysis model. These results suggest that there are at least two genetic loci involved in the determination of body size phenotypes that have effects large enough to allow their identification and mapping.

Linkage Analysis

Segregation analysis focuses on the phenotypes of family members and attempts to infer genetic effects by analyzing patterns of phenotypic segregation in families. Currently, the third step in scientific investigation is the major area of focus. Linkage analysis is used to find the physical location(s) in the genome relevant to the phenotype. Two basic strategies are employed to identify genes that influence complex phenotypes: candidate gene analysis and whole genome searches. The field has arrived at this final step largely because of the availability of huge numbers of polymorphic markers spread throughout the genome that allow more direct testing for specific genetic mechanisms.[33]

The challenge of the candidate gene approach is to identify appropriate candidate genes. A gene might be a candidate because it is expressed in adipose tissue [such as tumor necrosis factor-α (TNF-α)] or because of its homology to other genes such as the human homologues of mouse obesity genes, *LEP*, *LEPR*, *TUB*, or *ASP*. One problem with the candidate gene approach is that the more learned about the etiology of obesity, the longer the list of possible candidate genes grows.[29,34] A whole genome search involves a search for genetic effects at different locations along chromosomes, without regard to genetic candidates.

Traditional model-based linkage analysis involves tracing cosegregation and recombination between measured marker alleles and unmeasured disease alleles among members of nuclear families or multigenerational pedigrees.[35,36] The newer model-free methods of linkage analysis assess the number of marker alleles shared at a locus among relative pairs—most often sibling pairs. Affected children and their parents provide yet another sampling design that is used widely to study linkage disequilibrium or association. Regardless of the analytical approach that is used, mapping of any phenotype, whether simple or complex, involves the identification of chromosomal regions that tend to be shared among affected relatives and tend to differ between affecteds and unaffecteds.[37]

Linkage versus Linkage Disequilibrium

Although linkage analysis focuses on allelic associations within families, linkage disequilibrium analysis focuses on allelic associations across families. For example, suppose that at some point in the distant past, a disease-causing mutation M occurred on a chromosome that contained the allele X at a polymorphic marker locus (with alleles X, Y, and Z) close to the disease locus. Also suppose that allele S was present at a more distant polymorphic marker locus (with alleles R, S, and T) on the same chromosome. Over time, recombination occurs between homologous chromosomes and there is a greater chance for recombination the further apart the loci are on the chromosome. Recombination, in this example, results in some of the M chromosomes having an R or a T allele at the more distant marker locus. Suppose that each of three obese siblings in one family inherit a chromosome with the R-X-M haplotype, and that each of three obese siblings in a second family inherit a chromosome with the S-X-M haplotype. If we were to conduct a linkage analysis using the more distant marker, the fact that marker allele R is associated with obesity in one family and that marker allele S is associated with obesity in another family suggests genetic linkage. Usually, the allelic association is family specific, or stated differently, different marker alleles cosegregate or travel together with the unknown obesity susceptibility allele in different families. If this pattern is observed consistently across families, then genetic linkage is supported. To the contrary, if we study a number of families and find that there is nonrandom association of a specific marker allele and the unmeasured obesity susceptibility allele, the two loci are said to be in linkage disequilibrium. Therefore, continuing the example but focusing on the closer marker locus, there is an association between the X allele and obesity in both families, and if this association were to be observed consistently among a number of families, then the X allele actually may be the obesity susceptibility allele, if it is a functional mutation, or it may be in linkage disequilibrium with a nearby obesity susceptibility allele. Linkage disequilibrium usually exists only for closely linked markers because recombination, a constant feature of meiosis, destroys the allelic association with more distant markers over time. Thus, linkage disequilibrium (allelic association) exists when a specific marker allele is located so close to the susceptibility allele that they are inherited together over many generations and observed as such in many apparently unrelated families.

One approach that can be used to conduct an association analysis is a simple case-control study focusing on unrelated cases (eg, obese individuals) and controls (nonobese individuals). Individuals in these two groups would be genotyped at a candidate locus, and the allelic distributions (or genotype distributions) in the two groups would be compared using a chi-square test for association. A major concern with using this design is that if the case and control groups are not matched with respect to ethnicity, any results, positive or negative, could be confounded because of ethnic subgroups distributed differently in the case and control groups (population stratification) that may have different allele frequencies at the candidate locus. As an alternative to the case-control approach, family based methods have been developed that allow control for possible ethnic differences by comparing the alleles transmitted versus not transmitted from parents to children.

Transmission Test for Linkage Disequilibrium

The family based method that is used most frequently to investigate an association between the disease and a specific measured genetic factor, be it a specific allele at a genetic locus or a specific haplotype formed using the genotypes at several linked loci, is called the transmission-disequilibrium test (TDT).[38] The most common sampling design used to obtain data for a TDT analysis is the parent/affected child trio design. The affected children from different trios make up the case group for the association analysis, and the "controls" are contructed artificially from the alleles that the parents do not transmit to their affected children. Suppose our focus is on investigating the association between obesity and allele X at the measured genetic (marker) locus and that in one of the trios the father is heterozygous for the X and Y alleles at this locus. Suppose that he transmits the X allele to his affected daughter, his Y allele then is used as one of the alleles for the artificial control. Suppose that the mother has genotype ZZ at the locus. She will transmit one Z allele to her affected daughter and the other Z allele will serve as the second allele for the artificial control.

Results of transmission from a large number of parents heterozygous for the X allele are displayed in a table that focuses on the specific genetic factor of interest (see Table 1). Each of the case-artificial control pairs can be classified into one of the four cells in the table. Our example pair would be counted in the cell where the X allele (the genetic factor) was present in the case but absent in the control, that is, the B cell of this table. Because the A and D cells of this table do not provide any information regarding the difference between cases and controls in terms of transmission of the genetic factor, they do not enter

Table 1

Transmission Test for Linkage Disequilibrium

Genetic factor	Present in the control	Absent in the control
Present in the case	A	B
Absent in the case	C	D

the analysis. If there was no association between the genetic factor and case-control status, we would expect the counts in the B and C cells to be equal. The familiar McNemar's chi-square test [$\chi^2 = (B - C)^2/(B + C)$] is used to determine whether there is equality.

A study conducted at the University of Pennsylvania[39] determined haplotypes based on two polymorphic markers flanking the human *LEP* gene. Transmission of one particular haplotype from parents, heterozygous for the haplotype of interest, to their obese children was evaluated to determine whether transmission occurred more frequently than expected by chance (50%). There was excess transmission of the haplotype (58.7% of the time) when obesity was defined as a BMI of at least 30. The excess (65.7%) was significant ($P < 0.05$) when the BMI of the cases was at least 40. This suggests that there is a specific mutation in the *LEP* gene or some other gene very close to *LEP* that is associated with extreme obesity in some of these individuals.

Allele-Sharing (Model-Free) Methods of Linkage Analysis

Most of the recent investigations of genetic linkage of obesity and quantitative body size phenotypes have used methods that are based on the concept of sharing alleles that are identical by descent (IBD). Two copies of the same allele at a genetic locus, for example, allele R, in two different individuals (related or not) are identical by state (IBS). In two genetically related individuals, if the two copies of the same allele are inherited from a common ancestral source, they are IBD. Table 2 demonstrates three examples of allele sharing in two siblings. In the first example, the father has the RS genotype and the mother has the ST genotype at the marker locus. These parents have two obese children, both with the RT genotype. We know that they each had to inherit the R allele from their father and the T allele from their mother, so the probability that they share two alleles IBD is 1.0. This also can be expressed as a sharing of 100% of their alleles at that locus.

In the second example, we have two parents, each with the RS genotype at the marker locus. These parents have two obese children, one with genotype SS and one with genotype RS at the marker locus. The first child received an S allele from each parent, and the second child received one S allele but we cannot determine from which parent. However, we know that the S allele is IBD with one of the S alleles that the sibling received. So the probability that they share one allele IBD is 1.0. This also can be expressed as a sharing of 50% of their alleles at the locus.

Table 2

Sharing Genetic Material That Is IBD

Marker locus genotypes				Alleles IBD			
Father	Mother	Child 1	Child 2	Pr (0 IBD)	Pr (1 IBD)	Pr (2 IBD)	Sharing
$R_f S_f$	$S_m T_m$	$R_f T_m$	$R_f T_m$	0.0	0.0	1.0	100%
$R_f S_f$	$R_m S_m$	$S_f S_m$	$R_f S_m$ or $R_m S_f$	0.0	1.0	0.0	50%
$R_f S_f$	$S_{m1} S_{m2}$	$R_f S_{m1}$	$S_f S_{m1}$ or $S_f S_{m2}$	0.5	0.5	0.0	25%
		$R_f S_{m2}$	$S_f S_{m1}$ or $S_f S_{m2}$				

The final example is less definitive. In this example, the mother is homozygous for the S allele. The first child is RS and the second child is SS. The first child received the R allele from the father and one of the mother's S alleles. The second child received the father's S allele and one of the mother's S alleles. So it is only the S alleles from the mother that possibly can be IBD. The two obese offspring could share one allele IBD or they could share neither allele IBD; so the probability of sharing no alleles or one allele is 0.5. This is expressed as a 25% sharing of their alleles at the locus. When the genotype is unavailable for one or both parents, all possible genotypes at the marker locus for the missing parent(s) must be considered. Population marker allele frequencies then enter into the IBD calculations. Misspecification of these allele frequencies can produce false-positive linkage results. Specifically, underestimating the frequency of an allele will lead to overestimating the degree of IBD sharing at the locus.

Therefore, how is IBD information utilized to conduct a linkage analysis? The simplest use is in the conduct of an affected sib-pair analysis. The basic motivation of affected sib-pair analysis is that if an allele at a marker locus is cosegregating with a disease gene, then siblings who have the disease are more likely to receive the same marker allele IBD. This concept was first proposed by Penrose in 1935.[40]

The University of Pennsylvania study also included an affected sib-pair analysis that focused on the mean proportion of alleles shared IBD by obese sibling pairs for a marker near the human *LEP* gene locus.[39] If the definition of obesity was a BMI of at least 30, there was no evidence for excess sharing—the mean proportion was 0.51, when we would have expected 0.50 if there were no association. However, if the definition of obesity was a BMI of at least 40, then there was an excess of sharing at the marker locus close to the *LEP* gene, with a mean of 0.60 ($P < 0.05$). This again suggests the involvement of *LEP* or some nearby gene in the etiology of extreme obesity.

If the phenotype of interest is quantitative rather than qualitative, the analytical approach is altered slightly, but it still focuses on the principle of allele sharing. The basic motivation is this: if a marker locus is cosegregating with a locus affecting the quantitative trait, then the phenotypes of siblings that share more alleles at that locus should be more similar than the phenotypes of siblings that share fewer alleles at that locus—a concept again due to Penrose.[41]

The simplest type of sib-pair linkage analysis of a quantitative phenotype focuses on D, the difference in the phenotypes of two siblings after adjustment for differences due to, for example, age and gender. D^2 is then the phenotypic difference squared. If sibling pairs are genotyped at a marker locus that is linked to a genetic locus that plays a role in the etiology of this phenotype, we might expect that siblings who share 0% of their alleles at that locus IBD would have larger D^2 values, in general, than siblings who share 100% of their alleles IBD. The amount of allele sharing, is denoted on the x-axis of a scatter plot by π, and the squared phenotypic difference is on the y-axis. Thus if the marker locus is linked to a genetic locus that affects the phenotype, we will see a negative association between D^2 and π. Therefore, the hypothesis test focuses on the slope of a fitted line β. This approach was proposed by Haseman and Elston.[42]

Alternatively, maximum likelihood methods can be used to test whether the variance of the D's for sibling pairs who share no alleles IBD, is greater than the variance of the D's for sibling pairs who share one allele IBD, which in turn is greater than the variance of the D's for sibling pairs who share two alleles IBD.[43] These analysis methods now are being utilized in a number of different population studies that are focusing on obesity-related traits using multipoint linkage analysis to search the entire genome for linked genetic loci.

Multipoint Linkage Analysis—San Antonio Family Heart Study

The San Antonio Family Heart Study is investigating obesity-related phenotypes in Mexican American families.[44,45] Sib-pair linkage analyses have focused on individuals at least 18 years of age. A candidate gene analysis of the *LEP* region identified linkage of extremity skin folds, 32,33-split proinsulin level, and proinsulin level to markers in the *LEP* region.[44] These three suggestive linkages all had associated log odd (LOD) scores above 3.0, and the linked marker loci explained more than 50% of the variation in each of the three quantitative phenotypes. A whole-genome search identified linkage of leptin levels to a region of chromosome 2.[45] The LOD score is used as a measure of the strength of the evidence for linkage.[36] Lander and Kruglyak[37] have suggested that if you are conducting a whole-genome search, the value of the LOD score that should be used to indicate significant linkage is 3.6. The maximum LOD score for serum leptin levels from the genomewide search was 4.95 and was associated with a marker that mapped to chromosome 2p21. This locus accounted for nearly 50% of the variation in serum leptin levels. The next highest LOD score for serum leptin levels was just over 2.0 on chromosome 8. The results from the chromosome 2 linkage analysis of fat mass paralleled those of leptin but with lower LOD scores (all <2.0). Because leptin levels and fat mass are correlated very highly, this is not surprising, and is, in fact, encouraging. These results also may indicate that serum leptin levels are measured more precisely than is fat mass.

Multipoint Linkage Analysis—Pima Indians

The most extensive sib-pair linkage analyses to date have been conducted in the members of the Gila River Indian Community.[46-49] Again, these investigations have been conducted using adult siblings. Two of these analyses have used the candidate gene approach. TNF-α expression is increased in the adipose tissue of obese humans, which makes it a reasonable candidate. Linkage was detected between percent body fat and a marker near the TNF-α gene at 6p21.3.[47] However, no evidence of linkage between BMI, percent body fat, resting metabolic rate, 24-hour energy expenditure or 24-hour respiratory quotient, and markers at the *LEP, LEPR, TUB,* or *ASP* candidate loci was found.[46]

A whole-genome search in this population identified several suggestive linkages, although the LOD scores were 3.0 or less and thus did not meet the criterion for significant linkage.[37] These possible linkages were on chromosomes 3p24.2-p22 and 11q21-q22 with percent body fat,[48] chromosome 11q23-q24 with 24-hour energy expenditure, and chromosomes 1p31-p21 and 20q11.2 for 24-hour respiratory quotient.[49]

Multipoint Linkage Analysis—
Quebec Family Study

Sib-pair linkage analyses to date in the Quebec Family Study have focused on candidate regions that are suggested by their homology with mouse obesity regions. One analysis identified suggestive linkage of BMI, the sum of skin folds, and insulin area after an oral glucose tolerance test to a region on chromosome 1p32-p22 that is homologous with the leptin receptor locus and a mouse quantitative trait locus.[29,50] Another analysis identified suggestive linkage of BMI, percent body fat, and fasting insulin to a region of chromosome 20q that is homologous with another mouse quantitative trait locus.[51]

Summary of Multipoint Linkage Analysis Results

The most important human chromosomal regions exhibiting linkage from multipoint analyses using adult sibling pairs include 1p, 2p, 3p, 6p, 7q, 11q, and 20q. Preliminary multipoint analyses of younger sibling pairs (mean age 13.4) from unselected Muscatine, IA nuclear families identified five candidate regions on 1p, 2q, 3q, 7q, and 11p.[52] There actually may be a subset of genes whose effects can be identified only in a childhood population, because their genetic effects become obscured by environmental factors over time in individuals that carry them. Three possibilities, identified from the Muscatine Study, include genes in the candidate regions of 2q, 3q, and 11p.

The results from these ongoing investigations are encouraging with regard to the potential to eventually locate genes involved in the determination of body size phenotypes. Positioning of disease loci to chromosome intervals using genetic markers has become increasingly straightforward, particularly given the availability of genetic maps containing thousands of markers.[33] The major challenge will be the identification and evaluation of the genes within an implicated interval and the identification of specific disease-causing mutations.

The Changing Role of Genetic and Lifestyle Influences on Obesity

Environmental and lifestyle factors in modern life must be responsible for a large proportion of the obesity that currently exists, because the obesity epidemic is emerging within a relatively constant gene pool. However, this does not mean that genetic effects are unimportant. There is considerable evidence to suggest that some individuals and some groups, for example, the Pimas, are more susceptible genetically than other individuals. But the balance of genetic versus environmental influences is changing. Prentice[53] provides a schematic representation of the current epidemic in terms of the distribution of BMI. In the past, the average BMI was approximately 21 to 22 kg/m^2 and there was only a shallow right-hand tail to the BMI distribution. At that time, it would have been very likely that any seriously obese person would have a definite genetic susceptibility, perhaps resulting from a single major gene defect, or more likely arising from polygenic effects. However, we are now at a point where the individuals with genuine genetic susceptibilities are being obscured by the volume of individuals with lifestyle obesities. As more and more people become obese the concept of genetic susceptibility loses its value, and we may have to turn our attention to individuals who seem to be resistant genetically to weight gain.[53]

Genotype-Environment Interaction Effects

Ultimately, our focus will turn to the evaluation of genotype-environment interaction effects. We already know that the response of plasma lipid levels to alterations in the amount of fat in the diet and of blood pressure levels to the amount of salt in the diet vary considerably among individuals. Some individuals appear to be relatively insensitive (low responders) to dietary changes, while others appear to be relatively sensitive (high responders) to changes. It is reasonable to assume that this variability in response to dietary change is determined, at least in part, by genetic factors. Further, if the magnitude of the phenotypic response to dietary change depends on the genotype of an individual at a particular genetic locus or at several genetic loci, there are said to be genotype-environment interaction effects involved in determining the phenotypic response. Such interaction effects may help to explain the weight-gain variability among individuals in response to a high-fat diet or to low-physical activity.

Bouchard et al[54] have investigated possible genotype-environment interaction effects indirectly, by focusing on MZ twins subjected to a common intervention. In one study, 12 pairs of healthy male MZ twins with no family history of obesity, hyperlipidemia, or diabetes were given a 1000 kcal caloric surplus over a period of 100 days. At the end of the overfeeding period, there was nearly a threefold weight-gain difference between the lowest and the highest responder. The intraclass correlation coefficient,[3] which compares the variability in response between MZ pairs to the variability in response within MZ pairs, was 0.55 ($P < 0.05$) for body weight and ranged from 0.48 to 0.72 for several different body size and fat measures. This suggests that the response to dietary change was more homogeneous within MZ pairs than between MZ pairs.

In a second study,[54] seven pairs of healthy male MZ twins were subjected to a common negative energy balance protocol during which they exercised on cycle ergometers over a period of 93 days while their daily energy and nutrient intake was kept constant. Again, there were large differences in the magnitude of the weight loss across the participants, but the intraclass correlation coefficient was 0.74 ($P < 0.05$) for body weight and ranged from 0.72 to 0.87 for different body size and fat measures. The results from these studies suggest that genetic factors play a role in determining the phenotypic response to long-term alterations in energy balance.

Although most of the investigations of genotype-environment interaction effects in humans have been indirect because susceptibility loci have yet to be identified, investigations in mouse models may provide clues for future human investigations of genotype-environment interaction effects. West et al[55] compared the response of nine mouse strains to a high-fat diet and found an approximate sixfold difference in the level of adiposity between the dietary-fat–sensitive strain (AKR/J) and the dietary-fat–resistant strain (SWR/J). The segregation pattern of the adiposity phenotype in the progeny of crosses between the sensitive and resistant strains suggested a polygenic model of inheritance involving three or four loci.[55] Quantitative trait locus (QTL) analysis then was used to identify three dietary obese (Dob) loci[56,57] located on mouse chromosomes 4, 9, and 15, which map to human chromosomes 1p36.1-p35 for Dob1, 3p21 for Dob2, and 8q23-q24 for Dob3, respectively, based on the synteny homology between the mouse and human genomes. These Dob loci should be considered to be candidates for investigation of genotype-environment interaction effects in humans.

Mice are not men, or women; however, exploration of mouse obesity gene loci in humans is well underway. In humans, obesity is a heterogeneous disorder and it is unlikely that any single genetic mutation will describe the entire genetic contribution to obesity. Thus, whole-genome searches are being conducted to identify other candidate regions. A number of studies have found evidence for linkage of body size measures to markers in regions of mouse major genes and QTLs. The utility of using genetic mutations identified in the mouse to aid in our understanding of the pathogenesis of obesity in humans remains to be demonstrated; however, results are promising.

The most important resource for any etiologic investigation is the availability of a group of phenotypically well-characterized individuals or families. For example, participants in feeding studies or weight-reduction studies who show a dramatic response may help to identify families with a genetic predisposition to obesity or protection from obesity because of a specific gene in a biochemical pathway. Such individuals are invaluable to investigators trying to identify specific genetic defects involved in the etiology of obesity. Although the specific genetic defects that might explain susceptibility for large segments of the population have yet to be identified, there is still reason to be optimistic that advances in our understanding of the genetic and molecular causes of human obesity eventually will lead to an improved ability to treat or even prevent this increasingly prevalent condition.

References

1. Eckel RH, Krauss RM. American Heart Association call to action: Obesity as a major risk factor for coronary heart disease. *AHA Nutrition Committee Circulation* 1998;97:2099–2100.
2. King MC, Lee GM, Spinner NB, et al. Genetic epidemiology. *Annu Rev Public Health* 1984;5:1–52.
3. Snedecor GW, Cochran WG. *Statistical Methods.* Ames, IA: Iowa State University Press; 1967.
4. Meyer JM, Stunkard AJ. Twin studies of human obesity. In: Bouchard C, ed. *The Genetic of Obesity.* Boca Raton, Fla: CRC Press; 1994:63–78.
5. Neale MC, Cardon LR. *Methodology for Genetic Studies of Twins and Families.* Dordrect, The Netherlands: Kluwer Academic Publishers; 1992.
6. Bodurtha JN, Mosteller M, Hewitt JK, et al. Genetic analysis of anthropometric measures in 11-year-old twins: The Medical College of Virginia Twin Study. *Pediatr Res* 1990;28:1–4.
7. Jablon S, Neel JV, Gershowitz H, et al. The NAS-NRC twin panel: Methods of construction of the panel, zygosity diagnosis, and proposed use. *Am J Hum Genet* 1967;19:133–161.
8. Stunkard AJ, Foch TT, Hrubec Z. A twin study of human obesity. *JAMA* 1986;256:51–54.
9. Stunkard AJ, Harris JR, Pedersen NL, et al. The body-mass index of twins who have been reared apart. *N Engl J Med* 1990;322:1483–1487.
10. MacDonald A, Stunkard A. Body-mass indexes of British separated twins. *N Engl J Med* 1990;322:1530.
11. Allison DB, Kaprio J, Korkeila M, et al. The heritability of body mass index among an international sample of monozygotic twins reared apart. *Int J Obes Relat Metab Disord* 1996;20:501–506.
12. Stunkard AJ, Sorensen TI, Hanis C, et al. An adoption study of human obesity. *N Engl J Med* 1986;314:193–198.
13. Price RA, Cadoret RJ, Stunkard AJ, et al. Genetic contributions to human fatness: An adoption study. *Am J Psychiatry* 1987;144:1003–1008.
14. Heller R, Garrison RJ, Havlik RJ, et al. Family resemblances in height and relative weight in the Framingham Heart Study. *Int J Obes* 1984;8:399–405.
15. Perusse L, Leblanc C, Bouchard C. Inter-generation transmission of physical fitness in the Canadian population. *Can J Sport Sci* 1988;13:8–14.
16. Burns TL, Moll PP, Lauer RM. The relation between ponderosity and coronary risk factors in children and their relatives. The Muscatine Ponderosity Family Study. *Am J Epidemiol* 1989;129:973–987.
17. Elston RC, Stewart J. A general model for the genetic analysis of pedigree data. *Hum Hered* 1971;21:523–542.
18. Morton NE, MacLean CJ. Analysis of family resemblance. 3. Complex segregation of quantitative traits. *Am J Hum Genet* 1974;26:489–503.
19. Bonney GE. Regressive logistic models for familial disease and other binary traits. *Biometrics* 1986;42:611–625.

20. Bonney GE. On the statistical determination of major gene mechanisms in continuous human traits: Regressive models. *Am J Med Genet* 1984;18:731–749.

21. Hasstedt SJ, Ramirez ME, Kuida H, et al. Recessive inheritance of a relative fat pattern. *Am J Hum Genet* 1989;45:917–925.

22. Price RA, Ness R, Laskarzewski P. Common major gene inheritance of extreme overweight. *Hum Biol* 1990;62:747–765.

23. Province MA, Arnqvist P, Keller J, et al. Strong evidence for a major gene for obesity in the large, unselected, total Community Health Study of Tecumseh. *Am J Hum Genet* 1990;47:A143.

24. Moll PP, Burns TL, Lauer RM. The genetic and environmental sources of body mass index variability: The Muscatine Ponderosity Family Study. *Am J Hum Genet* 1991;49:1243–1255.

25. Bouchard C, Rice T, Lemieux S, et al. Major gene for abdominal visceral fat area in the Quebec Family Study. *Int J Obes Relat Metab Disord* 1996;20:420–427.

26. Comuzzie AG, Blangero J, Mahaney MC, et al. Major gene with sex-specific effects influences fat mass in Mexican Americans. *Genet Epidemiol* 1995;12:475–488.

27. Rice T, Despres JP, Perusse L, et al. Segregation analysis of abdominal visceral fat: The HERITAGE Family Study. *Obes Res* 1997;5:417–424.

28. Borecki IB, Bonney GE, Rice T, et al. Influence of genotype-dependent effects of covariates on the outcome of segregation analysis of the body mass index. *Am J Hum Genet* 1993;53:676–687.

29. Chagnon YC, Bouchard C. Genetics of obesity: Advances from rodent studies. *Trends Genet* 1996;12:441–444.

30. Rice T, Borecki IB, Bouchard C, et al. Segregation analysis of fat mass and other body composition measures derived from underwater weighing. *Am J Hum Genet* 1993;52:967–973.

31. Borecki IB, Blangero J, Rice T, et al. Evidence for at least two major loci influencing human fatness. *Am J Hum Genet* 1998;63:831–838.

32. Hasstedt SJ, Hoffman M, Leppert MF, et al. Recessive inheritance of obesity in familial non-insulin-dependent diabetes mellitus, and lack of linkage to nine candidate genes. *Am J Hum Genet* 1997;61:668–677.

33. Schuler GD, Boguski MS, Stewart EA, et al. A gene map of the human genome. *Science.* 1996;274:540–546.

34. Comuzzie AG, Allison DB. The search for human obesity genes. *Science* 1998;280:1374–1377.

35. Haldane JBS, Smith CAB. A new estimate of the linkage between the genes for color-blindness and haemophilia in man. *Ann Eugenics* 1947;14:10–31.

36. Morton NE. Sequential tests for the detection of linkage. *Am J Hum Genet* 1955;7:277–318.

37. Lander E, Kruglyak L. Genetic dissection of complex traits: Guidelines for interpreting and reporting linkage results. *Nat Genet* 1995;11:241–247.

38. Spielman RS, Ewens WJ. The TDT and other family-based tests for linkage disequilibrium and association. *Am J Hum Genet* 1996;59:983–989.

39. Reed DR, Ding Y, Xu W, et al. Extreme obesity may be linked to markers flanking the human OB gene. *Diabetes* 1996;45:691–694.

40. Penrose LS. The detection of autosomal linkage in data which consists of pairs of brothers and sisters of unspecified parentage. *Ann Eugenics* 1935;5:133–148.

41. Penrose LS. Genetic linkage in graded human characters. *Ann Eugenics* 1938;8:233–237.
42. Hasseman JK, Elston RC. The investigation of linkage between a quantitative trait and a marker locus. *Behav Genet* 1972;2:3–19.
43. Kruglyak L, Lander ES. Complete multipoint sib-pair analysis of qualitative and quantitative traits. *Am J Hum Genet* 1995;57:439–454.
44. Duggirala R, Stern MP, Mitchell BD, et al. Quantitative variation in obesity-related traits and insulin precursors linked to the OB gene region on human chromosome 7. *Am J Hum Genet* 1996;59:694–703.
45. Comuzzie AG, Hixson JE, Almasy L, et al. A major quantitative trait locus determining serum leptin levels and fat mass is located on human chromosome 2. *Nat Genet* 1997;15:273–276.
46. Norman RA, Leibel RL, Chung WK, et al. Absence of linkage of obesity and energy metabolism to markers flanking homologues of rodent obesity genes in Pima Indians. *Diabetes* 1996;45:1229–1232.
47. Norman RA, Bogardus C, Ravussin E. Linkage between obesity and a marker near the tumor necrosis factor-alpha locus in Pima Indians. *J Clin Invest* 1995;96:158–162.
48. Norman RA, Thompson DB, Foroud T, et al. Genomewide search for genes influencing percent body fat in Pima Indians: Suggestive linkage at chromosome 11q21–q22. Pima Diabetes Gene Group. *Am J Hum Genet* 1997;60: 166–173.
49. Norman RA, Tataranni PA, Pratley R, et al. Autosomal genomic scan for loci linked to obesity and energy metabolism in Pima Indians. *Am J Hum Genet* 1998;62:659–668.
50. Chagnon YC, Perusse L, Lamothe M, et al. Suggestive linkages between markers on human 1p32–p22 and body fat and insulin levels in the Quebec Family Study. *Obes Res* 1997;5:115–121.
51. Lembertas AV, Perusse L, Chagnon YC, et al. Identification of an obesity quantitative trait locus on mouse chromosome 2 and evidence of linkage to body fat and insulin on the human homologous region 20q. *J Clin Invest* 1997;100:1240–1247.
52. Burns TL, Donohoue PA, Lauer RM, et al. Loci linked to quantitative body size measures from a genomic scan: The Muscadine Study. *Circulation* 1998;98:I374.
53. Prentice AM. Obesity: The inevitable penalty of civilisation? *Br Med Bull* 1997;53:229–237.
54. Bouchard C, AT, Despres JP. The response to exercise with constant energy intake in identical twins. *Obes Res* 1994;2:400–410.
55. West DB, Boozer CN, Moody DL, et al. Dietary obesity in nine inbred mouse strains. *Am J Physiol* 1992;262:R1025–R1032.
56. West DB, Waguespack J, York B, et al. Genetics of dietary obesity in AKR/J eventually × SWR/J mice: Segregation of the trait and identification of a linked locus on chromosome 4. *Mamm Genome* 1994;5:546–552.
57. West DB, Goudey-Lefevre J, York B, et al. Dietary obesity linked to genetic loci on chromosomes 9 and 15 in a polygenic mouse model. *J Clin Invest* 1994;94:1410–1416.

Chapter 4

Developmental Aspects of Obesity: Nongenetic Influences

Laura L. Hayman, PhD, RN, FAAN

Introduction

The development and expression of obesity is influenced by the interaction of genetic and nongenetic factors. A review of the National Health and Nutrition Examination Surveys (NHANES) from 1963–1994 indicates a significant increase in overweight from the preschool years through adolescence.[1] The pattern and trend, similar to that observed for adults (see Chapter 1), suggest a fundamental shift in the determinants of energy balance in children and youth in the United States. Collectively, life span data point to the importance of population-based/public health strategies with emphasis on the nongenetic influences on obesity. Therefore, the purposes of this chapter are to (1) examine the nongenetic, potentially modifiable factors that contribute to the development and expression of obesity in childhood and adolescence; (2) examine developmental trends in the emergence of obesity-cardiovascular disease (CVD) risk factor associations; and, (3) identify specific areas for future research focused on individual and population-based approaches to primary prevention. In this chapter, nongenetic influences are defined as potentially modifiable behaviors and environments that contribute to the development and expression of obesity in childhood and adolescence. Conceptualized within a developmental-contextual life span framework,[2] emphasis is placed on individual behaviors relevant to obesity (ie, dietary intake and physical activity) and the environments (ie, family, school, and community) in which they develop and are maintained.

From: Fletcher GF, Grundy SM, Hayman LL (eds). *Obesity: Impact on Cardiovascular Disease.* Armonk, NY: Futura Publishing Co., Inc.; © 1999.

Partitioning the Genetic and Nongenetic Influences

Body mass index (BMI) frequently is used as a surrogate measure of obesity in epidemiological surveys of adults (see Chapter 1). Similarly, recent population-based surveys of children and adolescents, including the third NHANES (NHANES III), define overweight by the age- and sex-specific 95th percentile of BMI.[1] Very recent recommendations from a Pediatric Expert Committee support the use of BMI and suggest an in-depth health assessment for children and youth with BMI $\geq$ the 95th percentile for age and sex.[3] A comprehensive discussion of the methodological issues and challenges in defining and measuring obesity in children and youth is beyond the scope of this discussion. However, as illustrated in Table 1, in quantifying genetic and nongenetic influences, the method of measurement (ie, BMI, triceps skin fold) is an important consideration.

Substantial research has focused on quantifying the genetic influences on obesity using a variety of paradigms and methods.[4] Methodological limitations notwithstanding, twin and twin-family studies have been used extensively and provide most of the available data. By design, the results of these studies also provide indirect estimates of nongenetic influences. The classical and widely used approach to the analysis of twin data compares the similarity of identical or monozygotic (MZ) twins, who share all their genes, with fraternal or dizygotic (DZ) twins, who share (on average) half of their genes.[5] Based on this principle, the estimate of heritability (h^2) is calculated as twice the difference between the MZ and DZ intraclass correlation coefficients:

Table 1

Twin Correlations for Measures of Fat Patterning and Distribution

Study	Variable	r_{MZ}	r_{DZ}
Bouchard et al.[8]	BMI	0.88	0.34
($n_{MZ} = 87, n_{DZ} = 69$)	Sum of six skin folds	0.83	0.39
	Percentage body fat	0.73	0.21
	Fat mass	0.76	0.31
	Fat-free mass	0.93	0.53
	Extremity/trunk ratio	0.80	0.40
	Subcutaneous fat/FMR	0.61	0.15
Selby et al.[9]	Subscapular skin folds	0.76	0.34
($n_{MZ} = 134, n_{DZ} = 134$)	Triceps skin folds	0.70	0.38
	Triceps + subscapular skin fold	0.73	0.25
	Subscapular/triceps ratio	0.67	0.55

Abbreviations: MZ, monozygotic; DZ, dizygotic.
Adapted with permission from references 8 and 9.

$\{h^2 = 2(r_{MZ} - r_{DZ})\}$. In this approach, heritability (h^2) is defined as the proportion of variation in the characteristic accounted for by genetic factors in the population under study. Important to emphasize is that heritability estimates are specific to the population under study and must be viewed and interpreted accordingly. Across studies, these estimates have been shown to vary as a function of the sociodemographic characteristics of the population under study, the indicator and method of measurement of obesity, and analytic method used to quantify heritability.[4] Although minimal longitudinal data exist, estimates computed for the same population over time indicate that the magnitude of the estimate varies across the life span.[6,7] In addition, h^2 is based on the assumption that only additive genetic effects and shared common family environmental effects influence intrapair similarity. Thus, h^2, derived using the classical approach, is subject to biases in the presence of genetic dominance or epistasis (intraloci or interloci interactions).[4] Nonadditive genetic influences lower the DZ intraclass correlation to less than one half the MZ correlation; the end result is overestimation of the genetic influences.

Table 1 illustrates partial application of the classical twin approach and presents intraclass correlations by zygosity for measures of fat patterning and distribution. Data presented are part of the Quebec Family Study (QFS);[8] Bouchard and colleagues[8] examined genetic influences on BMI and measures of fat patterning and distribution in 87 MZ and 69 DZ twin pairs during the period of shared household environments. Selby and colleagues'[9] data are based on 134 MZ and 134 DZ veteran twin pairs (59–70 years of age) from the National Academy of Science-National Research Council registry. As can be noted, MZ correlations are quite high (0.61–0.93); DZ correlations range from 0.15 to 0.55. In the QFS data, MZ correlations exceed the DZ correlations by more than a twofold difference (except for fat-free mass); these results suggest genetic nonadditivity and/or an absence of family environmental effects. Heritability estimates calculated from these correlations, similar to other studies using the classical approach, indicate substantial genetic influences on most of these obesity-related characteristics. Particularly noteworthy, however, are the estimates derived by Bouchard[8] after extending the twin design to include other genetically informative relationships. The genetic component of the total transmissible variance in BMI and amount of subcutaneous fat were reduced to 5% while the genetic component of percent body fat and fat mass was 25%. These results suggest substantial nongenetic influences on these indicators of obesity in this population and point to the importance of methodological variation (ie, differences in research designs and indicators of obesity) as rationale for reported between-study variation in estimates of heritability.

One method for addressing some of the limitations in the classical twin approach and estimating nongenetic influences is the co-twin control or matched-pair analyses of MZ twins. Comparisons within genetically identical MZ twin pairs removes all genetic variability. Thus, if intrapair differences in a characteristic exist (ie, BMI), they must be attributable to environmental or potentially modifiable influences. Newman and colleagues[10] applied this approach in a matched co-twin analyses of 250 Caucasian, male MZ twins from the National Heart, Lung, and Blood Institute (NHLBI) Twin Study. The study was designed to examine the cross-sectional and longitudinal nongenetic influences of obesity (BMI) on risk factors for CVD (lipids and lipoproteins, blood pressure, and glucose intolerance). In both analyses, results indicated significant obesity-CVD risk factor associations. At midlife (42–55 years of age), heavier MZ co-twins had significantly higher levels of systolic and diastolic blood pressure, glucose (1-hour postload), total cholesterol (TC), low-density lipoprotein cholesterol (LDL-C), and triglycerides and lower levels of high-density lipoprotein cholesterol (HDL-C) than their genetically identical, lighter co-twin. Similar results were obtained in longitudinal analyses of weight change during adulthood (from mean age of 20 to mean age of 48 years) and risk factor status at middle age. These results suggest that associations between adult obesity and CVD risk are influenced by behaviors and environmental exposures that occur later in life and provide additional support for weight-reduction efforts during adulthood.[10]

Developmental Trends in Obesity-Cardiovascular Disease Risk Factor Associations

Application of the co-twin matched-pair analyses to data collected as part of the Delaware Valley Twin Study (DVTS)[11,12] provided a unique opportunity to examine developmental trends in the nongenetic influences of obesity on risk factors for CVD.[13] Specifically, the purpose of this longitudinal study was to examine the nongenetic influences of obesity (BMI and triceps skin folds) on risk factors for CVD (the lipid profile and systolic and diastolic blood pressure) during two phases of development: the school-age years (phase 1) and adolescence (phase 2). The influence of change in obesity (amount of gain in BMI from the school-age years to adolescence) on risk factors for CVD also was examined. The phase 1 sample consisted of a panel of 73 Caucasian, 6- to 11-year-old MZ twin pairs identified as potential participants for the longitudinal DVTS through public and private schools in the Philadelphia metropolitan area. Mean age of twin participants at phase 1 was 8.5 years; the mean age at phase 2 was 12.5 years. The median interval between phases was 40 months. In phase 2, 77% (*n* = 56 twin pairs) of the original phase 1 MZ cohort was retained in the study. Zygosity was determined on the basis of blood group antigens including Kell, Duffy, Kidd, ABO, Rh, MNSs, P, and Lewis. If co-twins were concordant on every antigen tested, they were classified as an MZ pair. Additional procedural and measurement details for the DVTS are described elsewhere.[11–14]

As illustrated in Table 2, significant mean intrapair differences in each of three measures of obesity were observed in both phases of development. In phase 1, the mean intrapair difference in weight was 2.4 kg and the mean intrapair difference in height was 0.635 cm. The lighter co-twin was, on average, slightly taller than the heavier co-twin. Similarly, in phase 2 (adolescence), significant mean intrapair differences in each of the measures of obesity was observed. The mean intrapair differences in weight and height were 2.38 kg and 0.33 cm, respectively. These results indicate significant environmental influences on obesity during the school-age years and adolescence. In previous analysis of MZ and DZ twins in this cohort at phase 1,[12] the

Table 2

t Statistics* for Differences between Heavier and Lighter MZ Co-Twins: Phase 1 and Phase 2 Obesity Variables; Delaware Valley Twin Study

	Heavier co-twin		Lighter co-twin				
	M	(SD)	*M*	(SD)	Difference	*t*	*P*
Phase 1	(*n* = 73)		(*n* = 73)				
Quetelet Index (kg/m²)	15.87	(2.06)	15.09	(1.68)	0.776	6.65	0.001
Rohrer Index (kg/m³)	12.17	(1.52)	11.53	(1.33)	0.640	5.66	0.001
Triceps skin fold (mm)	12.07	(5.03)	11.07	(4.40)	1.00	3.49	0.001
Phase 2	(*n* = 56)		(*n* = 56)				
Quetelet Index (kg/m²)	19.01	(2.91)	18.09	(2.74)	0.915	8.72	0.0001
Rohrer Index (kg/m³)	12.31	(1.81)	11.74	(1.67)	0.573	8.56	0.0001
Triceps skin fold (mm)	14.27	(6.26)	13.24	(5.75)	1.027	2.75	0.008

* Matched pairs.
Adapted with permission from reference 13.

amount of variance explained by genetic factors was slightly less than 50%. Considered together, these results suggest substantial environmental influences on obesity in this cohort at school age. Noteworthy, in both phases of development, obesity-CVD risk factor associations were observed. Specifically, in phase 1, intraindividual associations of obesity and atherogenic lipids emerged; heavier co-twins demonstrated higher (5 mg/dL) levels of TC and LDL-C and apolipoprotein-B than their lighter co-twin counterparts. The clinical significance remains to be determined; however, these results are consistent with studies of singletons.[15–17] However, the DVTS results suggest that nongenetic influences contribute to the emergence of obesity-CVD risk factor associations during this developmental period.

In adolescence, phase 2 of the DVTS, obesity-lipid associations also were observed. Specifically, in matched-pair regression analyses of phase 2 data,[13] obesity was defined as the intrapair difference (between heavier and lighter co-twins) in BMI (Rohrer Index). Dependent variables were the intrapair differences in levels of other CVD risk factors. Results indicated that nongenetic influences of obesity contribute to the nongenetic variability in HDL-C ($\beta = -0.33$, $P < 0.01$) and total triglyceride ($\beta = 0.31$, $P < 0.02$), accounting for 11% and 10%, respectively, of the nongenetic variance in these risk factors at phase 2. Adding to the environmental hypothesis were the results of the longitudinal analyses indicating significant intrapair differences in change in obesity (defined as the amount of gain in the Rohrer Index). This change in obesity was associated with total triglyceride ($P < 0.006$) accounting for 14% of the variance in this risk factor.[13] These results are consistent with Newman's observations regarding the nongenetic influences on obesity.[10] Taken together, the results support the matched-pair analyses as a viable approach for examining nongenetic influences. Most importantly, the results emphasize the role of potentially modifiable behaviors and environments in the development and expression of obesity across the life span and point to the importance of developmental transitions as critical periods for preventive interventions.

Additional longitudinal analyses of data collected from the DVTS cohort support the matched-pair results and emphasize obesity as part of the CVD risk profile.[18] Specifically, remeasurements of CVD risk factors were conducted later in adolescence (phase 3); the mean age was 15.5 years and the median P2–P3 interval was 30 months. Seventy-seven twin-pairs ($n = 154$ participants) were retained in the sample at P3. Stepwise regression analyses were conducted to determine the predictors of lipids and lipoproteins at phase 3. For these analyses, twin pairs were split and assigned randomly to group I or group II; this procedure allowed for independence of observations and provided the opportunity to cross-validate the findings. Obesity (BMI) or P1-P3 change in BMI and the respective P1 lipid values explained a significant portion of the variance in atherogenic lipids and HDL-C with R^2 ranging from 0.21 for HDL-C to 0.50 for TC and LDL-C. These results were consistent for both twin groups. As discussed by Obarzanek (see Chapter 2), these results are consistent with numerous observational studies of obesity-CVD risk factor associations in singletons.

Intraindividual clustering of risk factors in children and adults is well established; similarly, obesity and change in obesity are recognized determinants of adverse lipid profiles across the life span. From a developmental perspective, questions remain regarding the temporal sequence of obesity-CVD risk factor clustering. Toward that goal, in a very recent study, Tershakovec and colleagues[19] examined age-related changes in CVD risk factors of hypercholesterolemic (HC) children (nonfasting TC = 176 mg/dL; mean of two fasting LDL-C levels = ≥80th age- and sex-specific percentile). Specifically, the sample for this cross-sectional study of 4- to 10-year-old Caucasian children consisted of n = 227 HC and n = 80 nonhypercholesterolemic (NHC) children. In addition to the lipid profile, risk factors measured were skinfolds (biceps, triceps, suprailiac, and subscapular), percent weight-for-height median (WHM), systolic blood pressure, and insulin levels (HC only). Results indicated that HC had a greater percent WHM, greater skin fold thickness measures, and higher systolic blood pressure than their NHC counterparts. Analysis of variance (ANOVA) by age group with three interaction terms (age group, gender, and TC) was conducted for the anthropometric measures. A significant age interaction demonstrated that the HC group's larger suprailiac and sum of skin fold measures were expressed in the 8.0- to 9.9-year-old children but not in the 4.0- to 5.9-year olds. For both HC and NHC, systolic blood pressure was associated with the measures of adiposity; in the HC group, insulin levels also were associated with adiposity. As observed in a recent study of children with familial combined HC,[20] these results suggest that children with HC have greater body fat. The results also suggest that the expression of the HC precedes the expression of increased body fat; and altered insulin and blood pressure levels are expressed in association with increased body fat in children with HC. These results question the commonly held view that excess adiposity is a causative factor that precedes the phenotypic expression of dyslipidemias in children. As Tershakovec and colleagues[19] conclude, these results require replication with diverse samples and re-examination in longitudinal studies. As noted by Daniels,[21] if these results are confirmed, the mechanisms underlying the age-related differences in the TC-adiposity relationship still remain to be explicated.

Collectively, the results of the DVTS and epidemiological and clinical studies of children and adolescents suggest substantial nongenetic (potentially modifiable) influences on obesity, emphasize its importance as part of the CVD risk profile, and point to the need for individual and population-based approaches to primary prevention.

Health Behaviors: Modifiable Influences on Obesity

Health behaviors, particularly patterns of dietary intake and physical activity, generally are viewed as modifiable influences on obesity. These health behaviors develop within the context of the family environment and are influenced by many extrafamilial factors. Substantial research has examined the independent and combined influences of these health behaviors on the development and expression of obesity across the life span. Hill (see Chapter 15) presents an informative discussion on energy expenditure and obesity with emphasis on these modifiable influences. Although available data are equivocal, they do suggest that dietary intake and physical activity interact to influence the energy balance equation and the obesity-CVD risk profile in childhood and adulthood.[22–23]

Dietary Intake/Eating Behaviors

Consistent with the emphasis on primary prevention of obesity, recent research attention has focused on infancy, particularly the totality of infant feeding experiences including socialization of food preferences and self-regulation of eating behaviors. In a recent comprehensive review of this literature, Birch and Fisher[24] emphasize the importance of the family environment including the influence of parenting practices and eating behaviors on the development of these behaviors in their offspring. For example, food preferences as determinants of children's intake may be linked with early infant feeding practices that are under parental control.[25] Breast-feeding has been the recommended method of infant feeding because of the numerous, well-established physiological and psychological benefits. However, recent data suggest that early food preferences may be influenced by method of feeding.[24,25] Breast-fed infants have exposure to a variety of flavors reflecting maternal diet transmitted through human milk. In contrast, formula-fed infants have experience with a single flavor. Data from Sullivan and Birch,[25] consistent with other reports[26] suggest that breast-fed infants demonstrate greater acceptance of new foods during the transitional period of weaning. However, the long-term influences of these early infant feeding experiences remain to be clarified. Further, as Birch and Fisher[24] emphasize, whether infants differing in familial risk for obesity also differ in their responsiveness to flavors or in their responsiveness to solid food is unknown. This is a fertile area for future research. Using a gene-environment interaction paradigm, this type of inquiry could provide unique information regarding family focused modifiable influences in individuals at high risk for obesity.

As discussed by Obarzanek (see Chapter 2), familial aggregation of obesity has been investigated extensively. Similar to CVD, familial aggregation of obesity is attributed to both shared genes and shared (common) family environment. The mechanisms through which the family environment operates to influence health behaviors associated with obesity (including patterns of dietary intake and physical activity) remain to be clarified; however, available data provide some insight and direction for future research. In a recent review of the available literature on families and health actions, Baranowski[27] presents data to support a model of family reciprocal determinism. Derived from social cognitive theory and consistent with developmental contextualism,[2] this model emphasizes the dynamic interaction of person and environment in the development and acquisition of health behaviors, particularly eating behaviors. Applied to families and health actions, emphasis is placed on parental modeling and reinforcement of health behaviors as well as the influence of other important developmental contexts including school, peers, and the media. By definition and partially supported by available data, the model also suggests that children influence the health behaviors of their parents.[28,29]

Data from several sources support components of Baranowski's model and suggest the family as a unit of analysis and intervention. For example, data from several studies including the Framingham Children's Study[30] and the Princeton School District Study[31] indicate concordance in the dietary patterns of parents and children. Concordance, estimated by correlation analysis, is relatively low across studies and appears to vary as a function of age of the child, family role (ie, mother and father) ethnicity of the family, and nutrients or foods analyzed.[27,30,31] Results of a recent study of fat preferences and consumption in preschool children add to this database by demonstrating significant associations between parental BMI and children's fat preferences ($r = 0.75$).[32] In this study, Fisher and Birch[32] also observed significant associations between parental BMI and children's fat intake ($r = 0.67$). Noteworthy is that children were offered a single menu consisting of 32% energy as fat; children's fat intakes actually ranged from 25% to 41%.

Taken together and placed in the context of other recent studies,[33,34] these results suggest that children's preferences for and consumption of fat may be influenced by familial factors including the availability of and exposure to high-fat foods.[32]

In the context of modifiable influences on obesity, the family emerges as an important determinant of relevant health behaviors and should be considered as a unit of analysis in future research. Although familial patterns of dietary intake and eating behaviors have received more research attention than physical activity (discussed below), lacking are data on the specific mechanisms through which these behaviors are acquired and transmitted within multigenerational families. Further, most of the available data have been generated from studies of white, middle-class families. With emphasis on population-based approaches and primary prevention, future research should target families of diverse sociocultural economic backgrounds. Because obesity is influenced by energy intake and expenditure, future research on modifiable influences should have a conjoint focus (ie, patterns of dietary intake and physical activity).

Physical Activity

As discussed elsewhere in this volume, developmental trends in physical activity in children and adolescents in the United States argue convincingly for additional research on the determinants of this behavior. As illustrated in Figure 1, data from the 1992 National Health Interview Survey–Youth Risk Behavior Survey[35] indicate substantial declines in physical activity in both males and females during the

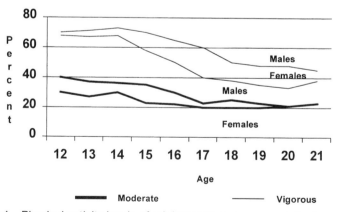

Figure 1. Physical activity levels of adolescents and young adults, by age and sex. Reproduced with permission from Reference 57.

transition from childhood to adolescence. This decrement has been observed in numerous studies and is pronounced particularly in females.[36-39]

Population-based data on temporal trends are lacking; however, the age-related downward trend in the prevalence of participation in physical activity combined with scattered data on the prevalence of sedentary activities[39] and potential benefits of decreasing these behaviors[40] underscore the need for additional research.

Individual and contextual/environmental factors have been linked with physical activity in children and adolescents. As Kohl and Hobbs[41] observed in a recent comprehensive review of this literature, most of the available data have been generated from cross-sectional studies. Thus, the temporal relationships between these factors and patterns of activity in children and adolescents remain to be clarified. In addition, between-study differences in operational definitions and methods of measurement of physical activity make it difficult to compare results across studies. These limitations notwithstanding, individual factors associated with physical activity include age, gender, physical fitness, health status, self-efficacy, knowledge and attitudes, education, and socioeconomic status.[36,41] Some of these factors (ie, self-efficacy)[42] are more amenable to modification than others (ie, age and gender). Data are inconclusive; however, they suggest that individual factors are influenced by developmental contexts/environments including the family (parental influences and competing attentions),[42-45] school (peer influences, programs, and policies),[46,49] and community (available facilities, safety issues, and policies).[48-50] Thus, using paradigms that allow for examination of individual and environmental factors (both main effects and interactions) would optimize the information yield and provide more specific direction for preventive interventions.

Daniels (see Chapter 5) argues convincingly for both individual and population-based approaches to increasing physical activity in children and youth with emphasis on some of these family and community factors. Adding to this database with implications for primary prevention of obesity are recent data from NHANES III[51] and accumulated data on the potential multidimensional role of schools in promoting healthy lifestyles and preventing obesity.[52,53] Specifically, Andersen and colleagues[51] used data from NHANES III to determine cross-sectional prevalence rates of daily television-watching habits and weekly bouts of vigorous physical activity in this nationally representative sample of US children aged 8 through 16 years. The relationship between BMI, body fatness, and bouts of vigorous activity and "television watching" also were examined. Eighty percent of children reported three or more periods of vigorous activity each week; however, the rate was lower in non-Hispanic black and Mexican American girls (69% and 73%, respectively). Twenty-six percent of US children watched 4 or more hours of television per day while 67% watched at least 2 hours per day. Most importantly, boys and girls who watched ≥4 or more hours per day had the highest skin fold thicknesses and BMIs while children who viewed ≤1 hour per day had the lowest BMIs. Non-Hispanic black children reported the highest prevalence rates (42%) of this sedentary activity. These population-based data confirm that vigorous activity among ethnic minority children is lower than among non-Hispanic white children. As Andersen and colleagues[51] conclude, these results have important implications for the design and implementation of school- and community-based interventions aimed at increasing physical activity in children and youth.

Schools have been suggested as critical, "captive" environments for promoting the adoption of healthy behaviors including patterns of physical activity and dietary intake. However, data from the Centers for Disease Control and Prevention (CDC and P) suggest[35] that substantial efforts are necessary for schools to optimize this potential. For example, as indicated in Figure 1, participation in all types of physical activity decreases as age or grade in school increases. CDC and P data also indicate that only 19% of all high school students are physically active for 20 minutes or more, 5 days a week. Further, daily enrollment in physical education classes declined from 42% to 25% among high school students during the period between 1991 and 1995.[35] School-based research initiatives including the Child and Adolescent Trial for Cardiovascular Health (CATCH)[54] and the Cardiovascular Health in Children (CHIC) Study[55] emphasize the school as a viable, feasible, and effective environment for changing health behaviors in ethnically diverse children and youth. The CATCH targeted the individual health behaviors and the modification of the school environment including the curriculum and educational materials, teacher training, and on-site consultation.[54] Students' moderate to vigorous physical activity (in school) increased from 37.4% at baseline to 51.9% post-intervention.[54] Thus, a major lesson learned from CATCH, supported by results of other school-based studies,[47,52,55] was demonstrating that changing school environments can result in changing health behaviors of children. Adding to this database, CHIC results also suggest that a short-term (8-week) classroom-based intervention can be effective in reducing cardiovascular risk factors (including levels of serum TC) in elementary school children.[55] However, longitudinal studies are necessary to determine adherence over time particularly throughout the adolescent transition.

Conclusions

Obesity is a highly prevalent chronic condition that results from an imbalance in energy intake and expenditure. Genetic and nongenetic factors interact across the life span to influence the development, expression, and maintenance of obesity. Developmental trends indicate the emergence of obesity-CVD risk factor associations early in life and point to the importance of an integrated profile approach to cardiovascular health with emphasis on primary prevention of obesity.[56,57] The current epidemic of obesity in the United States indicates an urgent need for effective high-risk and population-based approaches to prevention and management with emphasis on the potentially modifiable influences including health behaviors and the environments in which they develop and are maintained. Although many questions remain unanswered, available data emphasize the potential role of the family and school environments in the development and maintenance of health behaviors including patterns of dietary intake and physical activity. Developmentally appropriate and culturally competent, population-based strategies are recommended to reduce the public health burden of obesity. Toward that goal, a multidisciplinary research agenda that includes and emphasizes health behaviors and relevant sociocultural-environmental factors within and across diverse populations is suggested.

References

1. Troiano RP, Flegal KM. Overweight children and adolescents: Description, epidemiology and demographics. *Pediatrics* 1998;101:497–504.
2. Lerner RM. Theories of human development: Contemporary perspectives. In: Lerner RM, ed. *Theoretical Models of Human Development*. 5th ed. New York: Wiley, 1998:1–24.
3. Barlow SE, Dietz WH. Obesity evaluation and treatment: Expert committee recommendations [serial online]. *Pediatrics* 1998;102:E29.
4. Meyer JM, Stunkard AJ. Twin studies of human obesity. In: Bouchard C, ed. *The Genetics of Obesity*. Boca Raton, Fla: CRC Press, 1994:63–78.
5. Falconer DS. *Introduction to Quantitative Genetics*. New York: Wiley, 1989.
6. Meyer JM, Bodurtha JN, Eaves LJ, et al. Tracking genetic and environmental effects on adolescent BMI: The MCV Twin Study. Unpublished data.
7. Stunkard AJ, Foch TT, Hrubec Z. A twin study of human obesity. *JAMA* 1986;256:51–54.
8. Bouchard C, Perusse L, Leblanc C, et al. Inheritance of the amount and distribution of human body fat. *Int J Obes*. 1988;12:205–215.
9. Selby JV, Newman B, Quesenberry CP Jr, et al. Genetic and behavioral influences on body fat distribution. *Int J Obes* 1990;14:593–602.
10. Newman B, Selby JV, Quesenberry CP Jr, et al. Nongenetic influences of obesity on other cardiovascular disease risk factors: An analysis of identical twins. *Am J Public Health* 1990;80:675–678.

11. Hayman LL, Meininger JC, Stashinko EE, et al. Type A behavior and physiological cardiovascular risk factors in school-age twin children. *Nurs Res* 1988;37:290–296.

12. Meininger JC, Hayman LL, Coates PM, et al. Genetics or environment? Type A behavior and cardiovascular risk factors in twin children. *Nurs Res* 1988;37:341–346.

13. Hayman LL, Meininger JC, Coates PM, et al. Nongenetic influences of obesity on risk factors for cardiovascular disease during two phases of development. *Nurs Res* 1995;44:277–283.

14. Meininger JC, Hayman LL, Coates PM, et al. Genetic and environmental influences on cardiovascular disease risk factors in adolescents. *Nurs Res* 1998;47:11–18.

15. Webber LS, Voors AW, Srinivasan SR, et al. Occurrence in children of multiple risk factors for coronary artery disease: The Bogalusa heart study. *Prev Med.* 1979;8:407–418.

16. Khoury P, Morrison JA, Kelly K, et al. Clustering and interrelationships of coronary heart disease risk factors in schoolchildren, ages 6–19. *Am J Epidemiol* 1980;112:524–538.

17. Anonymous. Obesity and cardiovascular disease risk factors in black and white girls: The NHLBI Growth and Health Study. *Am J Public Health* 1992;82:1613–1620.

18. Hayman LL, Meininger JC, Gallager PR, et al. Tracking of the lipid profile from childhood to adolescence. *Circulation* 1995;92:767.

19. Tershakovec AM, Jawad AF, Stallings VA, et al. Age-related changes in cardiovascular disease risk factors of hypercholesterolemic children. *J Pediatr* 1998;132:414–420.

20. Shamir R, Tershakovec AM, Gallagher PR, et al. The influence of age and relative weight on the presentation of familial combined hyperlipidemia in childhood. *Atherosclerosis* 1996;121:85–91.

21. Daniels SR. Overweight and cholesterol elevation: Which is the chicken and which is the egg? *J Pediatr* 1998;132:383–384.

22. Epstein LH, Valoski A, Wing RR, et al. Ten-year outcomes of behavioral family-based treatment for childhood obesity. *Health Psychol* 1994;13:373–383.

23. Epstein LH, Kuller LH, Wing RR, et al. The effect of weight control on lipid changes in obese children. *Am J Dis Child* 1989;143:454–457.

24. Birch LL, Fisher JO. Development of eating behaviors among children and adolescents. *Pediatrics* 1998;101:539–548.

25. Sullivan SA, Birch LL. Infant dietary experience and acceptance of solid foods. *Pediatrics* 1994;93:271–277.

26. Capretta PJ, Petersik JT, Stewart DJ. Acceptance of novel flavours is increased after early experience of diverse tastes. *Nature* 1975;254:689–691.

27. Baranowski T. Families and health actions. In: Gochman DS, ed. *Handbook of Health Behavior Research.* New York: Plenum Press, 1997:179–206.

28. Nader PR, Perry C, Maccoby N, et al. Adolescent perceptions of family health behavior: A tenth grade educational activity to increase family awareness of a community cardiovascular risk reduction program. *J Sch Health* 1982;52:372–377.

29. Knight J, Grantham-McGregor S. Using primary-school children to improve child-rearing practices in rural Jamaica. *Child Care Health Dev* 1985; 11:81–90.

30. Oliveria SA, Ellison RC, Moore LL, et al. Parent-child relationships in nutrient intake: The Framingham Children's Study. *Am J Clin Nutr* 1992; 56:593–598.
31. Laskarzewski P, Morrison JA, Khoury P, et al. Parent-child nutrient intake interrelationships in school children ages 6 to 19: The Princeton School District Study. *Am J Clin Nutr* 1980;33:2350–2355.
32. Fisher JO, Birch LL. Fat preferences and fat consumption of 3- to 5-year-old children are related to parental adiposity. *J Am Diet Assoc* 1995;95:759–764.
33. Eck LH, Klesges RC, Hanson CL, et al. Children at familial risk for obesity: An examination of dietary intake, physical activity and weight status. *Int J Obes* 1991;16:71–78.
34. Michela JL, Contento IR. Cognitive, motivational, social, and environmental influences on children's food choices. *Health Psychol* 1986;5:209–230.
35. US Department of Health and Human Services. Physical activity and health: A report of the Surgeon General. Atlanta, Ga: Centers for Disease Control and Prevention; 1996.
36. Sallis JF. Epidemiology of physical activity and fitness in children and adolescents. *Crit Rev Food Sci Nutr* 1993;33:403–408.
37. Center for Disease Control, and Prevention. Youth risk behavior surveillance: United States, 1995. *MMWR* 1996.
38. Ross JG, Pate RR. The National Children and Youth Fitness Study II: A summary of the findings. *J Phys Educ Recr Dance* 1987;58:51–56.
39. Dietz WH, Strasburger VC. Children, adolescents, and television. *Curr Probl Pediatr* 1991;21:8–31.
40. Epstein LH, Saelens BE, Myers MD, et al. Effects of decreasing sedentary behaviors on activity choice in obese children. *Health Psychol* 1997;16:107–113.
41. Kohl HW, Hobbs KE. Development of physical activity behaviors among children and adolescents. *Pediatrics* 1998;101:549–554.
42. Reynolds KD, Killen JD, Bryson SW, et al. Psychosocial predictors of physical activity in adolescents. *Prev Med* 1990;19:554.
43. Biddle S, Goudas M. Analysis of children's physical activity and its association with adult encouragement and social cognitive variables. *J Sch Health* 1996;66:75–78.
44. Sallis JF, Patterson TL, Buono MJ, et al. Aggregation of physical activity habits in Mexican-American and Anglo families. *J Behav Med* 1988;11:31–41.
45. Zakarian JM, Hovell MF, Hofstetter CR, et al. Correlates of vigorous exercise in a predominantly low SES and minority high school population. *Prev Med* 1994;23:314–321.
46. Kelder SH, Perry CL, Peters RJ, et al. Gender differences in the Class of 1989 study: The school component of the Minnesota Heart Health Program. *J Health Educ* 1995;26:S36.
47. Arbeit ML, Johnson CC, Mott DS, et al. The Heart Smart cardiovascular school health promotion: Behavior correlates of risk factor change. *Prev Med* 1992;21:18–32.
48. Butcher J. Longitudinal analysis of adolescent girls' participation in physical activity. *Sociol Sport J* 1985;2:130–143.
49. Gottlieb NH, Chen MS. Sociocultural correlates of childhood sporting activities: Their implications for heart health. *Soc Sci Med* 1985;21:533–539.
50. Stucky-Ropp RC, DiLorenzo TM. Determinants of exercise in children. *Prev Med* 1993;22:880–889.

51. Andersen RE, Crespo CJ, Bartlett SJ, et al. Relationship of physical activity and television watching with body weight and level of fatness among children: Results from the Third National Health and Nutrition Examination Survey. *JAMA* 1998;279:938–942.
52. Resnicow K, Robinson TN. School-based cardiovascular disease prevention studies: Review and synthesis. *Ann Epid* 1997;7(suppl 7):S14–S31.
53. McGinnis JM. The year 2000 initiative: Implications for comprehensive school health. *Prev Med* 1993;22:493–498.
54. Luepker RV, Perry CL, McKinlay SM, et al. Outcomes of a field trial to improve children's dietary patterns and physical activity. The Child and Adolescent Trial for Cardiovascular Health. CATCH collaborative group. *JAMA* 1996;275:768–776.
55. Harrell JS, McMurray RG, Bangdiwala SI, et al. Effects of a school-based intervention to reduce cardiovascular disease risk factors in elementary-school children: The Cardiovascular Health in Children (CHIC) Study. *J Pediatr* 1996;128:797–805.
56. Strong WB, Deckelbaum RJ, Gidding SS, et al. Integrated cardiovascular health promotion in childhood. A statement for health professionals from the Subcommittee on Atherosclerosis and Hypertension in Childhood of the Council on Cardiovascular Disease in the Young, American Heart Association. *Circulation* 1992;85:1638–1650.
57. Gidding SS, Leibel RL, Daniels S, et al. Understanding obesity in youth. A statement for healthcare professionals from the Committee on Atherosclerosis and Hypertension in the Young of the Council on Cardiovascular Disease in the Young and the Nutrition Committee, American Heart Association. *Writing Group Circulation* 1996;94:3383–3387.

Chapter 5

Prevention of Obesity

Stephen R. Daniels, MD, PhD

Introduction

Much of medical care is focused on treatment of established disease. However, it should be clear that there are other important methods of intervention to improve health. One of the most important is to prevent the disease before it is established. This often is referred to as primary prevention and focuses on controlling risk factors for the disease.

Obesity occupies an interesting niche because it is considered a disease in its own right, but it also is a risk factor for some diseases and has an impact on risk factors for other diseases (Figure 1). Thus, obesity is in the middle of causal pathways leading to cardiovascular, pulmonary, orthopedic, psychological, and other diseases, such as diabetes mellitus.

In considering a preventive intervention, one must take several issues into consideration. This is similar to consideration of whether to implement a screening program in the health care setting (Table 1). First, the prevalence and severity of the disease should be evaluated. Is the disease common? Does the disease result in substantial discomfort, disability, and mortality? Second, the effectiveness of treatment of the disease should be considered. If treatment of the disease once it has developed is especially problematic, then prevention should be considered. Third, it is important to evaluate whether high-risk individuals can be identified. This allows preventive efforts to be focused on and helps to conserve resources. Finally, it must be determined whether appropriate preventive interventions are available. This involves consideration of the efficacy of the intervention, the likelihood of compliance, the appropriate timing of the intervention, and the possibility of side effects associated with the intervention.

From: Fletcher GF, Grundy SM, Hayman LL (eds). *Obesity: Impact on Cardiovascular Disease.* Armonk, NY: Futura Publishing Co., Inc.; © 1999.

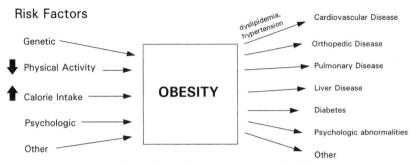

Figure 1. Obesity; both a risk factor and a disease.

This chapter will evaluate obesity as a candidate for prevention. The criteria listed above will be utilized in this evaluation.

The Problem of Obesity

Obesity is the most common,[1,2] frustrating, and costly nutritional problem in the United States. Health care costs for the sequelae of obesity amount approximately to $68 billion annually.[3]

There is a broad spectrum of sequelae of obesity. Overweight adults die from all causes at an earlier age than adults of normal weight. When suffering from a similar condition, adults who are overweight are sicker longer than those of normal weight.[4] Obesity has been shown to be associated with diabetes mellitus, cardiovascular disease, liver and gallbladder disease, pulmonary problems, orthopedic disorders, and a variety of psychological concerns.[5]

Obesity is the most powerful risk factor for non–insulin-dependent diabetes mellitus (NIDDM). In some populations, such as

---

Table 1

Principles of Prevention

1. Is the disease prevalent?
2. Is the disease associated with substantial morbidity and mortality?
3. Is the disease difficult to treat?
4. Is the treatment associated with important side effects?
5. Can a subset of the population who are at high risk of developing the disease be identified?
6. Are the determinants of the disease understood?
7. Is there an effective method to improve the risk?
8. Does the intervention strategy have minimal risk?
9. Is the preventive intervention cost-effective?

the Pima Indians, the incidence of NIDDM is related strongly to obesity. It has been reported that the likelihood of becoming diabetic more than doubles with every 20% excess in body weight.[6] In one study, when body mass index (BMI) was below 20 kg/m^2, the incidence of diabetes was 0.8 cases per 1000 person years. The incidence increased as BMI increased with an incidence of 72 cases per 1000 person years for BMI greater than 40 kg/m^2.[7]

Numerous cross-sectional studies have found relationships between obesity and adverse levels of cardiovascular risk factors.[8] The characteristic pattern of lipid and lipoproteins associated with obesity is elevation of triglycerides, decreased high-density lipoprotein cholesterol (HDL-C) and normal or marginally elevated low-density lipoprotein cholesterol (LDL-C).[9] People with increased visceral adiposity appear to be especially predisposed to lipid abnormalities.[9]

Hypertension also is associated with obesity. For example, the relative risk of hypertension for adults age 20–75 years in the United States is three times higher in overweight compared with nonoverweight individuals. This increased risk is pronounced even more in younger people (age 20–45) compared with older people.[10] In addition, obesity has been associated with left ventricular hypertrophy. Children and adults who are overweight have increased left ventricular mass and abnormal left ventricular geometry, which has been associated with increased risk of cardiovascular disease.[11]

It has been debated whether obesity has an impact on cardiovascular disease, which is independent of its effect on traditional risk factors. An overview of the evidence suggests that obesity is probably an independent risk factor for cardiovascular disease morbidity and mortality.[5] It remains to be determined whether there are differences in the impact of lifelong obesity compared with obesity that begins in adulthood and whether large fluctuations in weight are associated with an increased risk of cardiovascular disease.

Elevation of liver enzymes may be related to obesity in children.[12] This elevation has been shown frequently to be associated with fatty liver and, in some cases, cirrhosis. Gallbladder disease and cholelithiasis also are associated with obesity.[13] Obese women between 20 and 30 years of age have been reported to have a sixfold increase in the risk of developing gallbladder disease compared with normal weight women. Cholelithiasis may occur even more frequently with weight reduction in adults and in adolescents.[14] This suggests that prevention of obesity may be most helpful in preventing these problems.

Sleep apnea may be the complication of obesity that presents the most immediate risk for morbidity or mortality, especially for children and adolescents.[15] Sleep apnea has been reported to occur in approximately 7% of obese children.[16] One-third of children with body weight greater than 150% of ideal, who had a history of breathing problems during sleep, were found to have sleep apnea. Abnormalities in pulmonary function during the daytime also have been observed in obese subjects. The most extreme form of this abnormality is the obesity hypoventilation syndrome, which is characterized by obesity, somnolence, and alveolar hypoventilation.[17] In obese adults, there is a decrease in expiratory reserve volume as well as a tendency to an overall reduction in lung volumes. There also may be some degree of mismatch of ventilation and perfusion in the lungs of obese individuals.[18]

Several orthopedic problems have been associated with obesity, both in childhood and in adulthood. Obese children are at increased risk for slipped capital femoral epiphysis.[19] Approximately 40% of children with slipped capital femoral epiphysis are overweight. The mechanism is thought to be related to the mechanical effects of increased weight on the growth plate of the hip. When a young overweight patient has unilateral slipped capital femoral epiphysis, they are at risk to develop bilateral problems. Some studies have demonstrated an increased prevalence of osteoarthritis in obese adults.[20] The knee joint appears to be involved most frequently; however, there has not been uniformity on this issue in the literature.[20] Obese adults also are at increased risk of gout.[21]

There are some important psychological and social consequences of obesity in childhood and young adulthood. Overweight young children do not seem to have low self-esteem. However, obese adolescents do develop a negative self-image, which may persist. The National Longitudinal Survey of Youth evaluated a large population of individuals, age 16 to 24 years.[22] Women who were overweight as adolescents were more likely to complete less education, remain unmarried, and have lower income compared with women who were not obese. Of interest is the fact that similar relationships were not observed for young men. It is possible that low socioeconomic status (SES) is the cause of obesity. However, analyses controlling for parental education and family income suggest that obesity may be an antecedent rather than a consequence of low SES.

Prevalence of Obesity

Obesity probably is the most prevalent nutritional disorder in the United States. However, estimates of the incidence and prevalence of obesity vary. One reason for the variation is the fact that the estimation of the incidence and prevalence of obesity depends on both the method of measurement and the cut point used. Generally, published results of the prevalence of obesity have ranged from 5% to 25% in children and adolescents[23] and as high as 30% in adults.[24] A study of nursery school children revealed that 12% were greater than 120% ideal body weight based on height and 4.7% were greater than 130% ideal body weight.[25]

A number of factors have an influence on the amount of body fat, including age, sex, and race. At birth, the human body contains approximately 12% fat. This fat content at birth is higher than in any other mammals except the whale. The fat content rises during the newborn period, reaches a peak of approximately 25% at 5 months of age, and then declines to 15%–18% during the prepubertal years. BMI reaches a low point during childhood and then rises into adolescence and adulthood. This nadir is referred to as the point of adiposity rebound. During childhood, gender differences in body fat are minimal. However, there is a difference in body fat between boys and girls during adolescence.

Racial differences in fatness may exist in children and adolescents, but the explanation of these differences is debatable. It is difficult to separate genetic from environmental factors as an explanation for racial differences in obesity. SES and cultural factors probably play an important role in obesity development. For example, excess body weight is 7 to 12 times more frequent in women of lower SES compared with women of higher SES.[26] SES appears to have less of an impact on the occurrence of obesity in men.[27]

There may be important international differences in the prevalence of obesity in adults. The prevalence of adults with a BMI of 25–30 kg/m^2 appears to be similar in most western populations.[10,27–29] This represents a group of individuals who are mildly overweight and includes more men as the median BMI for women is 22 kg/m^2 compared with 25 kg/m^2 for men. However, the prevalence of adult individuals with a BMI above 30, indicative of definite overweight, is higher in the United States and Canada compared with Great Britain, The Netherlands, and Australia.[10,27–30]

In the United States, the incidence of becoming obese appears fairly uniform throughout childhood and adolescence with the exception of possibly increased incidence among adolescent girls.[31] The remission rate has an inverse relationship with age. This means that the earlier the onset of obesity in childhood, the greater the likelihood of spontaneous resolution with age. The later the onset of obesity, the higher the risk of persistence. These factors combine to result in the increasing prevalence of obesity observed with increasing age. One factor that has made it difficult to obtain valid estimates of the prevalence of obesity in the United States is the fact that most studies have included samples that are unrepresentative of the United States population.

Secular Trends

There has been concern that the prevalence of obesity has been increasing in children and adolescents over recent years. Dietz et al[32] analyzed data from national population studies. They defined obesity as a triceps skin fold greater than the 85th percentile for children or adolescents of the same age and sex sampled in cycles 2 and 3 of the National Health Examination Survey (NHES). The skin fold criteria then were used to examine changes in the national samples from the first and second National Health and Nutrition Examination Surveys (NHANESs I and II). They found that the prevalence of obesity increased by approximately 40% in both children and adolescents during the 15-year period of the surveys with more rapid increases in the prevalence among black than among white children.

Actually, this may be a trend that has been operative in adults for an even longer period of time. For example, data obtained for men in the United States at the time of evaluation for military service show that men inducted into the Army in 1950 were heavier than those inducted in 1918.[33] The Framingham Study has shown similar changes for men but has indicated that women may not be getting fatter.[34] Data from the NHANESs may provide important data concerning trends for obesity, because they are conducted periodically on probability samples of the population in the United States. Over the past 30 years, the mean and median BMI has increased consistently for adults. However, the trend for adolescents has been less consistent.[35] An important caveat is that estimates of central tendency, such as the mean and the median, may not provide the complete picture in determining whether or not there are secular trends for increasing obesity in the United States.

Gortmaker et al[36] used triceps skin fold thickness measurements of children obtained in four population surveys of the United States during the period of 1963 to 1980. They defined obesity as triceps skin folds ≥ 85th percentile of children of the same and sex in 1963–1970. Superobesity was defined as skin folds greater than the 95th percentile. Compared with the skin fold data from the 1963–1965 NHES cycle 2, skin fold data from the NHANES II survey (1976–1980) show a 54% increase in the prevalence of obesity among children 6–11 years old and a 98% increase in superobesity. Increases occurred among children of all ages, both genders, and for African and white American children.[36] Webber et al[37] also have presented data from the Bogalusa Study concerning secular trends in obesity.[37] They reported an increase in weight and ponderal index (weight/height^3) in 5- to 17-year olds over a 15-year period from 1973 to 1988. The ponderal index increased by approximately 5% during this period. The trend for increase in weight was most pronounced in the uppermost percentiles. These findings were consistent for both boys and girls in white and African American children.

Morrison et al[38] compared data on obesity from a group of children studied in Cincinnati, Ohio as part of the Lipid Research Clinics Prevalence Study from 1973 to 1975 with data from a second study performed in the same schools in 1989 and 1990. The school district has remained demographically stable during the 15 years between the studies. They found that students in 1990 had higher BMI, higher total cholesterol, and higher systolic blood pressure than students in 1975. Of interest is the fact that the increase in BMI occurred primarily in the upper six deciles of BMI (Table 2). This suggests that the children destined to be overweight are becoming even more overweight in recent years. This may be a harbinger of a major public health problem. Dietary data suggest that overall the consumption of calories has not changed from 1975 to 1990 and have, if anything, decreased in recent years.[38] The percent of calories from fat also has decreased in this time. These data appear to implicate dietary intake of simple carbohydrates and diminished physical activity as a determinant of observed trends in obesity. Webber et al[37] arrived at a similar conclusion from the study of children in Bogalusa.

It appears that the frequency of NIDDM also is increasing in adolescents. In one study, NIDDM accounted for one-third of all new cases of diabetes in Cincinnati in 1994.[39] The incidence of NIDDM among adolescents in Cincinnati appears to have increased by 10-fold

Table 2

Body Mass Index (BMI) for Third and Fifth Grade School Children in 1975 and 1990

BMI percentiles	BMI 1975 (kg/m^2)	BMI 1990 (kg/m^2)
95	22.3	25.4
90	20.7	23.1
80	18.9	20.5
70	18.1	19.0
60	17.2	17.9
50	16.6	17.2
40	16.2	16.5
30	15.7	15.9
20	15.1	15.5
10	14.6	14.8
5	14.1	14.2

since 1982. Most of these adolescents with newly diagnosed NIDDM were overweight. The mean BMI in this group was 37. These results suggest that the morbid effects of the trends in overweight have begun and that the sequelae of obesity may occur at increasingly younger ages as the prevalence and severity of obesity increase in childhood.

The reported trends in overweight have occurred over a 10–20 year period. This rapid change in the population strongly suggests an environmental rather than a genetic cause. It is unlikely that there could have been such a rapid, major change in the genes that cause or predispose to obesity. So although the search for genes that are related to obesity may have important biological and therapeutic conse- quences, there remains a large role for issues related to diet and physical activity in the prevention of obesity.

Difficulties with Treatment

There has been substantial interest in developing effective treat- ments for obesity. Much of the research in this area has focused on adults with obesity, but some work also has been done in treating children and adolescents. Generally, the aim of weight reduction should be to decrease morbidity rather than to achieve a cosmetic goal. A number of approaches have been proposed, including lifestyle mod- ification, drug therapy, and surgery. Unfortunately, even with modest goals for weight loss, many therapeutic approaches result in failure. Lifestyle approaches are more likely to be successful in persons with mild overweight rather than in those with severe obesity.[40] As indi- cated above, despite vigorous attempts at treatment of obesity since the 1950s, the prevalence of obesity continues to increase for both adults and children.[1] It is clear that in large part the results of treat- ment have been less than satisfactory.[3]

It has been shown that approximately two-thirds of people who lose weight will regain it in 1 year, and almost all will regain it within 5 years.[41] Many others who try cannot lose weight. The weight loss industry is estimated to generate $30–$50 billion annually without much success.[42] These failed attempts at weight loss may have an important negative psychological impact. There is social pressure to lose weight and failed attempts often leave patients with guilt and low self-esteem.

There also are important side effects of weight loss and the meth- ods used to accomplish it. Cholelithiasis occurs with increased fre- quency in association with weight reduction[43] and cholecystitis may occur with weight loss in both adults and children.[14] Some studies have suggested that frequent fluctuations in body weight also may be associated with adverse outcomes. For example, the Chicago Gas and Electric Study has shown that one cycle of weight loss and gain is a risk factor for coronary heart disease (CHD) mortality independent of high BMI.[44] In that study, the relative risk for CHD mortality was 1.8 for the gain-loss group compared with the no-change group, whereas no significant effects were seen in a weight gain and no-loss group. In addition, clinical studies suggest that weight gain after weight loss often results in a weight that exceeds the original weight.[45]

There are a variety of pharmacologic approaches to weight loss that have been proposed. Most of these approaches are directed at decreasing appetite, increasing energy expenditure, or both. Although some success with pharmacologic agents has been reported, most studies show a prompt regaining of weight once the drug is stopped.[46,47]

Questions also have been raised about the safety of drugs used to treat obesity. Serotonin reuptake inhibitors may increase the likelihood of the development of primary pulmonary hypertension.[48] A recent, uncontrolled case report suggests that valvular heart abnormalities might be related to treatment with a combination of fenfluramine and phentermine.[49] These findings have led to questions regarding the use of this combination and action by the Food and Drug Administration. New pharmacologic approaches are on the horizon, such as sibutramine, which has both catecholaminergic and serotonergic agonist effects, and lipase inhibitors, which prevent absorption of fats. These and other medications for treatment of obesity will need extensive testing before one can be sure they are safe and effective.

Surgery usually is recommended only for patients with morbid obesity. These procedures, such as jejunoileal shunts and gastroplasty, have been shown to be successful in some cases resulting in persistent weight loss and maintenance at least 10% below preoperative weight.[40] However, the jejunoileal shunt procedure may result in the blind loop syndrome and patients with either procedure must be followed for possible electrolyte disturbance or bowel obstruction.

There are reasons to be more optimistic about treatment of obesity in children and adolescents. Eating habits and patterns of physical activity may be established less firmly in children compared with adults. Treatment of pediatric obesity can utilize the growth of the child as an advantage.[50] Early treatment also may prevent the development of adipocytes. Nevertheless, many pediatricians have been frustrated in attempts to treat obesity in their patients. Pharmacologic agents and surgery usually are not recommended for children and adolescents. There also is a concern about the development of eating disorders, such as bulimia and anorexia nervosa in young patients.[50]

Identification of High-Risk Individuals

It would be of great utility to be able to identify those who are at increased risk of becoming obese. One concept that has been proposed is to focus intervention on children who are overweight. It has been hypothesized that children who are obese likely will be obese as adults. Whitaker et al[51] utilized records from individuals who were born under the care of a health maintenance organization (HMO) between 1965 and 1971 and remained in care at that HMO into young adulthood.[1] After adjustment for parental obesity, the odds ratio for obesity in adulthood associated with childhood obesity ranged from 1.3 (1 or 2 years of age) to 17.5 for obesity at 15–17 years of age. This demonstrates that younger children who are overweight, especially if their parents are not overweight, are a low risk for adult obesity. As children get older, obesity becomes an increasingly important predictor of adult obesity.

One problem with using childhood obesity as a risk indicator is that the obesity is already present. This means that the difficulties with therapy already will be operative. Other factors have been studied that may prove useful. Whitaker et al[51] found that parental obesity more than doubles the risk of adult obesity among both obese and nonobese children under the age of 10 years. This finding reflects both a genetic predisposition to obesity as well as the importance of shared lifestyle. Unfortunately, it remains unclear which environmental factors are most important in contributing to the expression of obesity.

It also has been suggested that maternal gestational diabetes may influence subsequent development of obesity in the child. Gestational diabetes affects 3%–5% of all pregnancies. The results of studies on this question have been conflicting. Some studies have suggested a relationship;[52,53] however, other studies have not supported this association.[54] Whitaker et al[54] found the prevalence of obesity was 19% in offspring of mothers treated for gestational diabetes and 24% in the offspring of mothers with negative glucose screens during pregnancy. This suggests that prenatal exposure to the effects of mild, diet-treated gestational diabetes does not increase the risk of childhood obesity.

Another factor that has been proposed as a method of predicting future obesity is the adiposity rebound. Changes in body composition are normal with growth and development. Children have a rapid increase in BMI during the first year of life. After 12 months BMI declines and reaches a minimum at, on average, 5 to 6 years. Then, BMI begins a gradual increase that continues through adolescence and most of adulthood. The nadir of BMI is called adiposity rebound.[55] An early (younger) adiposity rebound is associated with higher BMI in adolescence[55,56] and early adulthood.[57] Whitaker et al[58] examined whether a younger age of adiposity rebound was associated with an increased risk of adult obesity and if this risk was independent of parental obesity and the degree of fatness at age of adiposity rebound. They found the mean age at adiposity rebound was 5.5 years. The prevalence of obesity in adulthood was higher in those with early versus late adiposity rebound, those who were heavy versus lean at adiposity rebound, and those with heavy versus lean parents. After adjustment for parent BMI and the BMI at adiposity rebound, the odds ratio for adult obesity associated with early versus late adiposity rebound was 6.0 [95% confidence interval (CI) 1.3–26.6].

Siervogel and colleagues[56] used prospective data from the Fels Longitudinal Study to evaluate adiposity rebound. They found a significant inverse correlation between age at adiposity rebound and BMI at 18 years of age ($r = -0.46$ for boys and $r = -0.54$ in girls). The mechanism for adiposity rebound and the determinants of the timing remain unknown. In addition, interventions to alter the age of adiposity rebound have not been attempted. It is possible that the age of adiposity rebound could provide a useful marker to indicate children who are at high risk for future obesity and in whom preventive efforts should be focused. Future research should examine the biological and behavioral determinants of adiposity rebound and mechanisms through which an early age of adiposity rebound may influence the development of obesity.

Strategies for Prevention of Obesity

In theory, obesity should be easy to prevent. In practice, nothing could be further from the truth. Preventive efforts should focus on the environmental influences on obesity, such as diet, physical activity, and psychological factors. In addition, it appears reasonable to pursue two types of strategies to prevent obesity. The first would be a population-based, public health strategy. In this approach, attempts would be made to improve the diet and level of physical activity in all children and all families. A second approach would be more intensive and would focus on children who are found to be at high risk of developing obesity. It is likely that this approach would work most effectively in a clinical setting.

General Concepts

The composition of the most healthful diet for the prevention of obesity currently is not known. An appropriate diet for children must have the appropriate calories, nutrients, vitamins, and minerals to support normal growth and development. It is important to remember that slight deviations from caloric balance can result in significant changes in weight when they are continued over time. An excess of only 100 kcal/day will result in an approximate 10-lb weight gain over 1 year. Because it is difficult to count calories, it probably is better to focus on dietary patterns that emphasize more healthful foods. This approach most likely is to be successful if children are not made to feel hungry or deprived. It is likely that children will be more successful in adopting a diet to prevent obesity if the whole family participates in these changes.

The parents' role in preventing obesity is critical. Toddlers and preschoolers tend to regulate the amount of food and drink on their own. Children do not go to fast-food restaurants on their own—they must be taken. Food is not a bribe or a reward naturally. Unfortunately, there are numerous shortcuts available for parents to save time in feeding the family. This often ends up being detrimental to the diet of children. Children most often follow the actions rather than the words of their parents. Parents probably are the most important determinant of their children's eating behaviors. Parents must practice, not just encourage, healthful patterns of eating. This may be the only way to overcome a very powerful and alluring food industry.

There are numerous impediments to physical activity in childhood. Children in the United States average less than 15 minutes of physical activity each day.[4] On a normal school day, children sit down a minimum of 10 hours, including 6.5 hours in school, time riding to and from school, and time spent in front of the television or video games. Of the remaining 14 hours, 8 to 10 are spent asleep. Many children spend as much as 3–7 h/day watching television, playing video games, using the computer, or talking on the telephone.

Many parents point to their child's participation in organized sports as evidence of increased activity. Unfortunately, much inactive time is spent driving to and from these activities. Some of the time during practices is spent standing. Community sports programs often are focused on competitive sports, which may mean only a small proportion of the best athletes benefit. The most important concept is to encourage increased levels and duration of physical activity. Maximizing the time a child spends outside with friends may help to increase the level of activity. Intermittent bursts of intense physical activity actually may be more beneficial than prolonged low-level activity.[59,60] Children should come to see activity as fun rather than as "exercise." A useful concept may be to focus on reduction of inactivity rather than forcing children into exercise regimens. The child's safety may be an important factor in limiting the amount of physical activity.

Parents in the inner city may be afraid for their children to walk to school or play outside. One solution is for parents to participate in activities with children. Another would be for schools to develop after-hours programs that focus on activity in a safe environment. There are other benefits to increased levels of activity. Increased activity may help to promote improved diet by increasing the desire for foods high in carbohydrates rather than those high in fat.[60] Activity also may promote general health and well being. Parents should encourage a minimum of 30 minutes of sustained activity each day as recommended by the Surgeon General.[61]

Psychological factors may be both a determinant and an outcome of obesity. If successful prevention measures are to be implemented, which focus on lifestyle, it will be important to consider how psychological factors are likely to help or hinder such an intervention. Just as families who receive psychological intervention as part of treatment of obesity are more likely to be successful,[50] those who are able to deal with the psychological risk factors for obesity will be more likely to prevent it.

Behavioral approaches recognize that much of what is called lifestyle is based on behavioral issues. The use of behavioral change methods, such as self-management or self-control training or behavioral interventions directed at improving self-esteem have not been tested in a preventive setting. Epstein and colleagues[62] have used behavioral choice theory to target and reinforce overweight children for less sedentary behavior or greater activity. Behavioral choice therapy provides a framework for understanding the choice of behaviors. One way to increase physical activity is to increase the relative reinforcing value of physical activity. This can be accomplished by increasing the reinforcement for physical activity or decreasing the reinforcing value of sedentary activity.[50] One advantage of reinforcing reduction in sedentary activity to increase physical activity is the greater choice associated with this approach compared with approaches that directly reinforce increases in physical activity. Epstein et al[63] found that a group reinforced for less sedentary behavior showed a significantly larger decrease in the percent overweight and maintained their weight loss compared with a group reinforced for greater activity who lost less weight and regained what was lost.[63] There are many questions regarding the use of behavioral therapy in treatment of obesity. There is even less evidence concerning the most effective behavioral approaches in preventing obesity. It is likely that behavioral interventions should begin in childhood. However, many questions remain. Are these behavioral approaches applicable on a large scale outside the clinic setting? How should behavioral strategies be tailored to the developmental stage of the child or adolescent or adult? How should parents be involved in behavioral change for children? Can these behavioral interventions be implemented in schools, churches, community settings, or in the workplace? Future research should be directed at answering these questions.

Two Strategies for Prevention

There are two approaches that may be useful in the prevention of obesity. The first approach targets the population. It is directed at the following question: Why are there so many individuals who are overweight in our society? The second approach focuses on individuals. It is directed at the following questions: Is this person at risk for becoming obese and, if so, what can be done?

The aim of the population strategy is to seek methods to promote favorable shifts in the distribution of adiposity in the population. This approach has as an underlying principle that the population is "ill." It also suggests that the individuals at the tail of the distribution who are identified clinically as sick are just the extreme of a continuum. For example, the Intersalt Study collected information on BMI from 32 countries. It appears that these countries may be grouped and that the distributions for adiposity appear to shift up or down as a whole.[64,65] Even more important is the fact that the population shifts may important consequences for the prevalence of overweight. A downward shift in the mean and variation in skewness may result in a large proportion of the population who were classified as obese, now considered normal weight.[66]

The individual strategy is more clinical in nature. It allows for a more focused intervention and perhaps is better carried out in the context of the health care system. Such selective intervention may be more cost-effective than a population-based approach. However, most medical practices are not focused on prevention, and the resources and strategies for implementation of such an individual approach have not been established. In addition, there is little current evidence that such an approach will be successful.

Population Focus for Prevention

The population approach would have as its goal to lower the average level of adiposity among all children and adults in the United States. This would be accomplished by population-based changes in diet and physical activity. It should be expected that such a population-based approach would only result in a small decrease in the mean BMI. Modest population changes may mean that some individuals have avoided a level of obesity associated with severe metabolic consequence.

A population preventive approach must be multifaceted to be successful. It is likely that a coordinated effort from health professionals, government agencies, schools, the food industry, and the media will be needed.

Health professionals must promote prevention of obesity on a broad scale. They must serve as resources for the community as education and action programs are developed to change diet and physical activity. Nutrition education and counseling on physical activity should be part of ongoing health maintenance.

Government agencies should be involved in planning and implementing preventive strategies. Governmental subsidies should be directed at healthful foods through the school lunch programs and other assistance programs. Government efforts at food labeling should allow people to make informed choices. The government should support initiatives to increase the level of physical activity by supporting attractive, safe places for children, adolescents, and adults to be active.

The school occupies a central place in the lives of virtually all children in our country. During school, children often eat one or two meals each day[67] and spend lots of time in sedentary activity. If schools are committed to improving the bodies as well as the minds of children, then new programs must be implemented to encourage healthful eating patterns and physical activity. This approach has been shown to be successful. Whitaker et al[68] demonstrated that the availability of a low-fat entree at school lunch improved the diet of many students. Given the choice, these students selected low-fat items and the fat content of the average meal dropped from 36% to 30% of calories. Similar approaches to increasing physical activity both during school and after school will need to be evaluated. These may be difficult considerations at a time when the resource base for many schools is decreasing. It will be important to initiate frank discussion about appropriate priorities for schools given limited resources.

The food industry should redouble efforts to produce attractive, good tasting, healthful foods that can help reduce calorie consumption. Foods also should be labeled in a manner that allows informed choices. Finally, food marketing, including fast food, should be targeted to a more healthful diet.

The media must support all of these intervention strategies through news, educational, and entertainment programming. In addition, we must find ways to promote limitation of television watching and video game playing among children and adults. The media may be helpful in this area as well.

The Individual Approach

The individual approach aims to identify individuals who are at high risk of developing obesity and provide them with a targeted intervention. It is likely that the individual approach will be carried out in the context of ongoing health maintenance.

As indicated above, it may be difficult at the present time to identify with high sensitivity and specificity individuals who are destined to become obese prior to the development of obesity. Certainly, children of parents who are overweight will provide some focus. As research progresses, specific genetic markers may provide the basis for identifying individuals who are susceptible to obesity. Other approaches will likely include close follow-up of weight and body composition to evaluate whether children are becoming increasingly overweight compared with their peers. Evaluating the timing of the adiposity rebound may be helpful. It also may be important to focus on individuals who are more likely to have adverse sequelae from their obesity. This may involve better characterization of the distribution of fat. More research is needed in this area.

Once high-risk individuals are identified, intervention strategies should be implemented. Unfortunately, much research has focused on interventions to treat obesity and relatively few studies have been performed to evaluate preventive strategies. The advantage of the individual approach to intervention is that it allows for an individualized program based on interrupting specific pathways that may lead to obesity in a particular patient. It is likely that most interventions to prevent obesity will need to be aimed at families and will need to include a behavioral component. The intervention will be directed at decreasing intake of calories in the diet and expending additional calories by increasing physical activity. However, the successful intervention will have to target the behavioral determinants of diet and physical activity. It probably is optimum for the preventive intervention to begin as early in life as possible before behavioral patterns have become set. Another advantage of the individual approach is that it will allow close monitoring and readjustment of the intervention. The monitoring schedule must be organized to meet the needs of individual families.

The individual approach to prevention of obesity calls for the involvement of a multidisciplinary team of health care providers, including physicians, nurses, nutrition professionals, health educators, exercise specialists, and psychologists. The physician or nurse should be responsible for monitoring and coordination of the intervention. This approach also calls for a systems approach to better organize preventive care. This may include reminder systems, flow sheets, and telephone contact systems to ensure timely identification of appropriate patients and encourage compliance with intervention strategies.

Clearly, one potential difficulty with the individual preventive strategy is its cost. It will be focused on high-risk individuals, which will help, but it likely will be very labor intensive, which will be expensive. It seems likely that the long-term savings will be great if obesity and its attendant morbidity and mortality can be avoided. Nevertheless, an important aspect of the development of preventive approaches should include careful analysis of the costs and benefits. Such analysis will provide important backing for these interventions to be supported by third-party payers and managed care organizations.

Conclusions

Obesity is an important public health problem. The prevalence of obesity is increasing in both children and adults. The sequelae of obesity also appear to be increasing and probably are occurring earlier in life for many.

The treatment of obesity once it has been established is quite difficult. Although some can be successful in losing weight, most regain the weight within 1 year and almost all regain it within 5 years. The pattern of repeated weight gain and loss may result in even greater ultimate weight and may confer additional health risk.

Undoubtedly, the best public health approach is to develop methods to prevent obesity. Unfortunately, much remains to be learned about which preventive strategies are most useful and how to implement them. Much research has focused on how to treat obesity once it has developed. There are fewer data on the prevention of obesity.

It is likely that the prevention of obesity should take two forms, a population approach and an individual approach. The population approach would have as its goal the lowering of the population mean of BMI. This likely would reduce the number of individuals in the obese category. The population approach would involve health care providers, government agencies, schools, the food industry, and the media. It would include better education about healthful diets, labeling of foods, and strategies to promote patterns of diet that will result in lower consumption of calories. It also would include facilitating lifelong regular exercise starting in childhood. One appropriate focus would be to decrease physical inactivity, including television watching and video game playing.

The individual approach would target individuals at high risk of developing obesity. Unfortunately, at present it is difficult to identify such people with high sensitivity and specificity prior to the development of obesity. It will be important for research to focus on this question. It is possible that genetic studies will help to identify susceptible individuals. It is likely that the individual approach will work best if it is started early in life and involves the entire family. An advantage is that such strategies can be tailored for individual needs. However, at present effective strategies to prevent the development of obesity are not known. It is likely that they will include a behavioral component, but research in this area clearly is needed. The individual approach may be more costly and will need to be evaluated from a cost-effectiveness standpoint.

Given the public health importance of obesity and the widespread concern about it, this country should take on the challenge of preventing obesity. This effort is likely to involve commitment of substantial resources, but it is likely to be money well spent. This may be the only method for reversing the disturbing trend of increasing obesity, which, if unimpeded, may reverse the improvement in cardiovascular disease morbidity and mortality that has been a major triumph of public health in this century.

References

1. Kuczmarski RJ, Flegal KM, Campbell SM, et al. Increasing prevalence of overweight among US adults. The National Health and Nutrition Examination Surveys, 1960 to 1991 [see comments]. *JAMA* 1994;272:205–211.
2. Piscatella JC. *Fat-Proof Your Child*. New York: Workman Publishing, 1997.
3. Anonymous. Long-term pharmacotherapy in the management of obesity. National Task Force on the Prevention and Treatment of Obesity [see comments]. *JAMA* 1996;276:1907–1915.
4. Roberts WC. Floating in fat: Fat kids and fat adults. *Am J Cardiol* 1997;80: 1117–1119. Editorial.
5. Pi-Sunyer FX. Health implications of obesity. *Am J Clin Nutr* 1991;53: 1595S–1603S.
6. Department of Health Education and Welfare (DHEW). Report of the National Commission on Diabetes to the Congress of the United States. The long-range plan to combat diabetes. Washington, DC: DHEW; 1976:97. Publication NIH 76–1018.
7. Knowler WC, Pettitt DJ, Savage PJ, et al. Diabetes incidence in Pima Indians: Contributions of obesity and parental diabetes. *Am J Epidemiol* 1981;113:144–156.
8. Kissebah AH, Freedman DS, Peiris AN. Health risks of obesity. *Med Clin North Am* 1989;73:111–138.
9. Despres JP. Dyslipidaemia and obesity. *Baillieres Clin Endocrinol Metab* 1994;8:629–660.
10. Van Itallie TB. Health implications of overweight and obesity in the United States. *Ann Intern Med* 1985;103:983–988.
11. Daniels SR, Loggie JM, Khoury P, et al. Left ventricular geometry and severe left ventricular hypertrophy in children and adolescents with essential hypertension [see comments]. *Circulation* 1998;97:1907–1911.

12. Kinugasa A, Tsunamoto K, Furukawa N, et al. Fatty liver and its fibrous changes found in simple obesity of children. *J Pediatr Gastroenterol Nutr* 1984;3:408–414.
13. Bernstein RA, Giefer EE, Vieira JJ, et al. Gallbladder disease, II: Utilization of the life table method in obtaining clinically useful information. A study of 62 739 weight-conscious women. *J Chronic Dis* 1977;30:529–541.
14. Crichlow RW, Seltzer MH, Jannetta PJ. Cholecystitis in adolescents. *Am J Dig Dis* 1972;17:68–72.
15. Dietz WH. Health consequences of obesity in youth: Childhood predictors of adult disease. *Pediatrics* 1998;101:518–525.
16. Mallory GB Jr, Fiser DH, Jackson R. Sleep-associated breathing disorders in morbidly obese children and adolescents. *J Pediatr* 1989;115:892–897.
17. Sharp JT, Barrocas M, Chokroverty S. The cardiorespiratory effects of obesity. *Clin Chest Med* 1980;1:103–118.
18. Douglas FG, Chong PY. Influence of obesity on peripheral airways patency. *J Appl Physiol* 1972;33:559–563.
19. Kelsey JL, Acheson RM, Keggi KJ. The body build of patients with slipped capital femoral epiphysis. *Am J Dis Child* 1972;124:276–281.
20. Bray GA. Complications of obesity. *Ann Intern Med* 1985;103:1052–1062.
21. Rimm AA, Werner LH, Yserloo BV, et al. Relationship of obesity and disease in 73 532 weight-conscious women. *Public Health Rep* 1975;90:44–54.
22. Gortmaker SL, Must A, Perrin JM, et al. Social and economic consequences of overweight in adolescence and young adulthood [see comments]. *N Engl J Med* 1993;329:1008–1012.
23. Dietz WH Jr. Childhood obesity: Susceptibility, cause, and management. *J Pediatr* 1983;103:676–686.
24. Garn SM. Continuities and changes in fatness from infancy through adulthood. *Curr Probl Pediatr* 1985;15:1–47.
25. Ginsberg-Fellner F, Jagendorf LA, Carmel H, et al. Overweight and obesity in preschool children in New York City. *Am J Clin Nutr* 1981;34:2236–2241.
26. Goldblatt PB, Moore ME, Stunkard AJ. Social factors in obesity. *JAMA* 1965;192:1039–1044.
27. Bray GA, Gray DS Obesity, Part I: Pathogenesis. *West J Med* 1988;149:429–441.
28. Bray GA. Obesity: Definition, diagnosis and disadvantages. *Med J Aust* 1985;142:S2—S8.
29. Kluthe R, Schubert A. Obesity in Europe. *Ann Intern Med* 1985;103:1037–1042.
30. Baecke JA, van Staveren WA, Burema J. Food consumption, habitual physical activity, and body fatness in young Dutch adults. *Am J Clin Nutr* 1983;37:278–286.
31. Dietz WH. Obesity in infants, children and adolescents in the United States. I. Identification, natural history and aftereffects. *Nutr Res* 1981;1:117–137.
32. Dietz WH, Gortmaker SL, Sobol SM. Trends in the prevalence of childhood and adolescent obesity in the United States. *Pediatr Res* 1985;19:198A.
33. Bray GA. *The Obese Patient*. Philadelphia, PA: WB Saunders; 1976.
34. Kannel WB, Gordon T. Physiological and medial concomitants of obesity: The Framingham Study. In: Bray GA, ed. *Obesity in America*. Washington, DC: Department of Health, Education and Welfare; 1979. Publication NIH 79–359.

35. Harlan WR, Landis JR, Flegal KM, et al. Secular trends in body mass in the United States, 1960–1980 [see comments]; *Am J Epidemiol* 1988:128:1065–74.
36. Gortmaker SL, Dietz WH Jr, Sobol AM, et al. Increasing pediatric obesity in the United States. *Am J Dis Child* 1987;141:535–540.
37. Webber LS, Harsha DW, Nicklas TA, et al. Secular trends in obesity in children. In: Filer LJ, Lauer RM, Luepker RV, eds. *Prevention of Atherosclerosis and Hypertension Beginning in Youth*. Philadelphia, PA: Lea & Febiger;; 1994:194–203.
38. Morrison JA, James FW, Sprecher DL, et al. Sex and race differences in trends in cardiovascular disease risk factors in school children: The Princeton School Study 1975–1990. *Am J Public Health*. In press.
39. Pinhas-Hamiel O, Dolan LM, Daniels SR, et al. Increased incidence of non-insulin-dependent diabetes mellitus among adolescents. *J Pediatr* 1996; 128:608–615.
40. Eating Disorders and Obesity: A Comprehensive Handbook. New York: Guilford Press, 1995.
41. Anonymous. Methods for voluntary weight loss and control. NIH Technology Assessment Conference Panel. Consensus Development Conference, 30 March to 1 April 1992. *Ann Intern Med* 1993;119:764–770.
42. The painful business of losing weight. *The Economist* 1997;August:45–47.
43. Liddle RA, Goldstein RB, Saxton J. Gallstone formation during weight-reduction dieting. *Arch Intern Med* 1989;149:1750–1753.
44. Hamm P, Shekelle RB, Stamler J. Large fluctuations in body weight during young adulthood and twenty-five-year risk of coronary death in men. *Am J Epidemiol* 1989;129:312–318.
45. Johnson D, Drenick EJ. Therapeutic fasting in morbid obesity. *Arch Intern Med* 1977;137:1381–1382.
46. Rosenbaum M, Leibel RL, Hirsch J. Obesity. *N Engl J Med* 1997;337:396–407.
47. Weintraub M. Long-term weight control study: Conclusions. *Clin Pharmacol Ther* 1992;51:642–646.
48. Abenhaim L, Moride Y, Brenot F, et al. Appetite-suppressant drugs and the risk of primary pulmonary hypertension. International Primary Pulmonary Hypertension Study Group [see comments]. *N Engl J Med* 1996; 335:609–616.
49. Connolly HM, Crary JL, McGoon MD, et al. Valvular heart disease associated with fenfluramine-phentermine [see comments; published erratum *N Engl J Med* 1783]. *N Engl J Med* 1997;337:581–588.
50. Epstein LH, Myers MD, Raynor HA, et al. Treatment of pediatric obesity. *Pediatrics* 1998;101:554–570.
51. Whitaker RC, Wright JA, Pepe MS, et al. Predicting obesity in young adulthood from childhood and parental obesity. *N Engl J Med* 1997;337: 869–873.
52. Vohr BR, Lipsitt LP, Oh W. Somatic growth of children of diabetic mothers with reference to birth size. *J Pediatr* 1980;97:196–199.
53. Pettitt DJ, Baird HR, Aleck KA, et al. Excessive obesity in offspring of Pima Indian women with diabetes during pregnancy. *N Engl J Med* 1983;308: 242–245.
54. Whitaker RC, Pepe MS, Seidel KD, et al. Gestational diabetes and the risk of offspring obesity. *Pediatrics* 1998;101:E9.

55. Rolland-Cachera MF, Deheeger M, Bellisle F, et al. Adiposity rebound in children: A simple indicator for predicting obesity. *Am J Clin Nutr.* 1984; 39:129–135.

56. Siervogel RM, Roche AF, Guo SM, et al. Patterns of change in weight/ stature2 from 2 to 18 years: Findings from long-term serial data for children in the Fels longitudinal growth study [see comments]. *Int J Obes* 1991;15:479–485.

57. Rolland-Cachera MF, Deheeger M, Guilloud-Bataille M, et al. Tracking the development of adiposity from one month of age to adulthood. *Ann Hum Biol* 1987;14:219–229.

58. Whitaker RC, Pepe MS, Wright JA, et al. Early adiposity rebound and the risk of adult obesity. *Pediatrics* 1998;101:E5.

59. Tremblay A, Simoneau JA, Bouchard C. Impact of exercise intensity on body fatness and skeletal muscle metabolism. *Metabolism* 1994;43:814–818.

60. Tremblay A, Buemann B. Exercise-training, macronutrient balance and body weight control. *Int J Obes Relat Metab Disord.* 1995;19:79–86.

61. US Department of Health and Human Services. Physical activity and health: A report of the Surgeon General. Atlanta, GA: Centers for Disease Control and Prevention, National Center for Chronic Disease Prevention and Health Promotion; 1996.

62. Epstein LH. Application of behavioral economic principles to treatment of childhood obesity. In: Allison DB, Pi-Sunyer FX, eds. *Obesity Treatment: Establishing Goals, Improving Outcomes and Reviewing the Research Agenda.* New York: Plenum Press; 1995:113–119.

63. Epstein LH, Valoski AM, Vara LS, et al. Effects of decreasing sedentary behavior and increasing activity on weight change in obese children. *Health Psychol* 1995;14:109–115.

64. Anonymous. INTERSALT Study an international co-operative study on the relation of blood pressure to electrolyte excretion in populations. I. Design and methods. The INTERSALT Co-operative Research Group. *J Hypertens* 1986;4:781–787.

65. Rose G. *Strategies of Prevention: The Individual and the Population in Coronary Heart Disease Epidemiology from Aeteology to Public Health.* Oxford: Oxford University Press; 1992.

66. Law MR, Frost CD, Wald NJ. By how much does dietary salt reduction lower blood pressure? III: Analysis of data from trials of salt reduction [published erratum *BMJ* 939]. *BMJ* 1991;302:819–824.

67. Whitaker RC, Wright JA, Finch AJ, et al. School lunch: A comparison of the fat and cholesterol content with dietary guidelines. *J Pediatr* 1993;123:857–862.

68. Whitaker RC, Wright JA, Finch AJ, et al. An environmental intervention to reduce dietary fat in school lunches. *Pediatrics* 1993;91:1107–1111.

Part 2

Pathophysiology
of Obesity

Chapter 6

Obesity-Related Genes

Ronald M. Krauss, MD

Introduction

Advances in identifying genes contributing to regulation of body weight are of importance in understanding pathophysiological mechanisms and in developing improved therapies for obesity and its complications. The genetic contribution to obesity in most humans is caused by effects of genes that create susceptibility to increased body weight by interacting with diet and other environmental factors and with each other. Candidates for such obesity susceptibility genes can be selected by several approaches. First, a gene may be identified because a mutation in the gene influences obesity in a mendelian manner in humans or in an animal model, most commonly a rodent. Second, functional candidate genes may be examined because their products are suspected of being involved in the pathogenesis of obesity. Finally, there are positional candidate genes that are targeted primarily by association or linkage of a given obesity-related trait to a chromosomal locus.

Single Gene Models of Obesity

Currently, there are five single gene mouse models of obesity, and causative genes have been identified for each.[1] These models and genes are summarized in Table 1. The gene mutation that to date has had the greatest impact on our understanding of the pathophysiology of body weight regulation is that responsible for obesity in the ob mouse strain.[2] The ob gene product, designated leptin, is a cytokine-like protein secreted by adipocytes with multiple actions (see Figure 1). Effects on the central nervous system result in decreased energy intake

From: Fletcher GF, Grundy SM, Hayman LL (eds). *Obesity: Impact on Cardiovascular Disease.* Armonk, NY: Futura Publishing Co., Inc.; © 1999.

Table 1

Single Gene Mouse Models of Obesity

Mouse mutation	Human		Evidence from:	
	Chromosome	Gene product	Association	Linkage
Obese (ob)	7q31.1	Leptin	Yes	Yes
Diabetes (db)	1p31	Leptin receptor	Yes	NA
Agouti yel (Ay)	20q11.2	Agouti signaling protein	NA	ASIP
Fat (fa)	4q32	Carboxypeptidase E	NA	No
Tubby (tub)	11p15.5	Phosphodiasterase	NA	No

NA, information not available; ASIP, agouti signaling protein.

and increased energy expenditure. In addition, there are hormonal effects including increased production of gonadotropins. In adipose tissue, leptin has autocrine effects that include a decrease in fatty acid and triglyceride synthesis, as well as suppression of its own expression. Decreased fatty acid synthase is observed in both adipose tissue and skeletal muscle. In muscle there also is stimulation of free fatty

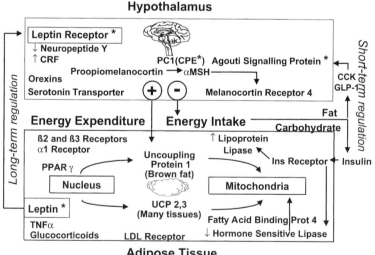

Figure 1.   Schematic representation of selected candidate gene products involved in the regulation of body fat and energy balance in the brain and adipose tissue. * Gene products shown to be affected by mutations in single gene mouse models of obesity (Table 1).

acid oxidation and levels of uncoupling protein. Finally, leptin has been found to suppress insulin release by pancreatic β-cells.

Two severely obese children, cousins in a consanguineous pedigree, have been found to have near-absence of leptin due to a homozygous leptin gene frame-shift mutation leading to a premature stop codon. However, in most obese humans increased leptin gene expression and plasma leptin levels have been observed, suggesting resistance to leptin action. Nevertheless, as described below, some studies have indicated linkage of the leptin gene locus to obesity in humans.

Earlier studies in the db mouse strain indicated that its defect was in responsiveness to the ob gene product. This has been documented with the identification of the leptin receptor and the finding of a splice defect in db mice resulting in loss of a signal region required for leptin receptor expression. A different mutation in the leptin receptor gene (proline for glutamine at residue 269) has been shown to be responsible for obesity in the Zucker fatty rat. This defect is associated with decreased leptin receptor expression and with markedly increased plasma leptin levels. There has been a recent report of a single case of severe obesity in a child with a mutant leptin receptor. In Pima Indians, three leptin receptor gene variants have been associated with obesity, but genetic linkage studies in humans have been negative.

Studies of a third mouse model of obesity, agouti yellow, led to the identification of an endogenous antagonist of melanocortin receptors [designated agouti signaling protein (ASIP)] that normally is expressed in the skin, where it results in yellow coat color. When expressed ectopically in the brain, it can antagonize the melanocortin 4 receptor, which is felt to block the anorexic action of α-melanocyte–stimulating hormone, resulting in the obese agouti yellow phenotype. An agouti-related protein, which has sequence homology with ASIP, also blocks melanocortin receptors and can result in obesity when expressed in transgenic mice.

Causative genes have been identified in two other mouse models. In the Fat strain, there is a mutation in carboxypeptidase E. It has been suggested but not documented that such a mutation may result in altered central nervous system processing of proopiomelanocortin or its products (Figure 1). The phosphodiesterase mutation responsible for Tubby has not been associated with a specific pathophysiologic effect yet. Neither of these two genes has been associated with obesity in humans, although severe obesity has been found in a compound heterozygote for mutations in the prohormone convertase 1 gene.

Prohormone convertase 1 acts proximally to carboxypeptidase E in the posttranslational processing of prohormones and neuropeptides, and thus this syndrome may be homologous to the Fat mouse phenotype. In addition, hypothalamic attenuation of the related prohormone convertase 2 gene has been found in two of seven patients with Prader-Willi syndrome, a Mendelian disorder associated with childhood obesity.[3] Although chromosomal sites have been identified for other Mendelian syndromes causing obesity in humans (eg, Ahlstrom, Bardet Biedl, and Cohen), causative genes have not been identified.[4]

Functional Candidate Genes

Searches for additional genes involved in human obesity have involved studies of association and linkage with candidate genetic loci. Association studies test for co-occurrence of an allele at a genetic locus with a trait in a population of unrelated individuals. Linkage studies test for cosegregation of an allele at a genetic locus with a trait in families. Candidate genes for association and linkage studies can be common polymorphisms or specific mutations. Alternatively, as described in the next section, linkage can be sought with anonymous polymorphic markers in a genomewide scan.

Functional Candidate Genes for Body Fat

Figure 1 presents a scheme for the involvement of a number of candidate gene products in the pathophysiology of obesity derived from studies in animal models and humans. In addition to the genes described above that are responsible for single gene obesity disorders in animal models and humans, there are a number of other candidate gene products for which there is evidence of involvement in regulation of body weight in animal models,[1,5] including those involving transgenic and gene knockout manipulations.[6] These include hypothalamic molecules that can act as signals for reduced food intake and adiposity (eg, corticotropin-releasing hormone, α-melanocyte–stimulating hormone, cholecystokinin, glucagonlike peptide-1, serotonin, neurotensin, and bombesin) and others that mediate increased food intake and adiposity (eg, neuropeptide Y, melanin concentrating hormone, orexins A and B, galanin, β-endorphin, dynorphin, norepinephrine, and growth hormone–releasing hormone). Recently, a mutant allele of the PPARλ2 gene has been found in 4 of 121 obese patients screened for mutations in this gene.[7] PPARλ is a member of a family of nuclear receptors, activated by fatty acid derivatives and other agents that can stimulate adipocyte differentiation from progenitor cells. Interestingly, mice with targeted inactivation of PPARα, a related receptor expressed primarily in liver, develop hypertriglyceridemia, hepatic steatosis, and delayed onset of obesity that is greater in females than males.[8]

Studies in humans have identified suggestive linkages of body fat variables with several candidate genes. Particularly strong linkages have been observed for leptin, tumor necrosis factor-α (TNF-α) and melanocortin receptors 3 and 5[4] (Table 2). Additionally, evidence for linkage or association has been reported for cholecystokinin, insulin, insulinlike growth factor 2, sulfonylurea receptor, glucocorticoid receptor, and intestinal fatty acid binding protein.

Finally, variants of both the apoB gene and the low-density lipoprotein (LDL) receptor have been associated with body fat and obesity, respectively (the latter in hypertensives), suggesting further that plasma lipid and lipoprotein transport may have a connection with pathways regulating adiposity.

Functional Candidate Genes for Energy Expenditure

Although a large number of proteins are of importance in regulating energy expenditure, including some of those described above, recent attention in humans has focused primarily on mitochondrial uncoupling proteins (UCPs) and adrenergic receptors. UCPs are proton transporters expressed in peripheral tissues that when activated can cause increased thermogenesis. UCP-1, the first of these proteins to be identified, is expressed in brown fat, a tissue found in very low levels in humans. Recently, however, UCP-2 and UCP-3 have been identified in other tissues including white adipose tissue and skeletal

Table 2
Genetic Loci with the Strongest Evidence for Linkage to Obesity in Humans

Chromosome	Locus/gene	Population
1p32-p22	D1S200 or LEPR	Quebec Family Study
2p21	D2S1788	San Antonio Heart Study
3p24.2-p22	D32432	Pima Indians
6p21.2	Tnfir 24 or TNFα	Pima Indians
7q31.3	D7S495 or LEP	Several studies
11q13	D11S911: UCP-2 or -3	Quebec Family Study
11q21-q22	D11S2000 to 2366	Pima Indians
18p11.2	MC5R	Quebec Family Study
20q12-q13.3	ASIP or MC3R	Quebec Family Study

muscle. A marker in the region of the UCP-2/UCP-3 genes has been found to be linked strongly to resting metabolic rate but not to adiposity. A large number of studies have addressed the possible association of obesity with variants of adrenergic receptors that may modulate storage and release of fatty acids by adipose tissue. While the β3-adrenergic receptor gene has attracted much interest in this regard, results of association and linkage studies involving this gene have been inconsistent.[9]

Recently, a protein polymorphism of the β2-adrenergic receptor has been associated with obesity in humans. Interestingly, a genetic marker on human chromosome 20q near the locus for adenosine deaminase, an α1-adrenergic agonist, has been linked to both body fat and insulin in humans, and as described below, a syntenic region in mice has been linked to body weight.[10] Finally, NaK–ATPase-α2 and -β have been associated with both respiratory quotient and percent body fat.

Genomewide Searches for Genes Linked to Obesity and Body Weight

Humans

Major genomewide linkage studies for obesity genes have been performed in three large studies to date. In the San Antonio Family Heart Study, involving 458 Mexican Americans from 10 pedigrees, a scan with 191 markers revealed the strongest linkage for body weight–related traits to a locus on chromosome 2p21.[11] This site showed particularly strong linkage to both serum leptin and fat mass.

In a group of 874 Pima Indians, a genomewide scan with more than 600 markers identified suggestive linkage [log10 of the odds ratio (LOD) scores × 2] of percent body fat to loci on chromosomes 11q and 3p24.[12] As with the chromosome 2 locus cited above, no specific candidate genes in these regions have been shown to contribute to the observed linkages.

Finally, in the Quebec Family Study, a study involving primarily French Canadians, two nearby markers on chromosome 1p, have been linked with body mass index (BMI), fat mass, and sum of skin folds.[9] These findings are of potential interest in light of the fact that this region is syntenic with the mouse db (leptin receptor) gene and as described below with the dietary obese 1 quantitative trait locus (QTL) in mice. A summary of the chromosomal loci with the strongest evidence of linkage to adiposity variables in humans is given in Table 2.

Mice

Numerous QTLs have been reported for indices of body fat and obesity in polygenic animal models, principally mice.[4] The large number of different obesity QTLs that have been described in mice and the relatively small effects contributed by individual loci suggests considerable genetic complexity. Moreover, there likely is to be considerable interaction among individual loci that may influence adiposity and body fat distribution through different mechanisms. In a multigenic obesity model,[13] four loci (on mouse chromosomes 6, 7, 12, and 15) that exhibited linkage with body fat or with the weights of four different fat depots differed with respect to their effects on the percent of body fat, specific fat depots, and plasma lipoproteins. A locus for hepatic lipase activity on chromosome 7 was coincident with loci affecting body fat and total cholesterol loci, providing a possible mechanism linking plasma lipoproteins and obesity. Notably, these four loci exhibited allele-specific, nonadditive interactions, indicating the value of inbred mice strains (as well as genetically manipulated animals) in investigating gene-gene interactions that likely are to contribute to common obesity phenotypes in animal models and in humans.

Mouse models also have been shown to be useful in identifying genes whose effects on adiposity are dependent on diet and for investigating diet-gene interactions in the pathogenesis of obesity. QTLs for diet-responsive obesity have been identified on mouse chromosomes 4, 9, and 15 in a cross between AKR/J (diet fat responsive) and SWR/J (resistant) mice.[14,15] Recently, an intercross between inbred mouse strains C57BL/6J (diet fat responsive) and CAST/Ei (lean and diet resistant) revealed highly significant linkage with loci on chromosomes 9 and 2 (three separate loci) that contribute to fat-pad mass for mice on a high-fat diet.[16] Two chromosomal 2 loci for body fat and lipoprotein levels coincided with a locus having strong effects on hepatic lipase activity, again suggesting an association of this enzyme with mechanisms affecting both adiposity and lipoprotein metabolism.

As described above, at least two of the following adiposity QTLs in mice appear to be syntenic to regions with loci linked to body fat variables in humans: (1) the dietary obese 1 QTL on mouse chromosome 4[15] is syntenic to the human chromosome 1p region linked to BMI, fat mass, and sum of skin fold[9] and (2) the multigenic obese 5 QTL on mouse chromosome 2 is syntenic to the region on human chromosome 20q linked to body fat.[10] Although these concordant linkage findings in humans and mice have not been shown to involve the same genes and could be caused by chance, they nevertheless indicate the potential value of a cross-species approach that could focus the search for genes of biological importance in the regulation of body fat and energy balance.

Acknowledgments: Claude Bouchard, Aldons Lusis, and David West are thanked for their helpful contributions to the preparation of this paper.

References

1. Campfield LA, Smith FJ, Burn P. Strategies and potential molecular targets for obesity treatment. *Science* 1998;280:1383–1387.
2. Campfield LA, Smith FJ, Burn P. The OB protein (leptin) pathway: A link between adipose tissue mass and central neural networks. *Horm Metab Res* 1996;28:619–632.
3. Gabreels BA, Swaab DF, de Kleijn DP, et al. Attenuation of the polypeptide 7B2, prohormone convertase PC2, and vasopressin in the hypothalamus of some Prader-Willi patients: Indications for a processing defect. *J Clin Endocrinol Metab* 1998;83:591–599.
4. Chagnon YC, Perusse L, Bouchard C. The human obesity gene map: The 1997 update. *Obes Res* 1998;6:76–92.
5. Woods SC, Seeley RJ, Porte D Jr, et al. Signals that regulate food intake and energy homeostasis. *Science* 1998;280:1378–1383.
6. Bray G, Bouchard C. Genetics of human obesity: Research directions. *FASEB J* 1997;11:937–945.
7. Ristow M, Muller-Wieland D, Pfeiffer A, et al. Obesity associated with a mutation in a genetic regulator of adipocyte differentiation. *N Engl J Med* 1998;339:953–959.
8. Costet P, Legendre C, More J, et al. Peroxisome proliferator-activated receptor alpha-isoform deficiency leads to progressive dyslipidemia with sexually dimorphic obesity and steatosis. *J Biol Chem* 1998;273:29577–29585.
9. Chagnon YC, Perusse L, Lamothe M, et al. Suggestive linkages between markers on human 1p32–p22 and body fat and insulin levels in the Quebec Family Study. *Obes Res* 1997;5:115–121.
10. Lembertas AV, Perusse L, Chagnon YC, et al. Identification of an obesity quantitative trait locus on mouse chromosome 2 and evidence of linkage to body fat and insulin on the human homologous region 20q. *J Clin Invest* 1997;100:1240–1247.
11. Comuzzie AG, Hixson JE, Almasy L, et al. A major quantitative trait locus determining serum leptin levels and fat mass is located on human chromosome 2. *Nat Genet* 1997;15:273–276.
12. Norman RA, Thompson DB, Foroud T, et al. Genomewide search for genes influencing percent body fat in Pima Indians: Suggestive linkage at chromosome 11q21–q22. Pima Diabetes Gene Group. *Am J Hum Genet* 1997;60:166–173.
13. Warden CH, Fisler JS, Shoemaker SM, et al. Identification of four chromosomal loci determining obesity in a multifactorial mouse model. *J Clin Invest* 1995;95:1545–1552.

14. West DB, Goudey-Lefevre J, York B, et al. Dietary obesity linked to genetic loci on chromosomes 9 and 15 in a polygenic mouse model. *J Clin Invest* 1994;94:1410–1416.
15. West DB, Waguespack J, York B, et al. Genetics of dietary obesity in AKR/J × SWR/J mice: Segregation of the trait and identification of a linked locus on chromosome 4. *Mamm Genome* 1994;5:546–552.
16. Mehrabian M, Wen PZ, Fisler J, et al. Genetic loci controlling body fat, lipoprotein metabolism, and insulin levels in a multifactorial mouse model. *J Clin Invest* 1998;101:2485–2496.

Chapter 7

Diet Drugs and Valvular Heart Disease

Gerard P. Aurigemma, MD

Introduction

Fenfluramine and dexfenfluramine, alone or in combination with phentermine, are appetite suppressants that have come into widespread use. It has been estimated that 1.2–4.7 million persons in the United States have been exposed to these drugs.[1] The use of the combinations of these medications has been stimulated partly by the work of Weintraub and coworkers[2] who showed that the combination of these medications permitted use of lower doses of individual agents and resulted in sustained weight loss. In early 1997, investigators at the Mayo Clinic became aware of an association between valvular heart disease and use of the combination of fenfluramine/phentermine. Much concern was generated by the subsequent publication of a series of 24 individuals with severe valvular disease and diet-drug usage[3] as well as data appearing on the World Wide Web, which suggested that the prevalence of valvular disease linked to these drugs approximated 30%.[1] The purpose of this chapter is to review the association between diet drugs and valvular heart disease.

Initial Description of Diet Drug Valvulopathy

In July 1997, researchers at the Mayo Clinic reported 24 cases of valvular heart disease in women who were given the combination of fenfluramine and phentermine.[3] These patients were treated for a mean duration of 12.3 months (range, 1–28 months). Twenty of the 24 patients had cardiovascular symptoms, and four had only a new heart

From: Fletcher GF, Grundy SM, Hayman LL (eds). *Obesity: Impact on Cardiovascular Disease.* Armonk, NY: Futura Publishing Co., Inc.; © 1999.

murmur. Both left- and right-sided valvular lesions were observed; either the mitral valve or the aortic valve was involved in all of the cases, and two or more valves were affected in 71% of the cases. The echocardiographic features of the valvulopathy included thickening and diastolic doming of the anterior mitral valve leaflet, thickening of the subvalvular apparatus, and tethering of the posterior leaflet. Both mitral and aortic regurgitation appeared to be the result of malcoaptation of the leaflets.

The histopathological features were similar to those seen in carcinoid valvular disease,[4] which usually affects the tricuspid and pulmonic valves, as well as what has been described in ergot alkaloid-induced valvular disease.[5] However, carcinoid heart disease usually affects right-sided heart valves and mitral and aortic valve involvement is distinctly unusual.[4] Connolly and coworkers[3] hypothesized that high-circulating levels of serotonin were related to the valvulopathy. In carcinoid heart disease, serum, blood, and platelet levels of serotonin have been shown to be elevated, and there are high-urine levels of serotonin metabolites.[4] However, to date, there is no evidence that serotonin levels are increased in patients with diet-drug valvulopathy.

The study, which represented the initial report identifying a link between diet drugs and valvulopathy, was a detailed series of case reports and did not address the issue of incidence or prevalence of valvulopathy, and the study was observational.

Prevalence of Diet-Drug Valvulopathy: Initial Estimates and Control Data

In September of 1997 data were made available on the World Wide Web by the Food and Drug Administration (FDA); these data apparently informed the FDA decision to seek withdrawal of fenfluramine and dexfenfluramine from the US market.[1] These data are taken from echocardiographic reports from five independent echocardiographic prevalence surveys of patients who had received dexfenfluramine or fenfluramine alone or in combination with phentermine. The criteria used by the FDA to classify subjects as having valvulopathy were based on estimates of valvular regurgitation in the healthy adults undergoing echocardiography in the Coronary Artery Risk Development in Young Adults (CARDIA) study[6] (Table 1). In this study of 4352 healthy adults aged 23 to 35 years, the prevalence of mitral regurgitation was 10.9% and was judged to be mild in 93.0%; the corresponding prevalence of aortic regurgitation was 1.2% (mild in 79.0%). It is important to note that very little published data exist

Table 1

Prevalence of Valvular Regurgitation by Color Flow Doppler in Normal Subjects

Author	N	Age (y)	AR	MR	TR
Reid[6]	4352	23–35	1.2%	10.9%	—
			79% mild	93% mild	
Singh[9]	3529	55 ± 10	10.5%	87%	76%
Klein[7]	61	20–49	0	39%	57%
	57	50–82	23%	58%	74%
			38% mild	64% mild	76% mild

AR, aortic regurgitation; MR, mitral regurgitation; TR, trivial regurgitation.

concerning the prevalence of Doppler abnormalities in obese subjects (see below). The FDA criteria for valvulopathy were greater than or equal to mild aortic regurgitation or greater than or equal to moderate mitral regurgitation. According to the FDA summary, the prevalence of patients with valvulopathy was 31.7% (range, 26.2% to 37.6%). The percentage of patients in these surveys with symptoms or signs of valvular disease accompanying echocardiographic abnormalities has not been made available. Because the data have not been published in a peer review journal, details concerning the grading scheme used by the investigators are not yet available.

The 31.7% prevalence of significant valvular regurgitation by the FDA criteria is considerably higher than what is expected in the general population. Although trivial (and likely clinically insignificant), valvular regurgitation by color flow Doppler is common; greater degrees are less common, particularly in subjects who are under 50 years of age. In the study of Klein and colleagues,[7] 61 normal volunteers aged 20 to 49 years were examined; mitral regurgitation graded as "trivial" was found in all subjects, but "mild" regurgitation was not encountered in any subject. No normal subject had any degree of aortic regurgitation. In the group of 61 normal subjects aged 50 to 82 years who were studied by the same authors, trivial degrees of regurgitation were much more common (64% for the mitral and 38% for the aortic valve) and mild regurgitation also was common (36% for mitral and 62% for aortic).[7] No normal subject was found to have regurgitation in excess of the "mild" grade.

More relevant to the present discussion are the preliminary data of Singh and coworkers[8] who examined the prevalence of valvular regurgitation in subjects in the Framingham Study; these subjects were free of prevalent cardiovascular disease. The mean age for the men in the series was 55 ± 10 and 54 ± 10 for women. As Table 1 shows, the prevalence of valvular regurgitation was high, particularly for the mitral and tricuspid valves. Aortic regurgitation, while not uncommon, was much less prevalent than regurgitation of other valves. Singh and coworkers[9] subsequently have examined the prevalence of valvular regurgitation by quintiles of body mass index (BMI) and have not found a correlation between prevalence of regurgitation and BMI.

Thus valvular regurgitation by the color Doppler technique is common and increases in prevalence with age. Most regurgitation detected by color Doppler is trivial or mild. Preliminary data does not suggest increasing prevalence of valvular regurgitation in obese individuals with no history of heart disease.

As noted above, the FDA data generated considerable response. By the fall of 1997 there was increasing concern regarding the prevalence of valvulopathy in subjects treated with these diet medications. It was unclear regarding subjects who should undergo echocardiography. Recent guidelines published by the American College of Cardiology/American Heart Association (AHA) Task Force on Echocardiography, a consensus panel, emphasizes that echocardiography is indicated in a patient with a heart murmur and cardiorespiratory symptoms or someone without symptoms who has a murmur if the clinical features indicate a moderate probability of cardiovascular disease.[10] However, according to the initial report,[1] murmurs were heard in only 17% of patients with valvular regurgitation meeting the FDA criteria for valvulopathy. This consideration led to the interim recommendation that individuals receive an antibiotic before undergoing dental or surgical procedures likely to introduce certain bacteria into the bloodstream[11] or to postpone elective procedures until the risk of endocarditis can be ascertained by examination or by echocardiography. For emergency procedures that must be performed before a cardiac evaluation is completed, it was recommended that empiric antibiotic prophylaxis should be administered according to AHA guidelines.[11]

More Recent Data

Two preliminary reports suggest that the FDA data overstated the prevalence of valvulopathy. Weissman and coworkers[12] recently reported data that suggests a much lower prevalence of valvular regurgitation in some patients treated with dexfenfluramine. These investigators reviewed echocardiograms on 1072 individuals who took part in a study of efficacy of dexfenfluramine as monotherapy. Subjects were randomized to either dexfenfluramine, sustained-release dexfenfluramine, or placebo. The average length of treatment was approximately 77 days. This efficacy study was halted prematurely in the fall of 1997 because of safety concerns, and subjects were offered echocardiograms to evaluate possible valvulopathy. These echocardiograms were performed at an average time of 33 days following cessation of treatment.

The incidence of significant mitral regurgitation (FDA criteria) was 1.7%–1.8% in the treatment groups and 1.3% in the placebo group ($P = 0.86$). For aortic regurgitation, the corresponding incidences were 5%–5.8% in the treatment groups and 3.6% in the placebo group ($P = 0.43$). Finally, multiple, significant valvular lesions were found in 6.5% in the immediate release group, 7.3% in sustained release, and 4.5% in placebo ($P = 0.3$). The odds ratios for combined valvular regurgitation for the treatment groups were 1.5 [95% confidence interval (CI) 0.7–3.0] and 1.7 (0.7–3.0) for immediate release and sustained release dexfenfluramine, respectively. However, there was a significant difference in posterior mitral valve leaflet abnormality, found in 1.5%–2.0% of active treatment subjects and 0.3% of placebo-treated subjects ($P = 0.045$ for the three-way comparison).

These results offer some reassurance, because they suggest that short-term treatment with dexfenfluramine is not associated with a significant increase in valvulopathy. Follow-up data is likely to be available soon, which help answer the question as to whether valvulopathy begins or progresses once treatment is discontinued.

Preliminary data from Riley and coworkers[13] also provide reassurance concerning the prevalence of new valve abnormalities in subjects treated with fenfluramine or dexfenfluramine. These investigators reviewed echocardiograms on 42 individuals (76% women, mean age 53 years) who had baseline echocardiograms prior to beginning treatment with fenfluramine or dexfenfluramine. Forty-eight percent of these individuals had been treated with the combination of fenfluramine and phentermine, and 26% had taken dexfenfluramine alone. The mean duration of treatment was 166 days. Only two individuals developed new or worsening valvular abnormalities; in one of these individuals a preexisting valvular abnormality appeared to progress. No patient treated with a single agent demonstrated new or worsening valvular abnormalities.

Summary

At this juncture, the following conclusions can be made concerning diet-drug valvulopathy. Most of these conclusions are based on preliminary data and no true epidemiological or case control studies in a large series of patients has been published yet. Left-sided valvulopathy has developed in association with treatment with dexfenfluramine and fenfluramine either alone or in combination with phentermine. Most reported cases are subjects treated with the combination of dexfenfluramine or fenfluramine in combination with phentermine; phentermine treatment alone does not appear to be associated with valvulopathy. However, more recent studies are reassuring; the incidence of valve regurgitation in association with dexfenfluramine alone, when prescribed for less than 3 months, appears to be modest, and one small study suggests that the incidence of new valve abnormalities is much lower than was feared initially. It also is reassuring that the prevalence of valvular regurgitation does not increase in proportion to BMI. Unfortunately, data do not yet exist concerning the nature of progression (or regression) of valvular lesions in affected individuals.

References

1. Anonymous. Cardiac valvulopathy associated with exposure to fenfluramine or dexfenfluramine: US Department of Health and Human Services interim public health recommendations. *MMWR Morb Mortal Wkly Rep* 1997;46:1061–1066.
2. Weintraub M, Hasday JD, Mushlin AI, et al. A double-blind clinical trial in weight control. Use of fenfluramine and phentermine alone and in combination. *Arch Intern Med* 1984;144:1143–1148.
3. Connolly HM, Crary JL, McGoon MD, et al. Valvular heart disease associated with fenfluramine-phentermine. *N Engl J Med* 1997;337:581–588.
4. Robiolio PA, Rigolin VH, Wilson JS, et al. Carcinoid heart disease. Correlation of high serotonin levels with valvular abnormalities detected by cardiac catheterization and echocardiography. *Circulation* 1995;92:790–795.
5. Redfield MM, Nicholson WJ, Edwards WD, et al. Valve disease associated with ergot alkaloid use: Echocardiographic and pathologic correlations. *Ann Intern Med* 1992;117:50–52.
6. Reid CL, Gardin JM, Yunis C, et al. Prevalence and clinical correlates of aortic and mitral regurgitation in a young adult population: The CARDIA Study. *Circulation* 1994;90:1619.
7. Klein AL, Burstow DJ, Tajik AJ, et al. Age-related prevalence of valvular regurgitation in normal subjects: A comprehensive color flow examination of 118 volunteers. *J Am Soc Echocardiogr* 1990;3:54–63.
8. Singh JM, Evans J, Levy D, et al. Prevalence of valvular regurgitation in a population-based cohort. *Circulation*. In press.
9. Singh J, Evans J, Levy D, et al. Obesity and valvular regurgitation: Is there an association? *J Am Soc Echocardiogr*. In press.
10. Cheitlin MD, Alpert JS, Armstrong WF, et al. ACC/AHA guidelines for the clinical application of echocardiography. A report of the American College of Cardiology/American Heart Association Task Force on Practice Guidelines. *Circulation* 1997;95:1686–1744.
11. Dajani AS, Taubert KA, Wilson W, et al. Prevention of bacterial endocarditis. Recommendations by the American Heart Association. *JAMA* 1997; 277:1794–1801.

12. Weissman N, Gottdiener JS. Prevalence of valvular abnormalities in patients exposed to dexfenfluramine: Result of a randomized, placebo-controlled trial. *N Engl J Med*. Submitted.
13. Riley M, Wee C, Phillips R, et al. New valvular abnormalities among fenfluramine and dexfenfluramine users with prior echocardiograms. *J Am Soc Echocardiogr*. In press.

Chapter 8

Mechanisms of Obesity Hypertension and Relevance to Essential Hypertension

John E. Hall, PhD, Michael W. Brands, PhD, Daniel W. Jones, MD, Eugene W. Shek, PhD, and Jeffrey Henegar, PhD

Introduction

Few medical problems have generated more interest or have been more intractable than obesity, the most common nutritional disorder in the United States and other industrialized countries. Growing evidence suggests that obesity is the prime cause of a cascade of cardiovascular, metabolic, and renal disorders including hypertension, diabetes, atherosclerosis, and chronic renal failure, many of which are interdependent. For example, abnormal kidney function plays a central role in the etiology of obesity hypertension, and the hypertension and metabolic abnormalities associated with obesity are important risk factors for end-stage renal disease (ESRD). Although this constellation of disorders often has been referred to as syndrome X, the insulin resistance syndrome, or the metabolic syndrome, obesity appears to be their central cause. (Figure 1).

Most Essential Hypertensive Subjects Are Overweight

Obesity hypertension often is considered to be a special form of hypertension. However, there is considerable evidence that excess

This research was supported by grant HL51971 from the National Heart, Lung, and Blood Institute and by the Renal Care Foundation, Inc.

From: Fletcher GF, Grundy SM, Hayman LL (eds). *Obesity: Impact on Cardiovascular Disease*. Armonk, NY: Futura Publishing Co., Inc.; © 1999.

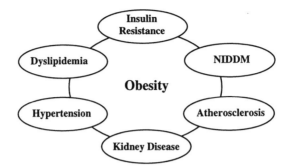

Figure 1. Obesity as a central cause of metabolic disorders, such as noninsulin-dependent diabetes mellitus (NIDDM), as well as hypertension and renal disease.

weight gain may be the most common cause of human essential hypertension. Currently, 30%–35% of the adult population in the United States is at least 20% overweight, with a body mass index (BMI) greater than 27 kg/m^2.[1,2] In some populations, such as elderly black women, the prevalence of obesity may be as high as 70%–80%, coinciding with a 70%–80% rate of hypertension.[3]

Because adverse cardiovascular events and total mortality increase substantially as BMI rises above 25 kg/m^2 (see review by Manson et al[4] and Wickelgren[5]), patients with BMIs greater than this value perhaps should be considered overweight. By this more stringent definition (BMI > 25 kg/m^2), over half of the adult population in the United States is overweight.[2] Similar statistics exist for other industrialized countries and the worldwide prevalence of obesity appears to be increasing steadily, leading many nutrition experts to declare an "epidemic" of obesity.[2]

An important consequence of excess weight gain is increased blood pressure. Population studies indicate that hypertension is virtually absent in very lean populations but is common among overweight groups.[6] Multiple studies have shown good correlations between BMI and blood pressure in normotensive and hypertensive subjects.[7,8] Risk estimates derived from the Framingham Study, for example, suggest that at least 78% of essential hypertension in men and 65% in women can be attributable directly to obesity.[9]

Blood Pressure Correlates with Body Mass Index in Lean or Obese Subjects

Figure 2 shows a linear relationship between BMI and blood pressure in over 22 000 Korean subjects, most of whom were not

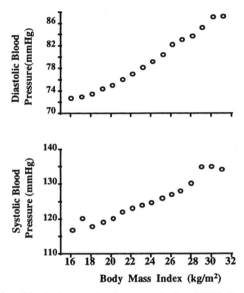

Figure 2. Relationship between body mass index (BMI) (kg/m²) and mean systolic and diastolic blood pressures (SBP and DBP, respectively) in 22, 354 Korean subjects. Adapted with permission from Reference 8.

overweight.[8] A similar relationship between BMI and blood pressure has been noted in other populations throughout the world.[6] This close association between BMI and blood pressure is somewhat surprising in view of the fact that BMI, although correlated with adiposity, is not a very direct marker of obesity. For example, people with marked increases in lean body mass (eg, body builders) may have increased BMI without increased adiposity. Also, older individuals in poor physical condition may have normal BMI but increased adiposity because of loss of skeletal muscle mass and replacement of muscle with adipose tissue. Also, BMI does not take into account variations of regional adiposity that may contribute to cardiovascular disease (CVD); hypertension and metabolic abnormalities such as insulin resistance are more prominent with central compared with lower body obesity.[10,11] These considerations suggest that the association between BMI and blood pressure found in many studies underestimates the impact of obesity in causing hypertension. However, the fact that there is an association between BMI and arterial pressure even in nonobese, lean populations indicates that the effect of weight gain on arterial pressure regulation may be more complex and can be explained simply by the level of increasing adiposity.

   The importance of excess weight gain as a factor in raising blood pressure is reinforced further by experimental studies in animals and in humans showing a rise in blood pressure with weight gain, even over a period of a few weeks.[12,13] Moreover, weight loss reduces blood pressure in normotensive and hypertensive subjects even when sodium intake does not decrease.[6,14,15] The therapeutic value of weight loss has been demonstrated repeatedly in multiple studies showing that even modest weight loss may lower blood pressure to near normal levels in many hypertensive patients.[2,6] Thus, experimental studies and observational studies support the conclusion that obesity may be the single most important risk factor for developing hypertension.

Why Are Some Overweight People Not Hypertensive?

The observation that obese subjects are not invariably hypertensive (according to the somewhat arbitrarily defined standard criteria of a systolic (SBP)/diastolic blood pressure (DBP) greater than 140/90), whereas some lean subjects are hypertensive, has led some investigators to discount the importance of excess weight as a major cause of human essential hypertension. One interpretation of this observation is that there are large, genetically determined variations in the blood pressure responses to weight gain. This concept would, at first glance, seem to be supported by the observation that some populations, such as the Pima Indians in the southwestern United States, have a high prevalence of obesity but may not have corresponding high rates of hypertension until diabetic nephropathy occurs.[16] Similarly, obesity has been suggested to confer a greater risk of hypertension in white females than black females.[16]These observations are consistent with the possibility that variable blood pressure responses to weight gain are determined genetically.

However, a more attractive explanation, is that most (if not all) individuals experience an increase in blood pressure with weight gain, but that the baseline blood pressure (ie, the blood pressure measured before weight gain) is variable, because of genetic differences or other factors that influence blood pressure regulation. Thus, a person with low baseline blood pressure may not be classified as "hypertensive" (greater than 140/90 mm), even though arterial pressure and risk for CVD would be higher than before the weight gain. On a population basis, weight gain would shift the frequency distribution so that a much greater fraction of obese subjects would be hypertensive in comparison with lean subjects (Figure 3). However, obese subjects with "normal" blood pressure (<140/90 mmHg) would be hypertensive relative to their baseline blood pressure, and candidates for therapy. In fact, much of the population risk for CVD occurs at

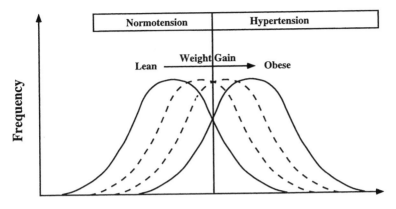

Systemic Arterial Blood Pressure

Figure 3. Postulated effect of weight gain to shift the frequency distribution of mean systemic arterial blood pressure to higher levels.

blood pressures much lower than 140/90 mmHg, and obesity adds to this risk.

This explanation fits with the finding that weight loss almost always reduces blood pressure in "normotensive" as well as hypertensive obese subjects.[6] Also, this is consistent with the observation that weight gain almost invariably increases blood pressure in humans and experimental animals. Thus, the observation that some obese subjects are not hypertensive (using the usual definition of hypertension) may be related mainly to their lower baseline blood pressure, rather than the absence of a rise in blood pressure with weight gain.

Mechanisms of Obesity Hypertension

Although there is clear evidence that obesity is a major factor in causing human essential hypertension, the mechanisms by which weight gain raises arterial pressure are not as well understood. Theoretical and experimental studies indicate that abnormalities of kidney function that cause a hypertensive shift of pressure natriuresis play a central role in all forms of hypertension.[17,18] Obesity hypertension is no exception, with studies in humans and experimental animals indicating that obesity impairs renal-pressure natriuresis.[19,20] Although multiple neurohumoral abnormalities have been proposed to alter renal function in obesity, it often is difficult in human studies to separate those changes that contribute to increased arterial pressure versus those changes that occur secondary to hypertension.

Experimental studies in animals allow a more mechanistic approach to the problem, but there are few animal models of obesity in which sequential changes in renal, cardiovascular, and endocrine functions have been examined during the development of hypertension before and after the suspected pressor systems have been inhibited. In recent years there has been a proliferation of rodent models of genetic obesity with rapid advances in our understanding of the molecular genetics of obesity. Unfortunately, in most of these genetic models, the cardiovascular and renal changes have not been well characterized. Those that have been studied often do not mimic the cardiovascular, renal, and neurohumoral changes found in obese humans. For example, the Zucker fatty rat, a widely used model of genetic obesity, has reduced plasma renin activity (PRA),[21] whereas obese humans often have increased PRA.[14] Also, increased sympathetic activity appears to play a significant role in causing hypertension in obese humans[22] but not in Zucker fatty rats.[21]

In contrast to genetic models of obesity, experimental animals fed high-fat diets have many of the abnormalities observed in obese humans. For example, obese dogs and rabbits fed high-fat diets exhibit endocrine, renal, sympathetic, cardiovascular, and metabolic changes very similar to those found in obese humans.[12,23–25] These observations lend credence to the hypothesis that dietary factors, especially a high-fat diet, play a dominant role in the etiology of human obesity.

Obesity Increases Regional Blood Flows, Cardiac Output, and Arterial Pressure

Studies in experimental animals and humans indicate that rapid weight gain increases and weight loss decreases regional blood flows, cardiac output, and arterial pressure. For example, in dogs placed on a high-fat diet for 5 weeks with a constant intake of sodium, protein, and carbohydrates, there were parallel increases in body weight and blood pressure, with arterial pressure increasing by approximately 15–20 mmHg[24] (Figure 4). This is similar to the modest changes in blood pressure observed in the first few weeks after rapid weight gain or weight loss in humans. A high-fat diet in dogs also markedly raised heart rate and cardiac output, in parallel with the weight gain. Total peripheral vascular resistance decreased during the high-fat diet, but when indexed for body weight (total peripheral vascular resistance index) there was a slight increase, similar to that observed in obese humans.[25,26]

Studies in humans also indicate that obesity is associated with volume expansion and increased regional blood flows, which sum-

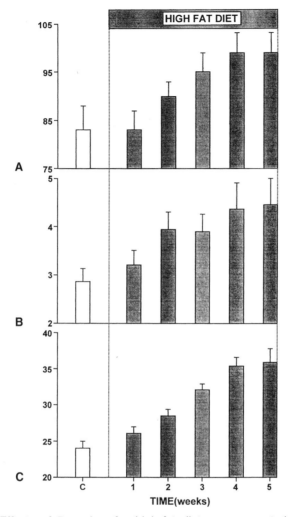

Figure 4. Effects of 5 weeks of a high-fat diet on mean arterial pressure, cardiac output, and body weight in dogs. (**A**), mean arterial pressure (mmHg); (**B**), cardiac output (L/min); (**C**), body weight (kg). Adapted with permission from Reference 24.

mate to give a rise in cardiac output. Part of the increased cardiac output observed with weight gain is caused by additional adipose tissue and the associated blood flow. However, blood flows in non-adipose tissue, including the heart, kidneys, gastrointestinal tract, and skeletal muscle, also increase with weight gain.[24-28] The mechanisms

responsible for increased regional blood flows have not been elucidated fully but are likely caused by, in part, increased metabolic rate
and local accumulation of vasodilator metabolites.

Despite the rise in cardiac output, there is evidence for impaired
cardiac function in obesity. In rabbits and dogs fed a high-fat diet for
5–12 weeks (Figure 5), there are increased intracardiac filling pressures
and impaired relaxation of the heart during diastole.[29,30] Clinical studies also suggest that cardiac hypertrophy is more severe in obese than
in lean subjects with comparable hypertension.[31] Furthermore, high-
sodium intake, which often coincides with high-caloric intake, exacer-
bates obesity-induced cardiac hypertrophy.[32] However, further studies
are needed to characterize more fully the impaired cardiac function
that occurs early in obesity, in the absence of overt cardiac failure, and
the mechanisms by which obesity initiates cardiac hypertrophy and
diastolic dysfunction.

Although cardiac systolic and diastolic functions are impaired in
obesity, stroke volume is maintained at a relatively constant level and
there is an increase in resting heart rate. Most available evidence in
obese humans and dogs indicates that the rise in the resting heart rate
primarily is caused by withdrawal of parasympathetic tone rather than
increased sympathetic activity or increased intrinsic heart rate.[33,34]

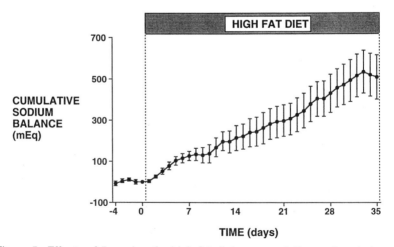

Figure 5. Effects of 5 weeks of a high-fat diet on cumulative sodium balance
in dogs. Adapted with permission from Reference 24.

Obesity Causes Impaired Renal-Pressure Natriuresis, Sodium Retention, and Increased Extracellular Fluid Volume

The fact that normal sodium excretion is maintained only at the expense of elevated arterial pressure indicates that obesity is associated with impaired renal-pressure natriuresis.[20] Normally, increased arterial pressure would raise sodium excretion above intake, thereby reducing extracellular fluid volume and eventually returning arterial pressure toward normal.[17,18] However, the attenuation of pressure natriuresis in obesity necessitates increased arterial pressure to maintain sodium balance in the presence of impaired renal excretory function.[20]

Figure 6 shows that during 5 weeks of a high-fat diet in dogs there was marked sodium retention, much more than can be accounted for by the increased adipose tissue. Extracellular fluid volume and plasma volume also are elevated markedly with dietary-induced obesity in experimental animals[23] as well as in obese humans.[26] Sodium retention and volume expansion in obesity are not caused by renal vasoconstriction or decreased glomerular filtration rate (GFR), because GFR and renal plasma flow are elevated in obese dogs,[24] rabbits,[27] and humans[28] when compared with lean control subjects. Thus, in the early phases of the obesity, before the onset of glomerular injury and loss of nephron function (discussed in a following section), sodium retention mainly is caused by increased renal tubular reabsorption (Fig. 6).

The precise causes of increased tubular reabsorption and impaired pressure natriuresis are not completely clear, but a role has been suggested for at least four factors: (1) insulin resistance and hyperinsulinemia, (2) activation of the renin–angiotensin system (RAS), (3) increased sympathetic nervous system activity, and (4) altered intrarenal physical forces caused by structural changes that compress the renal medulla.

Hyperinsulinemia Is Not a Primary Cause of Obesity Hypertension

Obesity is associated with glucose intolerance, fasting hyperinsulinemia, and an exaggerated insulin response to ingestion of meals or glucose loads.[35,36] The increased plasma insulin concentrations occur as a compensation for impaired metabolic effects of insulin, a condition known as "insulin resistance." However, not all tissues share in this insulin resistance, leading to the possibility of a supranormal insulin

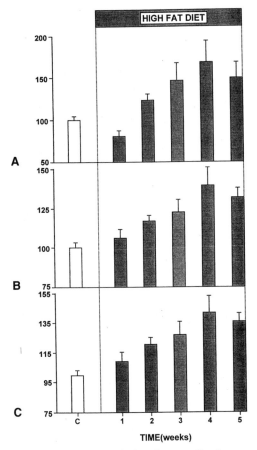

Figure 6. Effects of 5 weeks of a high-fat diet on effective renal plasma flow, glomerular filtration rate (GFR), and total sodium reabsorption in dogs. (**A**), effective renal plasma flow (% control); (**B**), glomerular filtration rate (% control); (**C**), sodium reabsorption (% control). Adapted with permission from Reference 24.

action in some tissues. Hypertension had been suggested as one of the unfortunate consequences of these increased levels of insulin.[36,37] Acute studies suggest that high-insulin levels may cause modest sodium retention and increased sympathetic activity, and these observations have been extrapolated to conclude that hyperinsulinemia may be an important cause of obesity hypertension.[36] However, as previously discussed in detail,[35,38,39] there is little evidence that chronic hyperinsulinemia causes hypertension. In dogs and humans acute or chronic hyperinsulinemia lasting for several weeks does not cause a hypertensive shift of pressure natriuresis or increased arterial pressure.[38,39] In fact, insulin infusions at rates that produce plasma concentrations similar to those found in obesity tend to reduce, rather than increase, arterial pressure because of insulin's vasodilator action, particularly in skeletal muscle.[38,39] In the kidney, the hemodynamic effects of insulin are minimal.[40]

Hyperinsulinemia not only fails to cause hypertension in humans or in dogs, but also does not potentiate the blood pressure or renal effects of other pressor substances such as norepinephrine or angiotensin II (AngII).[38,39] Moreover, hyperinsulinemia does not appear to increase arterial pressure even in obese subjects who are resistant to the metabolic and vasodilator effects of insulin.[41] Thus, multiple studies indicate that hyperinsulinemia cannot explain the increased renal tubular sodium reabsorption, the shift of pressure natriuresis, or the hypertension associated with obesity in humans or in dogs.

In contrast to the findings in humans and dogs, there is evidence in rats that chronic hyperinsulinemia causes small but significant increases in arterial pressure.[42] Insulin-induced hypertension in rats is associated with peripheral vasoconstriction and appears to be mediated through interactions with the RAS and thromboxane, because inhibition of thromboxane synthesis or angiotension converting-enzyme (ACE) inhibition abolished the rise in arterial pressure.[43,44] Moreover, blockade of endothelial-derived nitric oxide synthesis appears to greatly exacerbate insulin-induced hypertension in rats.[45] Whether these findings are relevant to obesity hypertension is unclear, but currently the available evidence suggests that in humans and dogs, hyperinsulinemia cannot account for the elevated arterial pressure associated with obesity. The close correlation between hyperinsulinemia and hypertension in obese subjects appears to be caused by the fact that obesity not only elevates arterial pressure but also causes insulin resistance and hyperinsulinemia through parallel but independent mechanisms.

Can Insulin Resistance Cause Hypertension Independently of Hyperinsulinemia?

There are other consequences of insulin resistance, besides hyperinsulinemia, that could conceivably cause hypertension. Numerous studies have shown that blood pressure is correlated with different measures of insulin resistance in hypertensive subjects.[36,37] However, insulin resistance usually occurs secondary to obesity and correlations may not imply necessarily a cause-and-effect relationship, similar to that described previously for hyperinsulinemia and hypertension.

Support for a role of insulin resistance comes from experimental studies demonstrating that improvement of insulin sensitivity with antihyperglycemic agents, such as thiazolidenediones, lowers arterial pressure.[46] However, these drugs also block L-type calcium channels and reduce arterial pressure in renovascular hypertension, which is not associated with insulin resistance or hyperinsulinemia.[46,47] Therefore, it is still unclear whether the blood pressure–lowering effects of these drugs are related to improvement of insulin sensitivity or to other actions.

Although a direct causal relationship between insulin resistance and hypertension has not been established, further investigation of this issue is warranted because of the well-recognized effects of insulin resistance on glucose and lipid metabolism. For example, insulin decreases mobilization of fatty acids and promotes fat storage via several mechanisms, including inhibition of hormone-sensitive lipase; thus, insulin normally decreases lipolysis of triglycerides and prevents release of fatty acids from adipocytes into the circulation. With resistance to insulin's actions, hormone-sensitive lipase activity would increase, thereby decreasing lipid storage and increasing plasma concentrations of fatty acids and lipids. These changes, if prolonged, could contribute to atherosclerosis of renal vessels or glomerulosclerosis and, therefore, increased arterial pressure. Also, with long-term obesity, glucose intolerance and hyperglycemia would become more and more severe, causing glycosylation of renal vascular and glomerular proteins, increased production of extracellular matrix, and loss of nephron function. Although glomerular hyperfiltration and increased renal plasma flow occur in the early phases of obesity, with chronic obesity and development of type II diabetes there often is progressive glomerulosclerosis, decreased renal blood flow and GFR, and loss of nephron function, which can progress to ESRD.

Renin–Angiotensin System Contributes to Increased Renal Tubular Reabsorption in Obesity

PRA is increased significantly in most obese subjects despite marked sodium retention and increased extracellular fluid volume.[14,20] Although the mechanisms by which obesity stimulates renin secretion have not been studied extensively, there are at least two likely explanations: (1) obesity may stimulate renin secretion by increasing loop of Henle sodium chloride reabsorption, thereby reducing sodium chloride delivery to the macula densa and (2) obesity may stimulate renin secretion by activation of the sympathetic nervous system. Both of these mechanisms appear to be involved in the pathogenesis of obesity hypertension, but their relative importance in stimulating renin release is unknown.

The possibility that the RAS contributes to increased sodium reabsorption in obesity hypertension is supported by our recent finding that treatment with an AngII antagonist blunted the sodium retention, volume expansion, and increased arterial pressure associated with a chronic high-fat diet in dogs.[48] Robles et al.[49] also found that ACE inhibition attenuated hypertension associated with 12 weeks of a high-fat diet in dogs. These observations suggest a role for AngII in stimulating sodium reabsorption, shifting pressure natriuresis, and causing hypertension during dietary-induced obesity. They also are consistent with a recent report by Reisin et al.[50] who found that ACE inhibitors were effective in reducing blood pressure in obese subjects, particularly in white and young patients.

Stimulation of the RAS also may contribute to the glomerular injury and nephron loss associated with obesity. Increased AngII formation, by constricting efferent arterioles, may exacerbate the rise in glomerular hydrostatic pressure caused by systemic arterial hypertension.[51] Although studies in type II diabetic patients, who are usually obese, support the view that treatment with ACE inhibitors may slow progression of renal injury, further studies are needed in nondiabetic, obese subjects to determine the efficacy of RAS blockers, compared with other antihypertensive agents, in lowering blood pressure and reducing the risk of renal injury.

Sympathetic Activation Contributes to Increased Renal Sodium Reabsorption in Obesity

Several sources of evidence suggest that sympathetic stimulation plays a major role in causing obesity-induced hypertension[13,22,52]: (1) high-caloric intake increases norepinephrine turnover, an index of sympathetic activity, in peripheral tissues and raises resting plasma norepinephrine concentrations; (2) high-caloric intake amplifies the rise in plasma norepinephrine that occurs with stimuli such as upright posture and isometric hand grip; (3) obese hypertensive subjects have increased sympathetic activity, measured directly with microneurographic methods, compared with lean subjects[53,54]; and (4) pharmacologic blockade of adrenergic activity markedly blunts the rise in blood pressure associated with obesity.[55]

Renal Sympathetic Nerves Mediate Increased Sodium Reabsorption and Hypertension in Obesity

Our previous studies indicate an important role for the renal sympathetic nerves in mediating obesity hypertension. For example, innervated kidneys retained almost twice as much sodium as denervated kidneys in unilaterally denervated dogs fed a high-fat diet for 5 weeks.[56] Moreover, bilateral renal denervation greatly attenuated the sodium retention and hypertension associated with a high-fat diet.[57] These findings indicate that increased renal tubular sodium reabsorption, impaired renal-pressure natriuresis, and hypertension associated with obesity are mediated, in part, by increased renal sympathetic nerve activity.

Leptin May Contribute to Sympathetic Activation in Obesity

The mechanisms by which sympathetic activation occurs in obesity are still unclear. Although the renal efferent sympathetic fibers contribute to sodium retention and hypertension, afferent pathways originating from renal mechano- or chemoreceptors do not appear to play a major role in stimulating sympathetic activity in obese dogs.[58] Moreover, the direct central nervous system (CNS) effects of insulin probably do not account for increased sympathetic activity, because increases in insulin concentration in the cerebral circulation, to values comparable to those found in obesity, do not elevate arterial pressure.[59]

More promising as a possible stimulus for increased sympathetic activity in obesity is leptin, the peptide product of the "obese gene," which is secreted by adipocytes in proportion to adiposity.[60,61] Leptin appears to play an important role in the regulation of energy balance by reducing appetite and increasing energy expenditure through sympathetic stimulation. Haynes et al.[62] reported that acute intravenous infusion of leptin increased sympathetic activity in the kidneys, the adrenals, and in brown adipose tissue. The possibility that leptin-mediated increases in sympathetic activity may contribute to obesity hypertension is consistent with our recent observation that chronic bilateral carotid artery infusion of leptin, at rates that raised plasma concentrations in the cerebral circulation to levels similar to those found in obesity, caused significant increases in heart rate and arterial pressure in rats.[63] However, further studies are needed to elucidate the physiological role of leptin and its interactions with other blood pressure control mechanisms in obesity.

Obesity Alters Intrarenal Physical Forces and Causes Structural Changes in the Kidneys

One striking feature of kidneys from obese subjects is that they are encapsulated almost completely with adipose tissue. Some of this fat penetrates the renal hilum into the sinuses surrounding the renal medulla and could, along with the fat around the capsule, act as a compressive force on the kidney. Chronic compression of the renal capsule (eg, perinephritic hypertension) consistently increases arterial pressure in direct proportion to the compressive force on the kidney.[64]

Obesity Causes Structural and Functional Changes in the Renal Medulla

In addition to compression of the renal capsule by extrarenal fat, there are also important changes in renal medullary histology, including increased interstitial cells and extracellular matrix between the tubules that could compress the renal medulla.[20,52] The increased extracellular matrix is composed of proteoglycans, rather than lipids. Also, total glycosaminoglycan content and hyaluronan, a major component of the renal medullar extracellular matrix, were elevated markedly in the inner medullas of obese dogs compared with lean dogs, but not in the outer medulla or the cortex.[65] Although the cause of this increased hyaluronan in the renal medulla is unknown, hyaluronan accumulation has been associated with increased interstitial fluid pressure and tissue edema in kidneys.[66] Further studies are needed to determine the mechanisms of hyaluronan accumulation in the renal medulla in obesity and the functional significance of this change.

The possibility that these observations in dogs are relevant to obese humans is supported by preliminary studies of kidneys from obese humans showing similar histological changes in the renal medulla.[67] However, further studies are needed to more fully characterize the histological and biochemical changes that take place in the renal medulla of obesity and the stimuli that initiate these changes.

One possible consequence of these structural changes in the renal medulla is that they could increase renal tissue pressure and compress the tubules and vasa recta. Because the kidney is surrounded by a tight capsule with a low compliance, increased interstitial cells or extracellular matrix would raise interstitial fluid hydrostatic and solid tissue pressures, causing compression of the delicate loops of Henle and vasa recta.[20,52] In support of this hypothesis, we found that renal interstitial fluid hydrostatic pressure was elevated to 19 mmHg in kidneys of obese dogs compared with only 9–10 mmHg in kidneys of lean dogs.[20,52] Although small increases in interstitial fluid pressure tend to inhibit tubular sodium reabsorption, large increases of the magnitude found in obese dogs would tend to reduce renal medullary blood flow, slow the flow rate in the renal tubules, and raise fractional sodium reabsorption.[20,52] These changes obviously cannot explain the initial rise in blood pressure associated with rapid weight gain, but they could contribute to the more sustained increases in tubular reabsorption and hypertension associated with chronic obesity.

Obesity Causes Early Structural Changes in the Glomeruli

Although obesity-induced type II diabetes is a well-recognized cause of renal disease, the mechanisms for progressive nephron loss are unclear and there are few clinical or experimental studies that have examined changes in glomerular structure and function in the early stages of obesity before major disturbances of glucose metabolism occur. However, there is evidence that obesity often is associated with microalbuminuria or even proteinuria, even before there are major histological changes in the glomerulus or evidence of glomerulosclerosis.[68] In dogs with dietary-induced obesity, we found significant histological changes in the glomeruli after only 5–6 weeks of a high-fat diet.[69] There was substantial enlargement of Bowman's space, increased glomerular cell proliferation, as evidenced by increased proliferating cell nuclear antigen (PCNA), increased mesangial matrix and thicker basement membranes, and increased expression of glomerular transforming growth factor-β (TGF-β). These early glomerular changes may be the precursors to development of proteinuria and glomerulosclerosis. Although the mechanisms that initiate these changes are unknown, it seems likely that the combined effects of neurohumoral factors (eg, AngII, insulin, and sympathetic activity) and changes in intrarenal physical forces may play a significant role in causing glomerular injury in obesity.

Glomerular Hyperfiltration May Contribute to Renal Injury in Obesity

The compensatory renal vasodilation and increased GFR, along with higher arterial pressure, are important in helping to overcome the renal medullary compression and increased sodium reabsorption associated with obesity. However, in the long-term, the renal vasodilation (which appears to occur mainly in afferent arterioles) may cause glomerular injury (Figure 7). Considerable evidence indicates that chronic glomerular hyperfiltration, especially in the presence of other risk factors such as hyperlipidemia, hyperglycemia, and systemic arterial hypertension, eventually may cause glomerulosclerosis and loss of functional nephrons. The quantitative importance of these stimuli and how they interact to cause proliferation of mesangial cells and increased extracellular matrix in the glomerulus are not well understood but likely involve a complex interplay of mechanical forces, vasoactive substances, cytokines, and growth factors.

Obesity May be the Most Common Cause of End-Stage Renal Failure

The two leading causes of ESRD are diabetes and hypertension.[70] Type II diabetes, which is caused primarily by obesity, accounts for at least 80%–90% of diabetes. Likewise, 70%–75% of essential hypertensive patients are overweight, and there is clear evidence that excess weight is a primary cause of human essential hypertension. These considerations suggest that obesity also may be one of the major causes

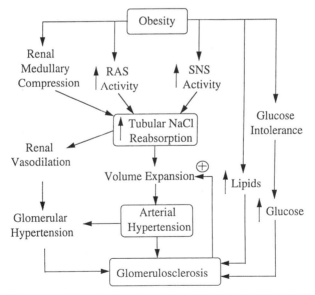

Figure 7. Summary of mechanisms by which obesity may cause hypertension and glomerulosclerosis by activation of the renin–angiotensin system (RAS) and sympathetic nervous systems, metabolic abnormalities, and compression of the renal medulla.

of ESRD. However, further epidemiological studies, especially in populations with high risk for developing ESRD, are needed to test this hypothesis.

Summary

Weight gain appears to be a major cause of increased blood pressure in many essential hypertensive patients and an important cause of ESRD. Although the precise mechanisms by which obesity raises blood pressure have not been elucidated fully, weight gain is associated with increased renal tubular reabsorption and a shift of pressure natriuresis toward higher blood pressures. The increased renal tubular reabsorption is compensated for, in part, by renal vasodilation, glomerular hyperfiltration, and increased blood pressure. However, chronic renal vasodilation and systemic hypertension also raise glomerular hydrostatic pressure and wall stress, which, along with activation of neurohumoral factors, hyperlipidemia, and hypoglycemia, may cause glomerulosclerosis and loss of nephron function in obese subjects. The mechanisms by which obesity increases renal tubular reabsorption and causes a hypertensive shift of pressure natriuresis are not understood completely but do not appear to be related directly to hyperinsulinemia. Activation of the sympathetic and RAS, as well as changes in intrarenal physical forces caused by renal medullary compression, appear to play an important role in the pathogenesis of obesity hypertension. However, the mechanisms that initiate these changes remain a fruitful area for further investigation, especially in view of the current "epidemic" of obesity in most industrialized countries and the key role of obesity in causing human essential hypertension and ESRD.

Acknowledgments: We thank Elaine Steed-Davis and Angela Engle for assistance in preparation of this manuscript

References

1. Najjar MF, Rowland M. Anthropometric reference data and prevalence of overweight, United States, 1976–80. *Vital Health Stat* 1987;11:1–73.
2. Stamler J. Epidemic obesity in the United States. *Arch Intern Med* 1993;153: 1040–1044.
3. Kumanyika S. Obesity in black women. *Epidemiol Rev* 1987;9:31–50.
4. Manson JE, Willett WC, Stampfer MJ, et al. Body weight and mortality among women. *N Engl J Med* 1995;333:677–685.
5. Wickelgren I. Obesity: How big a problem? *Science* 1998;280:1364–1367.
6. Alexander J, Dustan HP, Sims EAH, et al. *Report of the Hypertension Task Force*. Washington, D C : U S Government Printing Office; 1979.

7. Chiang BN, Perlman LV, Epstein FH. Overweight and hypertension. A review. *Circulation* 1969;39:403–421.
8. Jones DW, Kim JS, Andrew ME, et al. Body mass index and blood pressure in Korean men and women: The Korean National Blood Pressure Survey. *J Hypertens* 1994;12:1433–1437.
9. Garrison RJ, Kannel WB, Stokes JD, et al. Incidence and precursors of hypertension in young adults: The Framingham Offspring Study. *Prev Med* 1987;16:235–251.
10. Bjorntorp P. Metabolic implications of body fat distribution. *Diabetes Care* 1991;14:1132–1143.
11. Kissebah AH, Krakower GR. Regional adiposity and morbidity. *Physiol Rev* 1994;74:761–811.
12. Rocchini AP. The influence of obesity in hypertension. *News Physiol Sci* 1990;5:245–249.
13. Hall JE, Zappe DH, Alonso-Galicia M, et al. Mechanisms of obesity-induced hypertension. *News Physiol Sci* 1996;11:255–261.
14. Tuck ML, Sowers J, Dornfeld L, et al. The effect of weight reduction on blood pressure, plasma renin activity, and plasma aldosterone levels in obese patients. *N Engl J Med* 1981;304:930–933.
15. Reisin E, Abel R, Modan M, et al. Effect of weight loss without salt restriction on the reduction of blood pressure in overweight hypertensive patients. *N Engl J Med* 1978;298:1–6.
16. Berchtold P, Jorgens V, Finke C, et al. Epidemiology of obesity and hypertension. *Int J Obes* 1981;5:1–7.
17. Guyton AC. The surprising kidney-fluid mechanism for pressure control: its infinite gain. *Hypertension* 1990;16:725–730.
18. Hall JE, Mizelle HL, Hildebrandt DA, et al. Abnormal pressure natriuresis. A cause or a consequence of hypertension? *Hypertension* 1990;15:547–559.
19. Rocchini AP, Key J, Bondie D, et al. The effect of weight loss on the sensitivity of blood pressure to sodium in obese adolescents. *N Engl J Med* 1989;321:580–585.
20. Hall JE. Mechanisms of abnormal renal sodium handling in obesity hypertension. *Am J Hypertens* 1997;10:49S–55S.
21. Alonso-Galicia M, Brands MW, Zappe DH, et al. Hypertension in obese Zucker rats. Role of angiotensin II and adrenergic activity. *Hypertension* 1996;28:1047–1054.
22. Landsberg L, Krieger DR. Obesity, metabolism, and the sympathetic nervous system. *Am J Hypertens* 1989;2:125S–132S.
23. Hall JE. Renal and cardiovascular mechanisms of hypertension in obesity. *Hypertension* 1994;23:381–394.
24. Hall JE, Brands MW, Dixon WN, et al. Obesity-induced hypertension. Renal function and systemic hemodynamics. *Hypertension* 1993;22:292–299.
25. Rocchini AP. Cardiovascular regulation in obesity-induced hypertension. *Hypertension* 1992;19:I56–I60.
26. Messerli FH, Christie B, DeCarvalho JG, et al. Obesity and essential hypertension. Hemodynamics, intravascular volume, sodium excretion, and plasma renin activity. *Arch Intern Med* 1981;141:81–85.
27. Carroll JF, Huang M, Hester RL, et al. Hemodynamic alterations in hypertensive obese rabbits. *Hypertension* 1995;26:465–470.
28. Reisin E, Messerli FH, Ventura HO, et al. Renal hemodynamics in obese and lean essential hypertensive patients. In: Meserli FH, ed. *Kidney in Essential Hypertension*. Boston: Martinus Nihoff, 1948:125–129.

29. Carroll JF, Braden DS, Cockrell K, et al. Obese hypertensive rabbits develop concentric and eccentric hypertrophy and diastolic filling abnormalities. *Am J Hypertens* 1997;10:230–233.
30. Mizelle HL, Edwards TC, Montani JP. Abnormal cardiovascular responses to exercise during the development of obesity in dogs. *Am J Hypertens* 1994;7:374–378.
31. Lauer MS, Anderson KM, Levy D. Separate and joint influences of obesity and mild hypertension on left ventricular mass and geometry: The Framingham Heart Study. *J Am Coll Cardiol* 1992;19:130–134.
32. Carroll JF, Braden DS, Henegar JR, et al. Dietary sodium chloride (NaCl) worsens obesity-related cardiac hypertrophy. *FASEB J* 1998;12:A708.
33. Van Vliet BN, Hall JE, Mizelle HL, et al. Reduced parasympathetic control of heart rate in obese dogs. *Am J Physiol* 1995;269:H629–H637.
34. Arone LJ, Mackintosh R, Rosenbaum M, et al. Autonomic nervous system activity in weight gain and weight loss. *Am J Physiol* 1995;269:R222–R225.
35. Hall JE, Summers RL, Brands MW, et al. Resistance to metabolic actions of insulin and its role in hypertension. *Am J Hypertens* 1994;7:772–788.
36. Reaven GM, Hoffman BB. A role for insulin in the aetiology and course of hypertension? *Lancet* 1987;2:435–437.
37. Lucas CP, Estigarribia JA, Darga LL, et al. Insulin and blood pressure in obesity. *Hypertension* 1985;7:702–706.
38. Hall JE. Hyperinsulinemia: A link between obesity and hypertension? *Kidney Int* 1993;43:1402–1417.
39. Hall JE, Brands MW, Zappe DH, et al. Cardiovascular actions of insulin: Are they important in long-term blood pressure regulation? *Clin Exp Pharmacol Physiol* 1995;22:689–700.
40. Hall JE, Brands MW, Mizelle HL, et al. Chronic intrarenal hyperinsulinemia does not cause hypertension. *Am J Physiol* 1991;260:F663–F669.
41. Hall JE, Brands MW, Zappe DH, et al. Hemodynamic and renal responses to chronic hyperinsulinemia in obese, insulin-resistant dogs. *Hypertension* 1995;25:994–1002.
42. Brands MW, Hildebrandt DA, Mizelle HL, et al. Sustained hyperinsulinemia increases arterial pressure in conscious rats. *Am J Physiol* 1991;260: R764–R768.
43. Keen HL, Brands MW, Smith MJ Jr, et al. Inhibition of thromboxane synthesis attenuates insulin hypertension in rats. *Am J Hypertens* 1997;10: 1125–1131.
44. Brands MW, Harrison DL, Keen HL, et al. Insulin-induced hypertension in rats depends on an intact renin–angiotensin system. *Hypertension* 1997;29: 1014–1019.
45. Shek EW, Keen HL, Brands MW, et al. Inhibition of nitric oxide synthesis enhances insulin-hypertension in rats. *FASEB J* 1996;10:A556.
46. Dubey RK, Zhang HY, Reddy SR, et al. Pioglitazone attenuates hypertension and inhibits growth of renal arteriolar smooth muscle in rats. *Am J Physiol* 1993;265:R726–R732.
47. Zhang F, Sowers JR, Ram JL, et al. Effects of pioglitazone on calcium channels in vascular smooth muscle. *Hypertension* 1994;24:170–175.
48. Hall JE, Henegar JR, Shek EW, et al. Role of renin–angiotensin system in obesity hypertension. *Circulation* 1997;96:I33.
49. Robles RG, Villa E, Santirso R, et al. Effects of captopril on sympathetic activity, lipid and carbohydrate metabolism in a model of obesity-induced hypertension in dogs. *Am J Hypertens* 1993;6:1009–1015.

50. Reisin E, Weir MR, Falkner B, et al. Lisinopril versus hydrochlorothiazide in obese hypertensive patients: A multicenter placebo-controlled trial. Treatment in Obese Patients With Hypertension (TROPHY) Study Group. *Hypertension* 1997;30:140–145.
51. Hall JE. Control of sodium excretion by angiotensin II: Intrarenal mechanisms and blood pressure regulation. *Am J Physiol* 1986;250:R960–R972.
52. Hall JE, Brands MW, Henegar JR, et al. Abnormal kidney function as a cause and a consequence of obesity hypertension. *Clin Exp Pharmacol Physiol* 1998;25:58–64.
53. Jones PP, Davy KP, Alexander S, et al. Age-related increase in muscle sympathetic nerve activity is associated with abdominal adiposity. *Am J Physiol* 1997;272:E976–E980.
54. Grassi G, Seravalle G, Cattaneo BM, et al. Sympathetic activation in obese normotensive subjects. *Hypertension* 1995;25:560–563.
55. Hall JE, Van Vliet BN, Garrity CA, et al. Obesity hypertension: Role of adrenergic mechanisms. *Hypertension* 1993;21:528.
56. Kassab S, Wilkins C, Kato T, et al. Renal nerves play an important role in mediating the sodium retention in response to a high fat diet in conscious dogs. *Am J Hypertens* 1994;9:20A.
57. Kassab S, Kato T, Wilkins FC, et al. Renal denervation attenuates the sodium retention and hypertension associated with obesity. *Hypertension* 1995;25:893–897.
58. Zappe DH, Capel WT, Keen HL, et al. Role of renal afferent nerves in obesity-induced hypertension. *Am J Hypertens* 1996;9:20A.
59. Hildebrandt DA, Heath BJ, Hall JE. Systemic arterial pressure and heart rate responses to chronic carotid or vertebral artery insulin infusion. *FASEB J* 1994;8:A528.
60. Halaas JL, Gajiwala KS, Maffei M, et al. Weight-reducing effects of the plasma protein encoded by the obese gene. *Science* 1995;269:543–546.
61. Chua SC Jr, Chung WK, Wu-Peng XS, et al. Phenotypes of mouse diabetes and rat fatty due to mutations in the OB (leptin) receptor. *Science* 1996;271:994–996.
62. Haynes WG, Morgan DA, Walsh SA, et al. Cardiovascular consequences of obesity: Role of leptin. *Clin Exp Pharmacol Physiol* 1998;25:65–69.
63. Shek EW, Brands MW, Hall JE. Chronic leptin infusion increases arterial pressure. *Hypertension* 1998;31:409–414.
64. Brace RA, Jackson TE, Ferguson JD, et al. Pressure generated by scar tissue contraction: Perinephritis hypertension. *IRCS* 1974;2:1683.
65. Alonso-Galicia M, Dwyer TM, Herrera GA, et al. Increased hyaluronic acid in the inner renal medulla of obese dogs. *Hypertension* 1995;25:888–892.
66. Johnsson C, Tufveson G, Wahlberg J, et al. Experimentally-induced warm renal ischemia induces cortical accumulation of hyaluronan in the kidney. *Kidney Int* 1996;50:1224–1229.
67. Arnold MD, Brissie R, Soonz JS, et al. Obesity associated renal medullary changes. *Lab Invest* 1994;70:156A.
68. Wesson DE, Kurtzman NA, Frommer JP. Massive obesity and nephrotic proteinuria with a normal renal biopsy. *Nephron* 1985;40:235–237.
69. Henegar JR, Shek EW, Henegar L, et al. Renal functional and structural changes in the early stages of obesity. *Hypertension* 1997;30:474.
70. The National Institutes of Health. United States Renal Data System. 1994 Annual Report. Ann Arbor, MI: University of Michigan; 1994:xxi.

Chapter 9

Obesity and Lipoprotein Metabolism: Relationship to Cardiovascular Disease

Barbara V. Howard, PhD

Introduction

Rates of cardiovascular disease (CVD) are higher in obese individuals. Although the mechanism for this association is unclear, it must be related to the increases in CVD risk factors that are observed in obese individuals. One of the most likely metabolic alterations linking obesity to CVD is the effect of obesity on lipoproteins. The literature contains multiple reports on the diverse changes in lipoproteins that accompany obesity. This review examines the available population-based data on the associations of obesity and lipoproteins, summarizes possible metabolic mechanisms, and discusses the implications for weight-loss therapy.

Changes in Lipoproteins with Increasing Body Weight

Obesity almost universally is associated with increases in plasma triglycerides (TG)s. Analysis of the Second National Health and Nutrition Educational Survey (NHANES II) data set, which represents a random sample of American adults within a wide range of age and socioeconomic status, shows an increase in TG levels with increasing obesity in all age groups of white men and women. There is an approximately 100-mg/dL difference between normal-weight and obese men,[1] and an approximately 60-mg/dL difference in women

From: Fletcher GF, Grundy SM, Hayman LL (eds). *Obesity: Impact on Cardiovascular Disease*. Armonk, NY: Futura Publishing Co., Inc.; © 1999.

[Figure 1(a) and (b)].[2] These cross-sectional data are supported by longitudinal cohort data from the Coronary Artery Risk Development in Young Adults (CARDIA) Study showing that increasing weight is accompanied by increases in plasma TGs (CARDIA Study, unpublished data, May 1998) (Figure 2). Furthermore, several weight-loss studies of at least 1 year in duration show significant reductions in TGs (Table 1).[3-6] Although data are less complete in other ethnic groups, similar associations between body mass index (BMI) and plasma TGs have been reported in blacks,[7] Hispanics,[8] and American Indians,[9] which suggests that obesity may be associated with increases in TGs in all ethnic groups.

Obesity also appears to be associated consistently with decreases in high-density lipoprotein cholesterol (HDL-C) HDL-C. NHANES II data in white men and women show decreases in all age groups with increasing BMI.[1,2] There is an approximately 10-mg/dL difference between normal-weight and obese men and even greater decreases

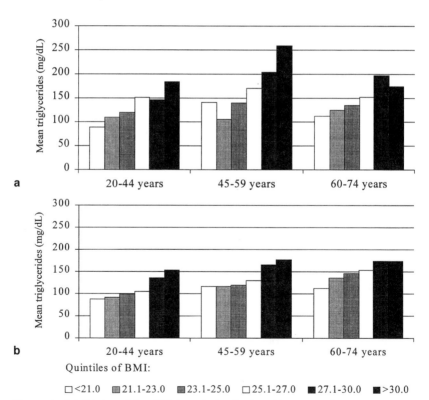

Quintiles of BMI:

□ <21.0   ▥ 21.1-23.0   ▤ 23.1-25.0   □ 25.1-27.0   ■ 27.1-30.0   ▪ >30.0

Figure 1. (a) Triglycerides (TGs) and obesity in white men: Second National Health and Nutrition Educational Survey (NHANES II) (b) TGs and obesity in white women: NHANES II Adapted with permission from References 1 and 2.

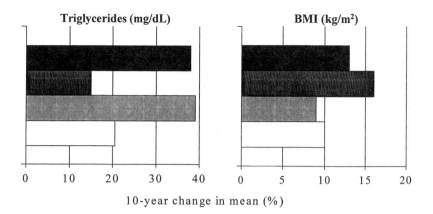

□ White women ▨ White men ▧ Black women ▨ Black men

Figure 2. Change in TGs with increase in weight: The Coronary Artery Risk Development in Young Adults (CARDIA) Study.

with obesity in women [Figure 3(a) and (b)]. Longitudinal data confirm this association, with an 8-year increase in BMI of 1 U associated with a decrease in HDL-C of approximately 3 mg/dL (Figure 4).[10] Weight-loss studies of longer than 1 year in duration show consistent increases in HDL (Table 1).[3–6,11] Again, there are fewer data available for other ethnic groups, but HDL concentrations are lower with obesity in blacks,[12] Hispanics,[8] and American Indians.[13] Thus, obesity appears to be associated consistently with lower HDL in all ethnic groups.

In contrast to the consistent changes in TGs and HDL, there appears to be less effect of obesity on low-density lipoprotein (LDL) concentrations. NHANES II data indicate that in young (20–44 years

Table 1

Weight Loss and Change in Lipoproteins

Study	N	No. months	% Change		
			TGs	HDL-C	LDL-C
Jalkanen[3]	24	12	−28	+8	NA
Karvetti and Hakala[11]	71F/22M	12	NA	+12	NA
Marniemi et al[4]	27F/10M	12	−41	+18	NA
Wood et al[5]	31F/40M	12	−5/−20	+6	−5
Wood et al[6]	42M	12	−22	+13	−3

TG, triglyceride; HDL-C, high-density lipoprotein cholesterol; LDL-C, low-density lipro-protein cholesterol; F, female; M, male; NA, not available.

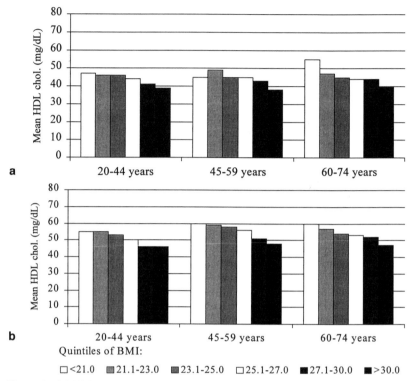

Figure 3. (a) High-density lipoprotein cholesterol (HDL-C) and obesity in white men: NHANES II (b) HDL-C and obesity in white women: NHANES II Adapted with permission from References 1 and 2.

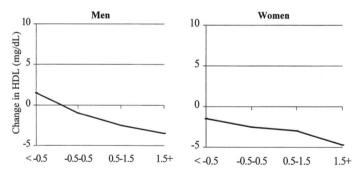

Figure 4. Change in HDL-C levels by change in body mass index (BMI): The Framingham Offspring. Study (aged 20–49 years). Adapted with permission from Reference 10.

old) white men, there is a significant increase in LDL concentration with increasing BMI. Obese young men had approximately 30 mg/dL higher LDL than did those of normal weight [Figure 5(a)].[1] However, in middle-aged and older men, there were only minimal differences in LDL cholesterol (LDL-C) between BMIs in the range of <21.1 kg/m^2 to >30 kg/m^2. In white women, there is again a significant increase in LDL-C with BMI in younger women (20–44 years old), with approximately 20 mg/dL difference between normal-weight and obese individuals [Fig. 5(b)].[2] A relationship also was seen in middle-aged women (45–59 years old), but the increase with increasing BMI was not as great and, in women over the age of 60, there was little association between BMI and LDL. Some longitudinal data show that increases in weight are accompanied by increases in LDL-C (Figure 6).[10] In one such study, a 1-U increase in BMI causes an approximate 5.5-mg/dL increase in LDL-C.[14] However, long-term weight-loss studies are less consistent, with only two[5,6] of five studies[3–6,11] showing significant

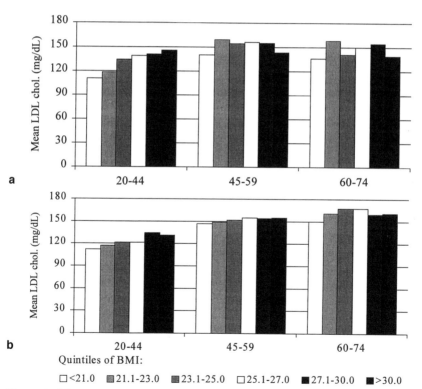

Figure 5. (a) Low-density lipoprotein cholesterol (LDL-C) and obesity in white men: NHANES II (b) LDL-C and obesity in white women: NHANES II. Adapted with permission from References 1 and 2.

decreases in LDL (Table 1). In other racial groups, there appears to be a complex relationship between LDL and obesity.[7] In American Indians, LDL increases over the first three quintiles of BMI and then decreases (Figure 7). Because the American Indian data in the last two quintiles reflect a much greater degree of obesity, it may be that increasing body fat influences LDL in a bimodal fashion, with very large amounts of fat causing decreases in LDL. This could be caused by LDL receptor activity in adipocytes or by dilution of body LDL pools by the increasing plasma volume of very obese subjects.

Despite the lack of consistent changes in LDL concentration with obesity, there is a decrease in LDL size in obese individuals, consistent with their higher TG and lower HDL concentrations. This decrease is observed in whites[15] as well as in other ethnic groups (R. S. Gray, R. R. Fabsitz, L. D. Cowan, unpublished manuscript, 1999).

In addition to the amount of body fat affecting lipoproteins, lipoprotein concentrations also appear to be influenced by the distribution or pattern of body fat. In a study of premenopausal women, adjusted for fat mass, very LDL (VLDL), TG, and HDL-C (inversely) were correlated significantly with fat mass and also with waist-to-hip ratio, an indicator of body fat distribution (Table 2).[16] Similar observations were recorded in a group of 38-year-old European men (Table 3).[17] Waist-to-thigh ratio adjusted for BMI was correlated significantly with TGs and HDL (inversely). Higher TGs and lower HDL concentrations also have been shown in black women with central fat distribution, although the changes do not appear to be as large as in white women.[18] Body fat distribution also is associated with higher TGs and lower HDL in Hispanics[8] and American Indians (R. S. Gray, R. R.

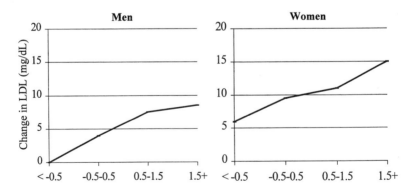

BMI change between Exam 1 (1971-75) and Exam 2 (1979-83)

Figure 6. Change in LDL-C levels by change in BMI: The Framingham Offspring Study (aged 20–49 years). Adapted with permission from Reference 10.

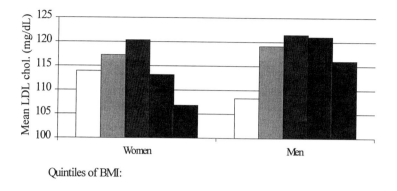

Quintiles of BMI:

☐ <25.1   ▨ 25.11-28.28   ☐ 28.28-31.21   ■ 31.21-35.44   ■ 35.44+

Figure 7. LDL-C and obesity in nondiabetic American Indians (aged 45–74 years): The Strong Heart Study.

Fabsitz, L. D. Cowan, unpublished manuscript, 1999). LDL-C concentration does not appear to be associated with body fat distribution in most studies in any ethnic group, but central body fat is associated with increases in small, dense LDL particles.[15] The combination of high TG concentrations; low HDL; and small, dense LDL is a metabolically interrelated dyslipidemia that has been associated with insulin resistance.[19] Thus, this obesity-associated pattern of dyslipidemia, particularly in those with central adiposity, is likely related to insulin resistance in obese individuals, especially those with a central fat distribution. Studies to date have not differentiated the extent of the effects of central versus peripheral fat on plasma lipoproteins.

Metabolism of Lipoproteins in Obesity

Studies of VLDL and LDL metabolism have provided a possible mechanism for the effects of obesity on lipoprotein concentrations (Table 4; Figure 8). There is a greatly increased production rate of VLDL apolipoprotein (apo)-B and VLDL TGs in obese individuals.[20,21] Thus, the rate of production of VLDL particles in obese individuals appears to be increased. One possible cause of this elevated VLDL production might be increased availability of substrates for TG synthesis, because free fatty acid concentrations tend to be elevated in obese individuals, particularly those with abdominal obesity. The increase in free fatty acids also could be caused by the lipolysis of larger amounts of postprandial particles. An increase in total body cholesterol synthesis in obese individuals provides larger hepatic cholesterol pools, which subsequently stimulate VLDL production (Figure 8).[22]

Table 2

Correlations Between Body Fat Distribution and Lipoprotein Levels in Premenopausal Women

Variable	Full correlations		Partial correlations	
	Fat mass	WHR	Fat mass*	WHR**
VLDL TGs	0.56§	0.49§	0.33‡	0.34‡
HDL-C	−0.47§	−0.45§	−0.27†	−0.30†
LDL-C/LDL TGs	−0.42§	−0.29†	−0.31†	−0.09
				−0.41§
HDL-C/HDL TGs	−0.27†	−0.46§	−0.01	

VLDL, very low-density lipoprotein. Reproduced with permission from Reference 17.
* Adjusted for waist-to-hip ratio (WHR).
** Adjusted for fat mass.
† $P < 0.05$.
‡ $P < 0.01$.
§ $P < 0.001$.

There does not appear to be impaired clearance of VLDL in obese individuals (Table 4). In fact, clearance rates can be higher, most likely a result of the larger VLDL pool.

Examination of LDL metabolism in obese individuals shows several competing changes. Fractional clearance rates of LDL are higher in obese subjects than in lean controls, and a smaller proportion of VLDL is converted to LDL.[20] Thus, despite a greater influx of apoB into the LDL compartment via increased VLDL synthesis, LDL levels may be

Table 3

Regression Coefficients (β) for Obesity Variables in Relation to Serum Lipids in Men Aged 38 Years

	BMI	Waist-to-thigh ratio
TGs	0.052‡	0.88‡
Total cholesterol	0.046†	1.03*
HDL-C	−0.020‡	−0.26†
LDL-C	0.032*	0.56

Adapted with permission from Reference 19.
Adjusted for body mass index (BMI).
* $P < 0.05$.
† $P < 0.01$.
‡ $P < 0.001$.

Table 4

Changes in Lipoprotein Metabolism in Obesity

Increases in

VLDL TG production
VLDL apoB production
VLDL remnant removal
LDL apoB production
LDL apoB clearance
ApoAI or apoAII clearance
Hepatic lipase

apo, apolipoprotein.

normal or even lower in obese individuals because of the increased clearance rate for both VLDL remnants and LDL particles. The change in LDL particle distribution also can be explained by the alterations in VLDL and LDL metabolism, because more rapid VLDL-to-LDL cascade and LDL clearance preferentially remove larger LDL particles.[23]

Fewer data are available on HDL metabolism in obese individuals. Obese women have less HDL_2 cholesterol[24] and smaller, denser HDL particles, and obese individuals have a higher level of hepatic lipase activity. The fractional clearance rate for apoAI, the primary determinant of HDL concentration, is positively associated with both BMI and waist-to-hip ratio.[25] Thus, the lower level of HDL in obesity appears to be attributable to increased catabolism, possibly mediated by greater activity of hepatic lipase.

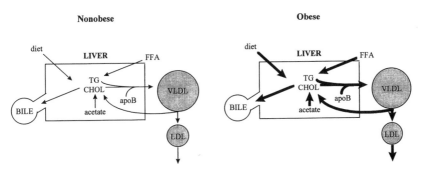

Figure 8. Differences in biliary cholesterol and lipoprotein metabolism between nonobese and obese individuals. Reproduced with permission from Reference 22.

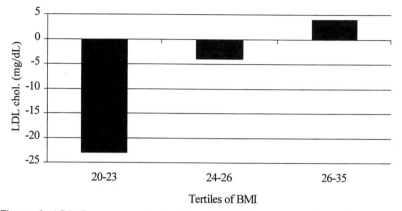

Figure 9. LDL-C response by tertiles of BMI in women. Reproduced with permission from Reference 28.

Cholesterol-Lowering Therapy in Overweight Individuals

Several small studies have shown an association between obesity and reduced response to cholesterol-lowering diets. In a study of obese men and women, there was no change in plasma cholesterol when eggs were removed from the diet as compared with lean subjects who responded with decreases in plasma cholesterol.[26] In a study of hypercholesterolemic women, leaner women had a greater reduction in cholesterol levels than did obese women in response to a very low fat, low-cholesterol [American Heart Association (AHA) phase 3]) diet.[27] In a larger study that compared AHA step I diets with different proportions of mono- and polyunsaturated fatty acids, there was an inverse correlation between BMI and LDL response (Figure 9).[28] This was seen in both white and African American participants. When men and women were analyzed separately, the negative association between obesity and LDL changes was observed in women, but only minimal differences between obese and lean men were seen. Obesity also may affect the response of LDL to pharmacologic intervention. In a study of 6003 individuals, overweight subjects had smaller decreases in cholesterol after treatment with gemfibrozil.[29]

Summary and Conclusions

Obesity in both genders and all ethnic groups studied is associated with a significant dyslipidemia consisting of higher TGs, lower

HDL concentration, and a preponderance of small dense LDL particles. This dyslipidemia is associated with increasing adiposity and, in studies where measures of body fat distribution are available, is associated even more strongly with central or abdominal adiposity. This dyslipidemia previously has been shown to be an essential component of the insulin resistance syndrome.[30] Obesity has been shown in many studies to be associated with increasing insulin resistance, particularly if body fat is distributed centrally or in the abdominal or truncal region. Thus, increasing adiposity, with the associated greater flux of free fatty acids, results in hepatic oversecretion of VLDL, increased clearance of HDL, and a preponderance of small dense LDL particles. The mechanism of these changes is a cholesteryl ester transfer protein (CETP)-mediated exchange of cholesterol and TGs, followed by depletion of the lipids and the LDL particle by hydrolysis.[30] All of the components of this dyslipidemia, including higher TGs, lower HDL, and increases in small dense LDL, have been shown to be atherogenic. Weight loss, even if it does not result in normalization of body weight, can improve this dyslipidemia and thus reduce CVD risk.

Obesity and its relation to LDL-C is more complex. In younger men and premenopausal women, increasing obesity is associated with higher levels of LDL. However, in older white men and women and in some ethnic groups, obesity, and even central fat distribution appear to have less effect on LDL concentrations, and extreme obesity may be associated with lower LDL. Weight loss has been shown to improve LDL concentrations in some and but not all studies. The variability—by gender, ethnicity, and amount of body fat—of the relations of LDL with obesity may explain the differing responses in weight-loss studies. Nevertheless, obese individuals appear to be less responsive to dietary approaches to cholesterol lowering and perhaps more resistant to the pharmacologic effect of lipid-lowering drugs. Thus, weight loss certainly should be included among the therapeutic strategies for all individuals with elevated LDL if they are above normal body weight.

Many unanswered questions remain concerning both the specific metabolic mechanisms of the dyslipidemia in obesity and the strategies and mechanisms of improvements that might be effected by weight loss or other therapeutic interventions. With the increasing rate of obesity in the United States and the increased CVD risk in these individuals, more studies are warranted.

References

1. Denke MA, Sempos CT, Grundy SM. Excess body weight. An underrecognized contributor to high blood cholesterol levels in white American men. *Arch Intern Med* 1993;153:1093–1103.

2. Denke MA, Sempos CT, Grundy SM. Excess body weight. An under-recognized contributor to dyslipidemia in white American women. *Arch Intern Med* 1994;154:401–410.
3. Jalkanen L. The effect of a weight reduction program on cardiovascular risk factors among overweight hypertensives in primary health care. *Scand J Soc Med* 1991;19:66–71.
4. Marniemi J, Seppanen A, Hakala P. Long-term effects on lipid metabolism of weight reduction on lactovegetarian and mixed diet. *Int J Obes* 1990;14: 113–125.
5. Wood PD, Stefanick ML, Williams PT, et al. The effects on plasma lipoproteins of a prudent weight-reducing diet, with or without exercise, in overweight men and women. *N Engl J Med* 1991;325:461–466.
6. Wood PD, Stefanick ML, Dreon DM, et al. Changes in plasma lipids and lipoproteins in overweight men during weight loss through dieting as compared with exercise. *N Engl J Med* 1988;319:1173–1179.
7. Folsom AR, Burke GL, Ballew C, et al. Relation of body fatness and its distribution to cardiovascular risk factors in young blacks and whites. The role of insulin. *Am J Epidemiol* 1989;130:911–924.
8. Haffner SM, Stern MP, Hazuda HP, et al. Do upper-body and centralized adiposity measure different aspects of regional body-fat distribution? Relationship to non-insulin-dependent diabetes mellitus, lipids, and lipoproteins. *Diabetes* 1987;36:43–51.
9. Howard BV, Bogardus C, Ravussin E, et al. Studies of the etiology of obesity in Pima Indians. *Am J Clin Nutr* 1991;53:1577S–1585S.
10. Anderson KM, Wilson PW, Garrison RJ, et al. Longitudinal and secular trends in lipoprotein cholesterol measurements in a general population sample. The Framingham Offspring Study. *Atherosclerosis* 1987;68:59–66.
11. Karvetti RL, Hakala P. A seven-year follow-up of a weight reduction programme in Finnish primary health care. *Eur J Clin Nutr* 1992;46:743–752.
12. Burke GL, Bild DE, Hilner JE, et al. Differences in weight gain in relation to race, gender, age and education in young adults: The CARDIA Study. *Coronary Artery Risk Development in Young Adults Ethn Health* 1996;1:327–335.
13. Howard BV, Davis MP, Pettitt DJ, et al. Plasma and lipoprotein cholesterol and triglyceride concentrations in the Pima Indians: Distributions differing from those of Caucasians. *Circulation* 1983;68:714–724.
14. Shekelle RB, Shryock AM, Paul O, et al. Diet, serum cholesterol, and death from coronary heart disease. The Western Electric Study. *N Engl J Med* 1981;304:65–70.
15. Williams PT, Krauss RM. Associations of age, adiposity, menopause, and alcohol intake with low-density lipoprotein subclasses. *Arterioscler Thromb Vasc Biol* 1997;17:1082–1090.
16. Despres JP, Moorjani S, Lupien PJ, et al. Regional distribution of body fat, plasma lipoproteins, and cardiovascular disease. *Arteriosclerosis* 1990;10: 497–511.
17. Seidell JC, Cigolini M, Deslypere JP, et al. Body fat distribution in relation to serum lipids and blood pressure in 38-year-old European men: The European Fat Distribution Study. *Atherosclerosis* 1991;86:251–260.
18. Dowling HJ, Pi-Sunyer FX. Race-dependent health risks of upper body obesity. *Diabetes* 1993;42:537–543.

19. Howard BV. Insulin actions in vivo: Insulin and lipoprotein metabolism. In: Alberti KGMM, DeFronzo RA, Keen H, eds. *International Textbook of Diabetes Mellitus.* 2nd ed. West Sussex, UK: John Wiley & Sons; 1995.

20. Egusa G, Beltz WF, Grundy SM, et al. The influence of obesity on the metabolism of apolipoprotein B in man. *J Clin Invest* 1985;76:596–603.

21. Kesaniemi YA, Beltz WF, Grundy SM. Comparisons of metabolism of apolipoprotein B in normal subjects, obese patients, and patients with coronary heart disease. *J Clin Invest* 1985;76:586–595.

22. Howard BV. Obesity, cholelithiasis, and lipoprotein metabolism in man. In: Grundy SM, ed. *Bile Acids and Atherosclerosis.* Vol 15. New York: Raven Press; 1986:169–186.

23. Gaw A, Packard CJ, Murray EF, et al. Effects of Simvastatin on apo B metabolism and LDL subfraction distrubution. *Arterioscler Thromb* 1993;13:170–189.

24. Howard BV, Xiaoren P, Harper I, et al. Lack of sex differences in high density lipoproteins in Pima Indians. Studies of obesity, lipase activities, and steroid hormones. *Arteriosclerosis* 1987;7:292–300.

25. Brinton EA, Eisenberg S, Breslow JL. Human HDL cholesterol levels are determined by apo A-1 fractional catabolic rate, which correlates inversely with estimates of HDL particle size: Effects of gender, hepatic and lipoprotein lipases, triglyceride and insulin levels, and body fat distribution. *Arterioscler Thromb* 1994;14:707–720.

26. Bronsgeest-Schoute DC, Hermus RJJ, Dallinga-Thie GM, et al. Dependence of the effects of dietary cholesterol and experimental conditions on serum lipids in man: The effect on serum cholesterol of removal of eggs from the diet of free-living habitually egg-eating people. *Am J Clin Nutr* 1979;32:2193–2197.

27. Cole TG, Bowen PE, Schmeisser D, et al. Differential reduction of plasma cholesterol by the American Heart Association Phase 3 diet in moderately hypercholesterolemic, premenopausal women with different body mass indexes. *Am J Clin Nutr* 1992;55:385–394.

28. Hannah JS, Jablonski KA, Howard BV. The relationship between weight and response to cholesterol-lowering diets in women. *Int J Obes* 1997;21:445–450.

29. Muls E, van Gral L, Vansant G. Effects of initial BMI and on-treatment weight change on the lipid-lowering efficacy of fibrates. *Int J Obes* 1997;21:155–158.

30. Howard BV. Insulin actions in vivo: Insulin and lipoprotein metabolism. In: Alberti KGMM, Zimmet P, DeFronzo RA, et al, eds. *International Textbook of Diabetes Mellitus,* Second Edition. West Sussex, UK: John Wiley & Sons, Ltd; 1995.

Chapter 10

Is Insulin Resistance an Independent Risk Factor for Coronary Heart Disease?

Scott M. Grundy, MD, PhD

Introduction

Insulin resistance is a condition characterized by multiple aberrations in the metabolism of carbohydrate and lipids. The defining feature of insulin resistance is reduced ability of insulin to exert its actions in various tissues and organs. The presence of insulin resistance often is reflected by hyperinsulinemia. There is a growing belief that the state of insulin resistance is a precursor for two major diseases: type II diabetes and coronary heart disease (CHD). In fact, many investigators hold the view that insulin resistance is a risk factor for CHD. The purpose of this discussion is to examine the question of whether insulin resistance is an "independent" risk factor for CHD. This is an important but exceedingly complex question. A simple answer may not be forthcoming. There seems to be little doubt that insulin resistance is "associated" with an increased risk for CHD, but the nature of this association is open to question. This discussion will examine the nature of this link.

Categories of Risk Factors

To understand the connection between various risk factors and risk for CHD an appropriate categorization of risk factors is required. Four major categories of risk factors are "causal," "conditional," "predisposing," and "coronary plaque burden." Two other characteristics

From: Fletcher GF, Grundy SM, Hayman LL (eds). *Obesity: Impact on Cardiovascular Disease*. Armonk, NY: Futura Publishing Co., Inc.; © 1999.

of risk factors are their "frequency" in the population and their "independence" from other risk factors. Causal risk factors that contribute importantly to CHD in a population because of their high frequency are called "major" risk factors. Those that exert their causality independently of other causes are called "independent" risk factors. Each of these categories of risk factors and their qualities deserve some attention.

Causal Risk Factors

Several factors raise the risk for CHD by their direct effects on the arterial wall. In so doing, they promote atherogenesis or in related ways bring about acute coronary events (unstable angina and myocardial infarction). The well-established causal risk factors include cigarette smoking, hypertension, elevated serum cholesterol [and low-density lipoprotein (LDL) cholesterol], reduced high-density lipoprotein (HDL) cholesterol, and diabetes mellitus.[1] The precise mechanisms whereby each of these factors contributes to the development of CHD are not understood fully; evidence for a direct influence on atherogenesis nonetheless is strong. In addition, these risk factors appear to be independent of one another in their atherogenic effect. The prime risk factor among the major risk factors is an elevated LDL cholesterol. LDL is necessary for atherogenesis; when LDL levels are low, rates of CHD likewise are low even when other risk factors are present.[2] In the presence of some elevation of LDL cholesterol, the other major risk factors assume increasing importance.

Conditional Risk Factors

These factors prospectively associate with CHD and may promote atherogenesis, although conclusive proof is lacking. Evidence supporting an independent role in atherogenesis for most of them is growing. They include high levels of triglyceride-rich lipoproteins (TGRLP), small LDL particles, lipoprotein (a) [Lp(a)], homocysteine, and various prothrombotic factors [eg, fibrinogen and plasminogen activator inhibitor-1 (PAI-1)]. Another conditional risk factor is impaired fasting glucose (IFG). The issue of independent atherogenicity of the conditional risk factors is important, especially because many of them are common in patients with insulin resistance.

Predisposing Risk Factors

This category includes factors that do not directly promote atherogenesis but do influence other causal (and conditional) risk factors.

They include obesity, physical inactivity, family history of premature CHD, and male sex. Besides affecting known causal risk factors, they may modify adversely "unidentified" causal risk factors. Some of the latter could be the conditional risk factors that have yet to be proven to be atherogenic; others may be truly unidentified. There has long been a dispute whether the predisposing risk factors also are independent risk factors. This question should be rephrased as follows: do the predisposing risk factors promote atherogenesis through unidentified risk factors in addition to affecting known causal risk factors? Prospective epidemiological studies indeed suggest that some of the predisposing risk factors act independently of the known causal risk factors, but the strength of this independence varies from study to study.

Atherosclerotic Plaque Burden

The presence of atherosclerotic plaques in the coronary arteries poses a threat for the occurrence of major coronary events (ie, unstable angina or myocardial infarction). These occur when plaques undergo rupture or erosion and produce an obstructing thrombus. Follow-up of patients undergoing angiographic studies shows that the probability of plaque rupture is proportional to the extent and severity of coronary lesions, or plaque burden.[3,4] One indicator of the plaque burden is a person's age. In most people, coronary atherosclerosis develops slowly but progressively throughout life; older people on the average have a greater plaque burden than do younger ones. Therefore, in assessment of coronary risk, the age factor is used as a surrogate for plaque burden. In the future, newer techniques of noninvasive assessment of subclinical atherosclerosis may be employed instead as an indicator of plaque burden.

Mechanisms of Insulin Action

To understand the effects of insulin resistance on coronary risk, it may be useful to review the essential actions of insulin on cellular function. The major sites of insulin action are skeletal muscle, adipose tissue, and liver, but other tissues also are insulin sensitive. In recent years, mechanisms whereby insulin exerts its actions have become better understood.[5–10] The action of insulin is initiated by the binding of insulin to the insulin receptor, a transmembrane glycoprotein possessing protein tyrosine kinase activity. Activation of receptor tyrosine kinase by insulin causes autophosphorylation of the receptor itself as well as phosphorylation of other proteins. Two of these other proteins are "docking proteins," insulin receptor substrate 1 (IRS-1) and substrate 2 (IRS-2). Phosphorylation of IRS-1 causes it to associate with other signaling molecules that contain SRC-2 homology domains. Two of the proteins that bind to IRS-1 are phosphatidylinositol-3 kinase (PI-3 kinase) and Ras protein. Progressive phosphorylations lead to activation of several more serine/threanine protein kinases leading to branching cascades. One protein in this sequence is the mitogen-activity protein (MAP) kinase. The spread of activation through these cascades is responsible for the pleiotrophic actions of insulin. Some of these pathways initiate short-term actions of insulin whereas others induce immediate metabolic reactions; yet others give long-term effects on cellular growth and differentiation.

One of the major outcomes of insulin action is an enhanced uptake of glucose by cells. This response appears to be mediated via activation of PI-3 kinase. The result is recruitment of vesicles containing a glucose transporter, GLUT-4, or recruitment of GLUT-4 from unique intracellular locations.[11-16] GLUT-4 transfers to the plasma membrane where it facilitates the transport of glucose into cells.

The number of other biochemical pathways influenced by insulin action is myriad. For present purposes, actions can be divided into stimulatory and inhibitory. Examples of these two categories are listed in Table 1. Besides stimulating the transport of glucose into cells, insulin promotes the synthesis of glycogen,[17-19] enhances the synthesis of fatty acids,[20,21] increases the synthesis of enzymes and other proteins,[21-27] and modifies differentiation and proliferation of cells. An inhibitory action of insulin is curtailment of hepatic gluconeogene-

Table 1

Categories of Insulin Action

Stimulatory Actions
- Promotes glucose transport into cells
- Enhances glycogen synthesis
- Increases fatty acid synthesis
- Promotes protein synthesis
- Modifies cellular differentiation and proliferation

Inhibitory Actions
- Inhibits gluconeogenesis
  Reduces hepatic glucose output
- Inhibits release of nonesterified fatty acids from adipose tissue
- Suppresses lipid-related factors
  Apolipoprotein-B-100
  Apolipoprotein-C-III
  Hepatic lipase

sis,[28–32] causing a reduction in hepatic glucose output. Insulin also inhibits the release of nonesterified fatty acids (NEFA) from adipose tissue[33]; during fasting, when plasma insulin levels are low, NEFA becomes a major source of energy, whereas in the postabsorptive state, when insulin levels are high, glucose is the predominant energy source.[34] Insulin action further inhibits a number of key pathways of related to lipid and lipoprotein metabolism[35–41]; for example, insulin action reduces the synthesis of apolipoprotein B and possibly apolipoprotein CIII and hepatic lipase.

Mechanisms of Insulin Resistance

The term "insulin resistance" implies an impaired cellular responsiveness to insulin. When insulin resistance is present, the stimulatory and inhibitory actions of insulin are impaired. Insulin resistance theoretically can exist at several levels (Table 2). First, the function of the insulin receptor could be defective, such that initiation of insulin signaling is impaired. Second, pathways of insulin-signaling cascades could be defective at multiple sites. Third, abnormalities may occur in ultimate targets of insulin action. Fourth, abnormalities in adipose tissue may lead to an elevated plasma NEFA, another putative cause of insulin resistance. Fifth, noninsulin regulators of metabolic processes may be abnormal causing insulin resistance as a secondary response. Finally, access of insulin to insulin receptors might be impaired because of circulating deficiencies or endothelial dysfunction. Examples of each of these forms for insulin resistance can be examined.

Defects at the level of the insulin receptor can cause insulin resistance. Several different types of defects occur. Multiple different mutations in the insulin receptor have been identified.[42–44] For example, genetic disorders named leprechaunism, Rabson-Mendenhall syndrome, and type A insulin resistance result from insulin receptor mutations; these disorders seemingly represent a spectrum of defects of the insulin receptor structure giving various severities of functional defects.[43] Mutations of the insulin receptor are of theoretical interest because they illustrate the metabolic consequences of severe insulin resistance; even so, they occur infrequently and thus account for only a small portion of the insulin resistance in the general population. Other abnormalities may impair the activation of the insulin receptor and also cause insulin resistance. One rare example is the presence of autoantibodies that block the insulin receptor (autoimmune insulin resistance). Recent studies[45,46] further show that tumor necrosis factor-α (TNF-α) can interfere with insulin action; this cytokine seemingly enhances the activity of protein kinase C (PKC), a kinase that phos-

Table 2

Candidates for Insulin Resistance

Defects in Insulin Receptor Function
- Mutations in the insulin receptor
- Antibodies to insulin receptor
- Impaired phosphorylation of insulin receptor
  Tumor necrosis factor-α (TNF-α)
  Protein Kinase C (PKC)

Defects in Insulin Signaling
- Insulin receptor substrates (IRS-1 and IRS-2)
- Other defects in phosphorylation cascade
  Phosphoinositide-3-kinase (PI-3 kinase)
  c-Cbl-associated protein (CAP)
- Excess intracellular fatty acids

Defects in Insulin Targets
- Glucose transporters (esp. GLUT-4)
- Glycogen synthase
- Lipid and lipoprotein regulators

Defects in Other Metabolic Regulators
- Uncoupling proteins (UCP-2 and UCP-3)
- Leptin
- β-3-adrenergic receptor

Causes of Elevated Plasma Nonesterified Fatty Acids (NEFA)
- Adipose tissue disorders
  Predominant truncal obesity
- Androgens
  Lipodystrophies
  Functional defect in NEFA release
- Excess glucocorticoids

Defects in Access of Insulin to Insulin Receptors
  Single gateway hypothesis

phorylates of serine residues of the insulin receptor.[47,48] Phosphorylation of serine on the insulin receptor at the expense of theronine apparently prevents the receptor from interacting normally with IRS-1 and IRS-2; this redirection of phosphorylation thus can induce insulin resistance.

A second set of abnormalities occurs in insulin-signaling pathways; these abnormalities theoretically could evoke insulin resistance.[49-56] For instance, mutations in the docking proteins, IRS-1 and IRS-2, like those of the insulin receptors, may produce insulin resistance. Indeed, polymorphisms in IRS-1 have been reported to associate with insulin resistance in humans;[57] whether these polymorphisms actually cause insulin resistance has been difficult to prove. Nevertheless, mice in which IRS-1 has been deleted manifest insulin resistance, as do those without IRS-2. Polymorphisms in other proteins of the insulin-signaling pathways theoretically could elicit insulin resistance.

However, such functional polymorphisms remain to be identified. One protein, c-Cbl–associated protein (CAP), appears to be involved in insulin signaling,[53] and its expression is enhanced by thiazolidinediones, an activator of the nuclear peroxicome proliferator activated receptor (PPAR)-γ. Thus, activation of this receptor could modulate the insulin-signaling pathways; if so, abnormalities in PPAR-γ function might be accompanied by insulin resistance.

The role that fatty acids plays in regulating insulin signaling and action has long been a topic of speculation. Randle[58] long ago proposed that high levels of circulating NEFA interfere with glucose oxidation and induce insulin resistance. Subsequent studies[59–61] support the concept that excess circulating NEFA reduce insulin sensitivity. Randle and associates[62,63] postulate that the presence of excess fatty acids in cells retards the oxidation of glucose by inactivating pyruvate dehydrogenase (PDH) complex, a key regulator of glucose oxidation. These workers[62,63] speculate that products of fatty acid oxidation enhance the activity of PDH kinase; the resulting phosphorylation of PDH inactivates the complex. In spite of long-term acceptance of the "Randle hypothesis," precise mechanisms whereby excess NEFA in cells reduce tissue sensitivity to insulin are not well understood. Moreover, some workers[64] suggest that high concentrations of intracellular fatty acid induce insulin resistance through other mechanisms. For instance, fatty acids can interact with PPARs and perhaps influence insulin sensitivity through this pathway. The interference of insulin signaling by excess intracellular NEFA appears to occur, but the mechanistic details remain to be elucidated.

One of the major actions of insulin is to promote the transport of glucose into cells. Should defects occur in the synthesis or function of glucose transporters (eg, GLUT-4), insulin function could be impaired.[65,66] Indeed, in mice, deletion of GLUT-4 engenders insulin resistance and diabetes.[65,66] Whether similar abnormalities in the function of GLUT-4 exist in humans remains unknown; however, this possible abnormality serves to illustrate how defects in targets of insulin action might produce insulin resistance or defective insulin action. For example, if defects were to exist in insulin-response elements in various insulin-sensitive genes, insulin action could be impaired. This possibility especially could occur in genes regulating the metabolism of lipids and lipoproteins.

Other candidates for contributors to insulin resistance include defects in noninsulin metabolic regulators, defects in adipose tissue leading to elevated plasma NEFA, and circulatory abnormalities causing reduced access of insulin to insulin receptors in cells of various tissues. Other metabolic regulators that may be abnormal include leptin,[67] uncoupling proteins,[68] and β-3-adrenergic receptors.[69] Potential causes of elevated plasma NEFA will be discussed later. Finally, insulin resistance theoretically could occur from a delay in transport of insulin across the endothelium of insulin-sensitive tissues, such as skeletal muscle.[70]

Major Factors Underlying Insulin Resistance

Obesity and Other Disorders of Adipose Tissue

One major contributor to insulin resistance is obesity. In fact, up to 50% of the variation in insulin sensitivity in populations can be explained by differences in body fat content of the individual.[71-73] The mechanisms whereby obesity influences insulin sensitivity in tissues throughout the body are not understood fully. The best-known hypothesis is that high levels of circulating NEFA resulting from obesity induce insulin resistance. Possible mechanisms for the NEFA influence at the cellular level were discussed previously.[58-63] Additionally, excess adipose tissue may release factors, such as TNF-α, that impair insulin sensitivity.[45,46] Without question the increasing prevalence of obesity in the United States augments the frequency of insulin resistance and enhances its severity among Americans.

Even mild obesity can worsen insulin resistance when it occurs in the presence of certain variations and/or disorders of adipose tissue. The most common variation is accumulation of fat predominantly in the body trunk. This condition is manifested by an increase in the ratio of waist-to-hip circumference and by an increase in waist circumference.[74-76] The latter increase depicts "abdominal obesity"; however, this term is somewhat of a misnomer, because excess fat is present subcutaneously over the whole trunk.[72,73] Abdominal obesity occurs commonly in overweight men; but approximately 20% of women also are susceptible to abdominal obesity with even moderate weight gain.[74-76] An excess of truncal fat is associated with increased concentrations of NEFA, and the latter probably account for the insulin resistance accompanying abdominal obesity. Seemingly, truncal adipose tissue has a more rapid turnover rate of fatty acids than does peripheral adipose tissue.[77] Androgens are a major factor responsible for the predominant deposition of fat in the trunk. This is shown by the tendency of men to develop abdominal obesity, whereas women typically manifest gluterofemoral obesity. In women with polycystic ovaries, which produce an excess of androgens, abdominal obesity and insulin resistance are common.[78,79] High levels of androgens consequently must be considered as one cause of insulin resistance, albeit through an indirect mechanism. Rare disorders of adipose tissue include "generalized lipodystrophy" and "partial lipodystrophy." The former is characterized by a complete absence of adipose tissue, the latter by a loss of adipose tissue in certain regions of the body, particularly the extremities. Lipodystrophy usually is accompanied by severe insulin resistance.[80] The causes of genetic forms of lipodystrophy are not known. Recently, the chromosomal location of the gene for familial partial lipodystrophy has been reported;[81] moreover, deletion of a transcriptional factor in mice results in a condition resembling the human disorder of familial generalized lipodystrophy.[82]

Finally, another disorder of adipose tissue could be one in which insulin signaling is defective in a way such that circulating insulin fails to suppress normally the release of NEFA. In other words, because of excessive release of NEFA, reduced insulin sensitivity in adipose tissue could elicit whole-body insulin resistance. It has been claimed that obesity itself is accompanied by insulin resistance in adipose tissue. This, however, may not be the case. In obese persons, elevated NEFA levels in the presence of hyperinsulinemia merely may reflect continued baseline release of NEFA secondary to an increased number of adipocytes. Still, truncal adipose tissue does appear to be more insulin resistant inherently than is gluterofemoral fat; this may explain why predominant truncal obesity causes whole-body insulin resistance. Moreover, excess circulating corticosteroids (or defective corticoid receptors in adipose tissue) may interfere with normal insulin signaling in adipose tissue and thereby cause excessive release of NEFA.[83–86] Also, a recent report from our laboratory indicated that many patients with endogenous hypertriglyceridemia have excessive release of NEFA independent of abdominal obesity.[87] Others report similarly for patients with familial combined hyperlipidemia.[88] Both forms of dyslipidemia typically are associated with insulin resistance. These findings suggest a primary defect in insulin signaling in adipose tissue.

Physical Inactivity

Another contributor to insulin resistance can be physical inactivity, an influence that can be reversed partially by physical activity.[89–91] The high prevalence of sedentary life habits among Americans consequently must be counted as another cause of insulin resistance in our society. Recent studies[92–94] have shown that physical activity increases the expression of GLUT-4 in skeletal muscle and thus may account for its ability to reduce insulin resistance. The potential for regular exercise to reduce insulin resistance is impressive;[95] this points to the need for increased physical activity as one approach to diminishing the burden of insulin resistance in the American population.

Aging

Several investigations[96–98] reveal that insulin resistance rises with advancing age. Undoubtedly, an increasing percentage of body fat in older people and reduced physical activity partially are responsible. Other factors may be at play as well. Cellular efficiency may decline with aging; if this is a general response, one of the pathways affected could be insulin signaling. Alternatively, a decline of muscle mass with advancing age should reduce overall metabolic efficiency and lead to cellular accumulation of energy sources; this accumulation could reduce insulin sensitivity. Still, the increase in insulin resistance with advancing age should be minimized by keeping total body fat content low and by exercise sufficient to maintain muscle mass.

Genetic Factors

The identification of rare genetic forms of insulin resistance raises the question of how much of the variation in insulin sensitivity in the general population can be explained by genetic factors. To date, this question has not been answered. A certain portion of this variation likely can be explained by genetic polymorphism in the insulin receptor, in the insulin-signaling pathway, and in insulin-response elements. But in addition, other genetic abnormalities could affect insulin sensitivity through various mechanisms. As already noted, several disorders of adipose tissue are known to produce insulin resistance; these include abnormalities in body fat distribution, different forms of lipodystrophy, and inherent variations in insulin sensitivity of adipose tissue. The search for common genetic causes of insulin resistance is important. If these could be identified, they might become targets for modification with drug therapy.

Metabolic Consequences of Insulin Resistance

The metabolic consequences arising out of a state of insulin resistance presumably can be explained by a reversal of the primary actions of insulin shown in Table 1. A complete absence of insulin secretion of course leads to the severe metabolic derangements found in type I diabetes. With insulin resistance, on the other hand, metabolic processes are deranged only mildly and do not threaten life immediately. Still, if sustained over a period of many years, they may predispose to certain chronic diseases, one of which is CHD. The metabolic abnormalities associated with chronic insulin resistance tend to cluster together in single individuals; this clustering has been called the "metabolic syndrome" (Table 3). Some of the risk factors of the metabolic syndrome are causal risk factors; others are the conditional risk factors that also may be directly atherogenic. Each category of risk factor can be reviewed briefly.

Atherogenic Dyslipidemia

This form of dyslipidemia is manifest by three lipoprotein abnormalities: elevated TGRLP, small LDL particles, and low-HDL levels. The majority of patients with atherogenic dyslipidemia have insulin resistance.[87,99] Two of the components of this dyslipidemia—elevated TGRLP and small LDL particles—are conditional risk factors; the third, a low-HDL level, is a documented causal risk factor. Indeed, there is growing evidence that all three abnormalities are atherogenic independently. As such they represent a set of lipoprotein abnormalities that promote atherosclerosis independently of an elevated LDL cholesterol.

Hypertension

Several reviews[100–102] summarize the relationship between insulin resistance and hypertension, the latter being one of the components of the metabolic syndrome. Hypertension has a multifactorial etiology; certainly, insulin resistance is only one of several conditions underlying an elevated blood pressure. The mechanisms whereby insulin resistance raises the blood pressure have been a matter for speculation.[100–102] Some investigators suggest that hyperinsulinemia enhances

---

Table 3

Metabolic Syndrome

Atherogenic Dyslipidemia
- Elevated TGRLP
- Increased small LDL particles
- Reduced HDL cholesterol

Hypertension

Glucose Intolerance
- IFG*
- Categorical hyperglycemia[†]

Prothrombotic State

---

* IFG: plasma glucose 110–125 mg/dL.

[†] Categorical hyperglycemia: plasma glucose ≥ 126 mg/dL.

the activity of the sympathetic nervous system that in turn raises the blood pressure. Others propose that elevated insulin concentrations promote sodium retention by the kidneys. Finally, it has been postulated that insulin resistance impairs normal transport of calcium across cellular membranes, which induces arteriolar vasoconstriction and raised blood pressure. Thus, the potential importance of insulin resistance in the etiology of "essential" hypertension is great but remains uncertain; the mechanisms underlying this association nonetheless are worthy of aggressive investigation.

Elevated Plasma Glucose

Fasting and postprandial glucose levels usually are normal for several years in patients with insulin resistance. This is because pancreatic β-cells normally can secrete enough insulin in response to insulin resistance to maintain glucose levels in the normal range. However, with aging, insulin secretion declines, and elevated glucose concentrations may appear in the face of insulin resistance. Before the onset of categorical hyperglycemia, the insulin-resistant patient usually manifests IFG, that is, a fasting plasma glucose of 110–125 mg/dL. This level of glucose, which is related closely to the category called impaired glucose tolerance (IGT), is a risk correlate of CHD. Certainly, once categorical hyperglycemia develops, the elevated glucose level is an independent risk factor for CHD. Whether IFG is truly an independent (or causal) risk factor for CHD or is only an indicator of the presence of insulin resistance remains uncertain.[103]

Prothrombotic State

Patients with insulin resistance often manifest several alterations in coagulation that may predispose acute thrombotic syndromes of coronary disease. Abnormalities that have been reported include increased serum fibrinogen,[104] increased pPAI-1,[105] and various platelet abnormalities.[106] The metabolic mechanisms underlying these abnormalities have not been elucidated.

Metabolic Syndrome and Coronary Heart Disease

Many patients with premature CHD have the clustering of metabolic risk factors that make up the metabolic syndrome. Because multiple risk factors often occur together, it has been difficult to define for individuals or for populations the specific contributions of individual risk factors to atherogenesis and to the development of CHD. This definition is confounded by the realization that some of the risk factors of the metabolic syndrome are conditional and have not been proven to be causal. Nonetheless, circumstantial evidence is growing that most of the risk factors play some role in atherogenesis; and ultimately, it is likely that the metabolic syndrome will be viewed as a constellation of risk factors acting independently but in concert to promote atherogenesis.

Insulin Resistance as a Predisposing Risk Factor

An important question is whether insulin resistance should be added to the list of predisposing risk factors? Several of the established predisposing risk factors—obesity, physical inactivity, family history, and possibly male sex—all can enhance insulin resistance. In fact, insulin resistance may be an intermediate link in the chain of causality between predisposing and causal risk factors. If insulin resistance per se is a true cause of the causal risk factors then it must be classified as a predisposing risk factor. There is no question that insulin resistance is associated strongly with causal risk factors. The strongest connections are with hypertension, low-HDL cholesterol concentrations, and hyperglycemia. The precise molecular mechanisms underlying these associations are not entirely clear, but there is little doubt that the metabolic alterations accompanying insulin resistance contribute in one or more ways to these risk factors.

In addition, insulin resistance is tied closely to several conditional risk factors: elevated TGRLP, small LDL particles, IFG, and a pro-thrombotic state. If these conditional risk factors prove to be atherogenic directly, insulin resistance will count as a predisposing risk factor for these factors as well. Finally, it is possible that insulin resistance underlies unidentified atherogenic factors that directly predispose to CHD. One possible factor is hyperinsulinemia, of which some investigators suggest an atherogenic potential. Another is an elevation in plasma NEFA, which could act at the level of the arterial wall to directly promote development of atherosclerosis. These possibilities among others remain the realm of speculation.

Insulin Resistance as a Causal Risk Factor

Also in the area of speculation is whether insulin resistance occurring in the cells of the arterial wall might modify the behavior of cells so as to promote atherogenesis. Studies on the pathogenesis of atherosclerosis are focusing increasingly on the role of local factors within the arterial wall. Three types of cells—macrophages, endothelial cells, and smooth muscle cells—have become the targets of intensive research. Each cell type is involved one way or another in atherogenesis. The extent to which the cellular defects of insulin resistance extend to these cells of the arterial wall is unknown; however, if their function is deranged in patients with insulin resistance, these derangements could promote atherogenesis. Investigation into the possibility that insulin resistance might have a direct atherogenic action, working through abnormalities in macrophages, endothelial cells, or smooth muscle cells, could prove to be fruitful.

Insulin Resistance as an Independent Risk Factor

If insulin resistance can be classified as a predisposing risk factor, its independence as a risk factor would depend on whether it acts through unidentified risk factors and beyond its action on the known causal risk factors. Indeed, the possibilities for independence are rich. In part this question is confounded by the apparent link between insulin resistance and conditional risk factors. If conditional risk factors are in fact unidentified causal risk factors, then independence would be enhanced. Should any of these conditional risk factors become accepted as causal risk factors, the independence of insulin resistance as a risk factor would be reduced accordingly. Even so, there are other possibilities for unidentified causal risk factors beyond current causal (and conditional) risk factors.

Any discussion of the independence of insulin resistance as a coronary risk factor may seem esoteric. However, this may not be the case. There seems to be a strong association between insulin resistance and CHD, particularly in some populations. For example, in South Asians, who have a high prevalence of insulin resistance, the risk for CHD appears to be much higher than can be explained through conventional risk factors.[107–109] The experience in this population raises the distinct possibility that the risk-enhancing actions of insulin resistance are acting through yet unidentified risk factors. Thus, epidemiological studies in various populations point in the direction of an independent relation between insulin resistance and CHD risk. This possibility raises the need for further investigation on the nature of the link. Indeed, the nature of the association between insulin resistance and CHD risk is one of the major unresolved issues in the overall field of atherogenesis.

References

1. Wilson PW, D'Agostino RB, Levy D, et al. Prediction of coronary heart disease using risk factor categories. *Circulation* 1998;97:1837–1847.
2. Grundy SM, Wilhelmsen L, Rose G, et al. Coronary heart disease in high-risk populations: Lessons from Finland. *Eur Heart J* 1990;11:462–471.
3. Ringqvist I, Fisher LD, Mock M, et al. Prognostic value of angiographic indices of coronary artery disease from the Coronary Artery Surgery Study (CASS). *J Clin Invest* 1983;71:1854–1866.
4. Emond M, Mock MB, Davis KB, et al. Long-term survival of medically treated patients in the Coronary Artery Surgery Study (CASS) Registry. *Circulation* 1994;90:2645–2657.
5. Myers MG Jr, Sun XJ, White MF. The IRS-1 signaling system. *Trends Biochem Sci* 1994;19:289–293.
6. Myers MG Jr, White MF. Insulin signal transduction and the IRS proteins. *Annu Rev Pharmacol Toxicol* 1996;36:615–658.
7. Kasuga M. Role of PI3-kinase and SH-PTP2 in insulin action. *Diabet Med* 1996;13:S87–S89.
8. Saltiel AR. Diverse signaling pathways in the cellular actions of insulin. *Am J Physiol* 1996;270:E375–E385.
9. Moule SK, Denton RM. Multiple signaling pathways involved in the metabolic effects of insulin. *Am J Cardiol* 1997;80:41A–49A.
10. White MF. The insulin signalling system and the IRS proteins. *Diabetologia* 1997;40:S2–S17.
11. Cushman SW, Simpson IA. Integral membrane protein translocations in the mechanism of insulin action. *Biochem Soc Symp* 1985;50:127–149.
12. Holman GD, Cushman SW. Subcellular localization and trafficking of the GLUT4 glucose transporter isoform in insulin-responsive cells. *Bioessays* 1994;16:753–759.
13. Ebeling P, Koistinen HA, Koivisto VA. Insulin-independent glucose transport regulates insulin sensitivity. *FEBS Lett* 1998;436:301–303.
14. Kahn BB. Lilly lecture 1995. Glucose transport: Pivotal step in insulin action. *Diabetes* 1996;45:1644–1654.
15. Rea S, James DE. Moving GLUT4: The biogenesis and trafficking of GLUT4 storage vesicles. *Diabetes.* 1997;46:1667–1677.
16. Cushman SW, Goodyear LJ, Pilch PF, et al. Molecular mechanisms involved in GLUT4 translocation in muscle during insulin and contraction stimulation. *Adv Exp Med Biol* 1998;441:63–71.
17. Azpiazu I, Saltiel AR, DePaoli-Roach AA, et al. Regulation of both glycogen synthase and PHAS-I by insulin in rat skeletal muscle involves mitogen-activated protein kinase-independent and rapamycin-sensitive pathways. *J Biol Chem* 1996;271:5033–5039.
18. Lawrence JC Jr, Roach PJ. New insights into the role and mechanism of glycogen synthase activation by insulin. *Diabetes* 1997;46:541–547.
19. Srivastava AK, Pandey SK. Potential mechanism(s) involved in the regulation of glycogen synthesis by insulin. *Mol Cell Biochem* 1998;182:135–141.
20. Goodridge AG. Regulation of the gene for fatty acid synthase. *Fed Proc* 1986;45:2399–2405.
21. Moule SK, Edgell NJ, Welsh GI, et al. Multiple signalling pathways involved in the stimulation of fatty acid and glycogen synthesis by insulin in rat epididymal fat cells. *Biochem J* 1995;311:595–601.

22. Pause A, Belsham GJ, Gingras AC, et al. Insulin-dependent stimulation of protein synthesis by phosphorylation of a regulator of 5'-cap function. *Nature* 1994;371:762–767.
23. Proud CG, Denton RM. Molecular mechanisms for the control of translation by insulin. *Biochem J* 1997;328:329–341.
24. Kimball SR, Jurasinski CV, Lawrence JC Jr, et al. Insulin stimulates protein synthesis in skeletal muscle by enhancing the association of eIF-4E and eIF-4G. *Am J Physiol* 1997;272:C754–C759.
25. von Manteuffel SR, Dennis PB, Pullen N, et al. The insulin-induced signalling pathway leading to S6 and initiation factor 4E binding protein 1 phosphorylation bifurcates at a rapamycin-sensitive point immediately upstream of p70s6k. *Mol Cell Biol* 1997;17:5426–5436.
26. Kimball SR, Horetsky RL, Jefferson LS. Signal transduction pathways involved in the regulation of protein synthesis by insulin in L6 myoblasts. *Am J Physiol* 1998;274:C221–C228.
27. Rother KI, Imai Y, Caruso M, et al. Evidence that IRS-2 phosphorylation is required for insulin action in hepatocytes. *J Biol Chem* 1998;273:17491–17497.
28. Pilkis SJ, Granner DK. Molecular physiology of the regulation of hepatic gluconeogenesis and glycolysis. *Annu Rev Physiol* 1992;54:885–909.
29. Groop LC, Ferrannini E. Insulin action and substrate competition. *Baillieres Clin Endocrinol Metab* 1993;7:1007–1032.
30. Scheen AJ, Lefebvre PJ. Insulin action in man. *Diabetes Metab* 1996;22:105–110.
31. Wise S, Nielsen M, Rizza R. Effects of hepatic glycogen content on hepatic insulin action in humans: Alteration in the relative contributions of glycogenolysis and gluconeogenesis to endogenous glucose production. *J Clin Endocrinol Metab* 1997;82:1828–1833.
32. Yki-Jarvinen H. Action of insulin on glucose metabolism in vivo. *Baillieres Clin Endocrinol Metab* 1993;7:903–927.
33. Groop LC, Bonadonna RC, DelPrato S, et al. Glucose and free fatty acid metabolism in non-insulin-dependent diabetes mellitus. Evidence for multiple sites of insulin resistance. *J Clin Invest* 1989;84:205–213.
34. DeFronzo RA, Ferrannini E. Regulation of intermediary metabolism during fasting and feeding. In: DeGroot LJ, ed. *Endocrinology*. Philadelphia, Pa: WB Saunders, 1995:1389–1410.
35. Adeli K, Theriault A. Insulin modulation of human apolipoprotein B mRNA translation: Studies in an in vitro cell-free system from HepG2 cells. *Biochem Cell Biol* 1992;70:1301–1312.
36. Salhanick AI, Schwartz SI, Amatruda JM. Insulin inhibits apolipoprotein B secretion in isolated human hepatocytes. *Metabolism* 1991;40:275–279.
37. Sparks CE, Sparks JD, Bolognino M, et al. Insulin effects on apolipoprotein B lipoprotein synthesis and secretion by primary cultures of rat hepatocytes. *Metabolism* 1986;35:1128–1136.
38. Chen M, Breslow JL, Li W, et al. Transcriptional regulation of the apoC-III gene by insulin in diabetic mice: Correlation with changes in plasma triglyceride levels. *J Lipid Res* 1994;35:1918–1924.
39. Talmud PJ, Humphries SE. Apolipoprotein C-III gene variation and dyslipidaemia. *Curr Opin Lipidol.* 1997;8:154–158.
40. Surguchov AP, Page GP, Smith L, et al. Polymorphic markers in apolipoprotein C-III gene flanking regions and hypertriglyceridemia. *Arterioscler Thromb Vasc Biol* 1996;16:941–947.

41. Li WW, Dammerman MM, Smith JD, et al. Common genetic variation in the promoter of the human apo CIII gene abolishes regulation by insulin and may contribute to hypertriglyceridemia. *J Clin Invest* 1995;96:2601–2605.
42. Taylor SI, Accili D, Haft CR, et al. Mechanisms of hormone resistance: Lessons from insulin-resistant patients. *Acta Paediatr Suppl* 1994;399:95–104.
43. Krook A, O'Rahilly S. Mutant insulin receptors in syndromes of insulin resistance. *Baillieres Clin Endocrinol Metab* 1996;10:97–122.
44. Kadowaki H, Takahashi Y, Ando A, et al. Four mutant alleles of the insulin receptor gene associated with genetic syndromes of extreme insulin resistance. *Biochem Biophys Res Commun* 1997;237:516–520.
45. Schreyer SA, Chua SC Jr, LeBoeuf RC. Obesity and diabetes in TNF-alpha receptor- deficient mice. *J Clin Invest.* 1998;102:402–411.
46. Halle M, Berg A, Northoff H, et al. Importance of TNF-alpha and leptin in obesity and insulin resistance: A hypothesis on the impact of physical exercise. *Exerc Immunol Rev* 1998;4:77–94.
47. Donnelly R, Qu X. Mechanisms of insulin resistance and new pharmacological approaches to metabolism and diabetic complications. *Clin Exp Pharmacol Physiol* 1998;25:79–87.
48. Roth RA, Liu F, Chin JE. Biochemical mechanisms of insulin resistance. *Horm Res* 1994;41:51–55.
49. Muller-Wieland D, Streicher R, Siemeister G, et al. Molecular biology of insulin resistance. *Exp Clin Endocrinol.* 1993;101:17–29.
50. Haring HU. The insulin receptor: Signalling mechanism and contribution to the pathogenesis of insulin resistance. *Diabetologia* 1991;34:848–861.
51. Haring HU, Mehnert H. Pathogenesis of type 2 (non-insulin-dependent) diabetes mellitus: Candidates for a signal transmitter defect causing insulin resistance of the skeletal muscle. *Diabetologia* 1993;36:176–182.
52. Dib K, Whitehead JP, Humphreys PJ, et al. Impaired activation of phosphoinositide 3-kinase by insulin in fibroblasts from patients with severe insulin resistance and pseudoacromegaly. A disorder characterized by selective postreceptor insulin resistance. *J Clin Invest* 1998;101:1111–1120.
53. Vered R, Johnson JH, Camp HS, et al. Thiazolidinediones and insulin resistance: Peroxicome proliferator activated receptor Y activation stimulates expression of the CAP gene. *Cell Biol* 1998;95:14751–14756.
54. Rondinone CM, Wang LM, Lonnroth P, et al. Insulin receptor substrate (IRS) 1 is reduced and IRS-2 is the main docking protein for phosphatidylinositol 3-kinase in adipocytes from subjects with non-insulin-dependent diabetes mellitus. *Proc Natl Acad Sci U S A* 1997;94:4171–4175.
55. Withers DJ, Gutierrez JS, Towery H, et al. Disruption of IRS-2 causes type 2 diabetes in mice. *Nature* 1998;391:900–904.
56. Paz K, Hemi R, LeRoith D, et al. A molecular basis for insulin resistance. Elevated serine/threonine phosphorylation of IRS-1 and IRS-2 inhibits their binding to the juxtamembrane region of the insulin receptor and impairs their ability to undergo insulin-induced tyrosine phosphorylation. *J Biol Chem* 1997;272:29911–29918.
57. Imai Y, Philippe N, Sesti G, et al. Expression of variant forms of insulin receptor substrate-1 identified in patients with noninsulin-dependent diabetes mellitus. *J Clin Endocrinol Metab* 1997;82:4201–4207.

58. Randle PJ, Garland PB, Hales CN, et al. The glucose-fatty acid cycle: Its role in insulin sensitivity and the metabolic disturbances of diabetes mellitus. *Lancet* 1963;I:785–789.
59. Boden G. Role of fatty acids in the pathogenesis of insulin resistance and NIDDM. *Diabetes* 1997;46:3–10.
60. McGarry JD. Glucose-fatty acid interactions in health and disease. *Am J Clin Nutr* 1998;67:500S–504S.
61. Le Marchand-Brustel Y, Gremeaux T, Ballotti R, et al. Insulin receptor tyrosine kinase is defective in skeletal muscle of insulin-resistant obese mice. *Nature* 1985;315:676–679.
62. Randle PJ, Priestman DA, Mistry SC, et al. Glucose fatty acid interactions and the regulation of glucose disposal. *J Cell Biochem.* 1994;55:1–11.
63. Randle PJ, Priestman DA, Mistry S, et al. Mechanisms modifying glucose oxidation in diabetes mellitus. *Diabetologia* 1994;37:S155–S161.
64. Wolfe RR. Metabolic interactions between glucose and fatty acids in humans. *Am J Clin Nutr* 1998;67:519S–526S.
65. Kahn BB. Alterations in glucose transporter expression and function in diabetes: Mechanisms for insulin resistance. *J Cell Biochem.* 1992;48:122–128.
66. Mueckler M. The molecular biology of glucose transport: Relevance to insulin resistance and non-insulin-dependent diabetes mellitus. *J Diabetes Complications* 1993;7:130–141.
67. Girard J. Is leptin the link between obesity and insulin resistance? *Diabetes Metab* 1997;23:16–24.
68. Krook A, Digby J, O'Rahilly S, et al. Uncoupling protein 3 is reduced in skeletal muscle of NIDDM patients. *Diabetes* 1998;47:1528–1531.
69. Arii K, Suehiro T, Yamamoto M, et al. Trp64Arg mutation of beta 3-adrenergic receptor and insulin sensitivity in subjects with glucose intolerance. *Intern Med* 1997;36:603–606.
70. Bergman RN. New concepts in extracellular signaling for insulin action: the single gateway hypothesis [see discussion 385–387]. *Recent Prog Horm Res* 1997;52:359–385.
71. Bogardus C, Lillioja S, Mott D, et al. Relationship between obesity and maximal insulin-stimulated glucose uptake in vivo and in vitro in Pima Indians. *J Clin Invest* 1984;73:800–805.
72. Abate N, Garg A, Peshock RM, et al. Relationships of generalized and regional adiposity to insulin sensitivity in men. *J Clin Invest* 1995;96:88–98.
73. Abate N, Garg A, Peshock RM, et al. Relationship of generalized and regional adiposity to insulin sensitivity in men with NIDDM. *Diabetes* 1996;45:1684–1693.
74. Kissebah AH. Intra-abdominal fat: Is it a major factor in developing diabetes and coronary artery disease? *Diabetes Res Clin Pract* 1996;30:25–30.
75. Bjorntorp P. Adipose tissue distribution, plasma insulin, and cardiovascular disease. *Diabete Metab* 1987;13:381–385.
76. Despres JP. Abdominal obesity as important component of insulin-resistance syndrome. *Nutrition* 1993;9:452–459.
77. Jensen MD, Haymond MW, Rizza RA, et al. Influence of body fat distribution on free fatty acid metabolism in obesity. *J Clin Invest* 1989;83:1168–1173.

78. Rosenfield RL. Current concepts of polycystic ovary syndrome. *Baillieres Clin Obstet Gynaecol* 1997;11:307–333.
79. Dunaif A. Insulin resistance and the polycystic ovary syndrome: Mechanism and implications for pathogenesis. *Endocr Rev* 1997;18:774–800.
80. Jackson SN, Howlett TA, McNally PG, et al. Dunnigan-Kobberling syndrome: An autosomal dominant form of partial lipodystrophy. *QJM* 1997;90:27–36.
81. Peters JM, Barnes R, Bennett L, et al. Localization of the gene for familial partial lipodystrophy (Dunnigan variety) to chromosome 1q21–22. *Nat Genet* 1998;18:292–295.
82. Shimomura I, Hammer RE, Richardson JA, et al. Insulin resistance and diabetes mellitus in transgenic mice expressing nuclear SREBP-1c in adipose tissue: Model for congenital generalized lipodystrophy. *Genes Dev* 1998;12:3182–3194.
83. Brindley DN. Role of glucocorticoids and fatty acids in the impairment of lipid metabolism observed in the metabolic syndrome. *Int J Obes Relat Metab Disord* 1995;19:S69–S75.
84. Bjorntorp P. Body fat distribution, insulin resistance, and metabolic diseases. *Nutrition* 1997;13:795–803.
85. Phillips DI, Barker DJ, Fall CH, et al. Elevated plasma cortisol concentrations: A link between low birth weight and the insulin resistance syndrome? *J Clin Endocrinol Metab* 1998;83:757–760.
86. Walker BR. Abnormal glucocorticoid activity in subjects with risk factors for cardiovascular disease. *Endocr Res* 1996;22:701–708.
87. Mostaza JM, Vega GL, Snell P, et al. Abnormal metabolism of free fatty acids in hypertriglyceridaemic men: Apparent insulin resistance of adipose tissue. *J Intern Med* 1998;243:265–274.
88. Aitman TJ, Godsland IF, Farren B, et al. Defects of insulin action on fatty acid and carbohydrate metabolism in familial combined hyperlipidemia. *Arterioscler Thromb Vasc Biol* 1997;17:748–754.
89. Wallberg-Henriksson H. Interaction of exercise and insulin in type II diabetes mellitus. *Diabetes Care* 1992;15:1777–1782.
90. Ruderman NB, Schneider SH. Diabetes, exercise, and atherosclerosis. *Diabetes Care* 1992;15:1787–1793.
91. Henriksson J. Influence of exercise on insulin sensitivity. *J Cardiovasc Risk* 1995;2:303–309.
92. Starke AA. The influence of diet and physical activity on insulin sensitivity. *Wien Klin Wochenschr* 1994;106:768–773.
93. Hayashi T, Wojtaszewski JF, Goodyear LJ. Exercise regulation of glucose transport in skeletal muscle. *Am J Physiol* 1997;273:E1039–E1051.
94. Goodyear LJ, Kahn BB. Exercise, glucose transport, and insulin sensitivity. *Annu Rev Med* 1998;49:235–261.
95. Perseghin G, Price TB, Petersen KF, et al. Increased glucose transport-phosphorylation and muscle glycogen synthesis after exercise training in insulin-resistant subjects. *N Engl J Med* 1996;335:1357–1362.
96. Rowe JW, Minaker KL, Pallotta JA, et al. Characterization of the insulin resistance of aging. *J Clin Invest* 1983;71:1581–1587.
97. Muller DC, Elahi D, Tobin JD, et al. The effect of age on insulin resistance and secretion: A review. *Semin Nephrol* 1996;16:289–298.
98. Couet C, Delarue J, Constans T, et al. Age-related insulin resistance: A review. *Horm Res* 1992;38:46–50.

99. Karhapaa P, Malkki M, Laakso M Isolated low HDL cholesterol. An insulin-resistant state. *Diabetes* 1994;43:411–417.
100. Edelson GW, Sowers JR. Insulin resistance in hypertension: A focused review. *Am J Med Sci* 1993;306:345–347.
101. Sowers JR. Insulin resistance and hypertension. *Mol Cell Endocrinol* 1990; 74:C87–C89.
102. Reaven GM, Lithell H, Landsberg L. Hypertension and associated metabolic abnormalities: The role of insulin resistance and the sympathoadrenal system. *N Engl J Med* 1996;334:374–381.
103. Stern MP. Impaired glucose tolerance: Risk factor or diagnostic category. In: Lefoith, Taylor SI, Olefsky JM, eds. *Diabetes Mellitus*. Philadelphia, Pa: Lippincott-Raven Publishers; 1996:467–474.
104. Imperatore G, Riccardi G, Iovine C, et al. Plasma fibrinogen: a new factor of the metabolic syndrome. A Population-Based Study. *Diabetes Care* 1998;21:649–654.
105. Byberg L, Siegbahn A, Berglund L, et al. Plasminogen activator inhibitor-1 activity is independently related to both insulin sensitivity and serum triglycerides in 70-year-old men. *Arterioscler Thromb Vasc Biol* 1998;18:258–264.
106. Trovati M, Anfossi G. Insulin, insulin resistance and platelet function: similarities with insulin effects on cultured vascular smooth muscle cells. *Diabetologia* 1998;41:609–622.
107. McKeigue PM, Ferrie JE, Pierpoint T, et al. Association of early-onset coronary heart disease in South Asian men with glucose intolerance and hyperinsulinemia. *Circulation* 1993;87:152–161.
108. Williams R, Bhopal R, Hunt K. Coronary risk in a British Punjabi population: Comparative profile of non-biochemical factors. *Int J Epidemiol* 1994;23:28–37.
109. Pugh RN, Hossain MM, Malik M, et al. Arabian Peninsula men tend to insulin resistance and cardiovascular risk seen in South Asians. *Trop Med Int Health* 1998;3:89–94.

Chapter 11

Obesity and Postmenopausal Hormones

Katherine M. Newton, PhD

Introduction

The associations between obesity and female reproductive hormones are complex. Both obesity and hormones influence the risk for diseases that affect older women. In this chapter the associations between obesity and estrogen, changes in hormones associated with menopause, and interactions between obesity and hormone replacement therapy (HRT) with coronary heart disease (CHD), breast cancer, and osteoporosis, will be described briefly. The implications for decision making about HRT also will be discussed.

Endogenous Estrogen and the Influence of Body Weight

Women experience profound changes in endogenous estrogens as they pass from their reproductive years through menopause. Estradiol is the principle estrogen in premenopausal women, and estrone predominates in postmenopausal women.[1] Prior to menopause, the ovarian follicle and the corpus luteum it forms after ovulation are responsible for 95% of circulating estradiol.[1] Estrone, present in far smaller amounts, is produced during the metabolism of estradiol and by the aromatization of androstenedione in peripheral adipose tissue. The peripheral aromatization of testosterone also produces small amounts of estradiol and estrone.[1,2] As women pass through menopause the levels of endogenous estrone and estradiol decrease dramatically. The major source of endogenous estrogens shifts from ovarian production

From: Fletcher GF, Grundy SM, Hayman LL (eds). *Obesity: Impact on Cardiovascular Disease*. Armonk, NY: Futura Publishing Co., Inc.; © 1999.

to the aromatization of androstenedione to estrone in adipose tissue and the peripheral conversion of estrone to estradiol.[1,2] Estrogen levels in premenopausal women vary throughout the menstrual cycle from 40 to 250 pg/mL for estradiol and 40 to 170 pg/mL for estrone. With menopause, estrogen levels fall to below 15 pg/mL for estradiol and 30 pg/mL for estrone.[1] With 0.625 mg of oral estrogen replacement therapy estradiol levels increase to 30 to 50 pg/mL and estrone levels increase to 153 pg/mL.[1]

Both the degree of adiposity,[3] and the distribution of body weight, affect endogenous estrone and estradiol levels in postmenopausal women. Circulating estrogens increase with body weight[3] because of increased secretion of androgen precursors by the adrenal gland, increased conversion of androstenedione to estrogen in peripheral adipose tissue, and decreased levels of sex hormone binding globulin (SHBG) associated with obesity.[4-6] Estradiol binds strongly to SHBG, and lower levels of SHBG leave larger amounts of unbound estradiol to be converted to estrone.[1,4] Serum estrone levels are as much as 40% higher in obese than nonobese postmenopausal women.[3]

Body weight distribution also affects circulating estrogen levels. Women with lower-body obesity (measured by waist-to-height ratio) have higher levels of estrone from peripheral aromatization of androstenedione.[7] Women with upper-body obesity have higher androgen production rates and free testosterone levels, lower levels of SHBG, and higher free estradiol levels.[7]

Body Weight, Menopause, and Hormone Replacement Therapy

There is conflicting data about the relative effects of aging, menopause, and HRT on changes in body weight and body fat distribution as women pass through their middle years. The prevalence of obesity increases with age, peaking at approximately ages 50–59 years in US women, (Figure 1). It is unclear whether this increase in obesity with age is strictly an effect of aging[8] or if the hormonal changes associated with menopause contribute to weight gain in midlife.[9] Whatever the cause, weight gain with aging is associated with unfavorable changes in CHD risk factors, including increases in blood pressure, total cholesterol, low-density lipoprotein cholesterol (LDL-C), triglycerides, and fasting insulin and a decrease in high-density lipoprotein cholesterol (HDL-C).[10] These risk factor changes result not only from weight gain, but also from the change in body fat distribution associated with aging. As women progress through menopause there is an increase in intra-abdominal fat and a decrease in lower-body fat.[11] Intra-

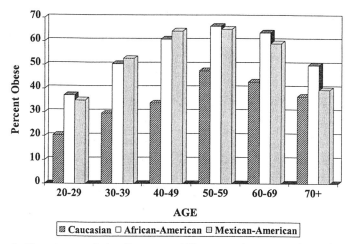

Figure 1. Prevalence of obesity among US women by age and race/ethnicity. Body mass index (BMI) $\geq$ 27.3 kg/m^2. [National Center for Health Statistics., Third National Health and Nutrition Examination Survey, 1988–1994. Data based on weighted sample size (N = 83 508 950) and unweighted sample size (N = 9036)].

abdominal obesity is correlated more strongly with insulin resistance, hypertension, and lipid abnormalities than lower-body obesity.[12]

The common belief that HRT causes weight gain has not been confirmed in observational studies or randomized trials.[13–16] In the Postmenopausal Estrogen and Progestin Study (PEPI) women were assigned randomly to placebo or one of four estrogen and progestin treatment arms.[14] Although body weight increased in all groups during this 3-year trial, weight gain was significantly less in women assigned to any of the estrogen treatment arms compared with the placebo group (Figure 2). In a smaller randomized double-blind crossover study, there were no short-term (6 month) changes in body weight associated with HRT use in perimenopausal women.[15] And after 15 years of follow-up in the Rancho Bernardo cohort, there were no differences in change in weight, body mass index (BMI) (= weight in kilograms/height in square meters), or fat mass between women who used HRT and those who did not.[16] Thus weight gain does not seem to be associated with HRT use, and HRT may lessen weight gain in postmenopausal women.

Body fat distribution may be affected by HRT use, but the findings are contradictory. In a 2-year trial of HRT in 62 early postmenopausal women, intra-abdominal fat was measured by dual energy X-ray absorptiometry. Intra-abdominal fat increased significantly more in women taking a placebo than in those taking estrogen plus progestin,

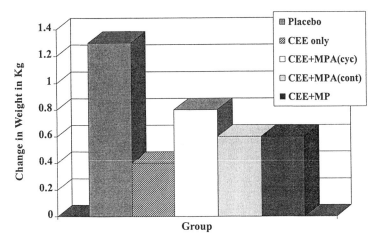

Figure 2. Change in body weight, in kilograms, over years, by treatments regimen. Postmenopausal Estrogen and Progestin Study (PEPI). Adapted with permission from Reference 14.

(Figure 3).[17] In contrast, in the PEPI study, waist-to-hip ratio increased equally in the placebo and intervention groups,[14] and in the Rancho Bernardo cohort, waist-to-hip ratio did not differ between women who did and did not use HRT.[16] It is possible that differences in the findings of these studies are caused by the methods used to assess abdominal fat. Unlike dual energy X-ray absorptiometry, waist-to-hip ratio does

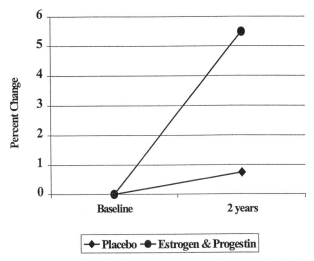

Figure 3. Change in abdominal fat percent, over 3 years, by treatment regimen. Adapted with permission from Reference 17.

not distinguish between intra-abdominal fat and subcutaneous abdominal fat.

There is evidence from observational studies that HRT users are leaner than women who had never used HRT (Table 1).[18–23] For example, in the Nurses Health Study, 31.8% of current HRT users had a BMI greater than 24.6 compared with 41.6% of never users.[19] In the First National Health and Nutrition Examination Study (NHANES I) Epidemiological Follow-up Study, 28% of non-HRT users with a nat-

Table 1

Studies Showing Hormone Replacement Therapy (HRT) by Measures of Body Weight and Adiposity

Study, design, population	Findings		
	Among controls, percent with ≥5 years of HRT use by BMI		
	BMI		
Massachusetts Women Case-Control Study, 858 controls aged 45–69[24]	<24		8%
	24–28		6%
	29+		5%

		Relative odds of HRT use		
	BMI	GHC women 1975–1984	German CVD study	Prevention Survey 1984–1986 and Steroid Study 1980–1982
Replacement estrogen use and body mass index[25]	<20	2.3 (1.0–5.0)	0.91 (0.21–4.0)	1.20 (0.85–1.7)
	20–24	1	1	1
	25–29	0.7 (0.45–1.36)	0.49 (0.27–0.87)	0.77 (0.56–1.1)
	30+	0.41 (0.18–0.93)	0.30 (0.13–0.7)	0.69 (0.43–1.1)

	BMI	Relative odds of HRT
EnPower Women's Survey, 1180 GHC women, 1995*	<20	1.5 (0.7–3.4)
	20–24	1.0
	25–29	1.1 (0.7–1.5)
	30+	0.9 (0.6–1.4)

* K. M. Newton and A. Z. La Croix, unpublished data, 1995.
BMI, body mass index (kg/m²); GHC, Group Health Cooperative of Puget Sound; CVD, cardiovascular disease.

ural menopause had a BMI greater than 29.5 compared with 15.4% of current HRT users.[21] There also is evidence that leaner women are more likely to use HRT.[24,25] However, in other studies, including data from the Lipid Research Clinics[26] and our own data from population-based studies at Group Health Cooperative of Puget Sound (K. M. Newton and A. Z. LaCroix, unpublished data, 1995), there was no association between HRT use and weight or BMI.

The association between lower weight and HRT use found in some studies has been implicated as a possible source of healthy user bias. This bias would occur if women who use HRT are inherently healthier than those who do not, leading to the appearance of a beneficial effect of HRT on health. This bias partially may account for the decrease in CHD risk that is associated with HRT in observational studies.[27] However, data from two cohorts of women in southeastern New England revealed no differences in prior BMI, blood pressure, or total and HDL-C between women who did and did not initiate HRT, though HRT users were less likely to smoke and more likely to exercise regularly.[28]

Obesity and Risk for the Common Diseases That Affect Older Women

Obesity is an important risk factor for three of the major diseases that affect older women. These diseases, CHD, osteoporosis, and breast cancer, account for a large proportion of disability and death in older women.[29–34]

Body weight is associated positively with CHD risk.[29–34] In the NHANES I Epidemiologic Follow-up Study, women aged 65 to 74 with BMI of 29 or greater experienced a 50% increase in CHD risk compared with women with BMI less than 21.[30] In the Nurses Health Study, increasing BMI was associated with increasing risk of fatal and nonfatal first myocardial infarction (MI), with more than a threefold increase in risk for those women with a BMI ≥ 29.[31] This association was attenuated but not eliminated after controlling for hypertension, diabetes, and hypercholesterolemia. These findings highlight the independent contribution of BMI to CHD risk. Even within the range of weight considered "normal," higher levels of body weight were associated with increased CHD risk.[32] In the Framingham Study metropolitan relative weight was associated independently with a 26-year incidence of MI, in both men and women,[34] and in a study of prognosis in women who survived a first MI, a 1-U increase in BMI was associated with a 3% increase in the risk of reinfarction.[35] The distribution of body fat appears to contribute to these associations. Waist-to-hip ratio is associated positively with the incidence of MI, angina pectoris, stroke, and death in women.[36]

The positive association between body weight and breast cancer risk also is well established. The Collaborative Group on Hormonal Factors in Breast Cancer reanalyzed data from 51 epidemiological studies, including a total of 52 705 women with breast cancer and 108 411 women without breast cancer. In their analyses, breast cancer risk increased 3.1% for every one-point increase in BMI (kg/m^2).[37] Five years after the cessation of HRT, breast cancer risk in past users equaled that of never users. Breast cancer risk gradually decreases with increasing time since menopause.[37] However, this relationship is greater for women of low BMI <25 kg/m^2 than for women whose BMI is ≥25 kg/m^2, (Figure 4).[37] For example, with premenopausal risk as the baseline, by 10 to 14 years after menopause the relative risk for breast cancer in women with BMI less than 25 is 0.55, while for a woman with BMI greater than 25 the relative risk is only 0.72.[37] Differences in endogenous estrogen levels with body weight and the decrease in endogenous estrogen with menopause may explain these findings.

Fracture and osteoporosis risks decrease as body mass increases.[38] The Study of Osteoporotic Fractures (SOF) was a prospective cohort study of 6754 women aged 65 and older who were followed for a mean of 5.7 years.[39] In this cohort, regardless of the body weight measure used (BMI, total body weight, and percent weight change since age 25),

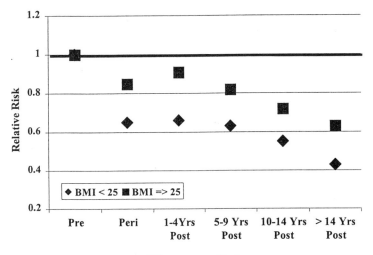

Figure 4. Change in relative risk for breast cancer after menopause, by BMI. Collaborative Group on Hormonal Factors in Breast Cancer, 1997. Adapted with permission from Reference 38.

women in the lowest weight quartile had a 1.8% to 2.7% increase in risk of hip fracture compared with women in the highest quartile. This protective effect of increasing body weight probably results from the greater amounts of circulating estrogen in heavier women.[40] Weight gain also is associated with a decrease in risk of fractures. For every 20% increase in weight since age 25, risk of hip fracture decreases by 40%.[41,42] And in the SOF study there was a 32% increase in risk of nonspine fracture for every 10% loss of body weight.[39]

The relative contributions of HRT on CHD, osteoporosis, and breast cancer risk have been portrayed using life table analysis.[43] For 50-year-old women not using HRT the lifetime probability of CHD was 46.1/100 women, the lifetime probability of hip fracture was 15.3/100 women, and the lifetime probability of breast cancer was 10.2/100 women. For 50-year-old women treated with long-term HRT, the lifetime probability of CHD was 34.2/100 women, the lifetime probability of hip fracture was 12.7/100 women, and the lifetime probability of breast cancer was 13.0/100 women.[43]

Do Obese and Lean Women Accrue Similar Benefits From Hormone Replacement Therapy?

Because obesity is a risk factor for three of the major diseases thought to be affected by HRT, we must consider obesity when counseling women about the risks and benefits of HRT. It is important to understand the contributions of HRT to osteoporosis and CHD prevention, and increased breast cancer risk in obese versus lean women.

Data suggest that obese women who use HRT gain similar cardioprotective benefits as lean women (Table 2). In the Nurses Health Study, the relative risk for CHD was similar in women regardless of their BMI, and the absolute rate difference for CHD was greater for women of higher BMI.[18] Unpublished data from a case-control study of HRT and incident MI[44] show that HRT was equally protective among nonsmoking women regardless of BMI; and among postmenopausal women who survived a first MI, HRT offered similar protection against reinfarction regardless of their BMI (K. M. Newton and A. Z. LaCroix, unpublished data, 1995).

Women at increased risk of breast cancer have been encouraged to refrain from HRT[45] because imposing a given relative risk on a higher baseline risk theoretically increases the absolute risk of breast cancer. However, data from the Collaborative Group on Hormonal Factors in Breast Cancer lead to a different conclusion. The risk for breast cancer associated with HRT decreased with either higher BMI or higher absolute body weight (Figure 5).[37] Thus women who are already at

Table 2

Studies Showing the Effects of Hormone Replacement Therapy (HRT) on Coronary Heart Disease Risk, Stratified by BMI

Study	Design/subjects	Findings		
		BMI	R (95% CI)	Rate difference*
Nurses Health Study[18]	Cohort study, 16 years follow-up, 59 337 women	<23.0	0.52 (0.33–0.84)	45
		23.0–28.9	0.67 (0.46–0.98)	36
		≥29.0	0.67 (0.40–1.13)	65

Study	Design/subjects	BMI	Never used	Ever used†
Leisure World Study[48]	Cohort study, 8881 postmenopausal women, 7.5 years follow-up	<35	1.14	0.92
		≥35	1.0	0.72

Study	Design/subjects	BMI	Nonsmokers OR (95% CI)	Smokers OR (95% CI)
Group Health Cooperative†	Case control study of HRT and CVD, N = 502 cases and 1193 controls	<24	0.74 (0.42–1.31)	0.95 (0.46–1.93)
		24–28	0.51 (0.30–0.87)	2.31 (0.76–7.01)
		≥28	0.57 (0.33–0.99)	0.94 (0.29–3.05)

Study	Design/subjects	Findings	BMI < 30	BMI 30+
Group Health Cooperative§	Cohort study of 726 women who survived first MI to hospital discharge, 2–13 years follow-up	Reinfarction	0.8 (0.4–1.8)	0.3 (0.4–2.2)
		Death	0.5 (0.2–1.1)	0.7 (0.2–2.5)

* Relative risk of coronary heart disease current vs. never used HRT and rate difference (cases prevented/100 000 women/year).

† B. M. Psaty and SR Heckbert, unpublished data, 1994. All cause mortality by even use of HRT.

§ K. M. Newton and A. Z. La Croix unpublished data, 1995. HRT and incident myocardial infarction by BMI and smoking.

RR, relative risk; CI, confidence interval; CVD, cardiovascular disease; OR, odds ratio; MI, myocardial infarction.

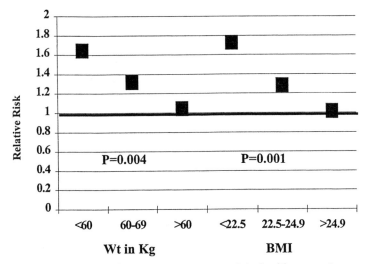

Figure 5. Relative risk of breast cancer associated with current or recent (within the last 4 years) use of hormone replacement therapy (HRT), by weight in kilograms and BMI. From the Collaborative Group on Hormonal Factors in Breast Cancer, 1997. Adapted with permission from Reference 38.

increased risk for breast cancer due to obesity may not add further risk by using HRT.

Data about the association between hormones and osteoporosis also come from the SOF study. HRT was associated with a 40% decrease in risk of hip fracture [relative risk (RR) 0.60 and 95% confidence interval (CI) 0.36–1.02] and a 60% decrease in risk of wrist fracture (RR 0.39 and 95% CI 0.24 to 0.64).[39] Estrogen's greatest effect in protecting against hip fracture was seen in women older than age 75; those who were current users and started HRT within 5 years of menopause had a relative risk of hip fractures of 0.29 (95% CI 0.09 to 0.92) compared with never users.[39] In the Framingham Study, the relative risk for hip fracture among women who had used HRT at any time was 0.65 (95% CI 0.44 to 0.98) compared with women who had never used HRT, and the risk for those who had used HRT in the previous 2 years was 0.34 (95% CI 0.12 to 0.98).[46] We were unable to identify any analyses that stratified the effects of HRT on risk of osteoporosis and fracture by levels of BMI.

Data From a Population-Based Managed Care Setting

Little is known about the factors that drive the HRT decision in obese versus lean women. HRT decision making involves a woman's personal preferences, menopausal symptoms, and attitudes about the use of HRT for long-term prevention of osteoporosis and cardiovascular disease and fears about the potential increase in risk for breast cancer.[47] Health care providers should counsel women about the risks and benefits of HRT and the impact of obesity on their risk for these diseases.

EnPower (Encouraging Prevention in Older Women) is an ongoing study at Group Health Cooperative of Puget Sound, a staff model Health Maintenance Organization (HMO) with over 500 000 enrollees in western Washington state. Preventive health practices, including factors associated with the use of HRT, are being investigated in this study. A telephone survey of 1180 randomly selected women aged 50 to 80 (80.3% response rate) and a mailed survey of all Group Health providers (family practice, internal medicine, obstetrics and gynecology, cardiology, nurse practitioners, and physician's assistants) who provide women's health care (82% response rate) have been completed.[47]

Unlike many other studies, there was only a weak association between HRT use and BMI in women in the EnPower survey (Table 1). However, results from both the EnPower women's survey and the EnPower provider's survey suggest that information given to women about HRT by their provider varies with body weight. Compared with leaner women, women with BMI > 30 were less likely to receive information about the possible health benefits of HRT from their provider (Figure 6) and were less likely to receive encouragement to take HRT (Figure 7). When asked how the presence of major risk factors associated with CHD affects whether they would encourage or discourage the use of HRT for prevention purposes for women over the age of 50, only 50% of providers indicated they would encourage or encourage strongly an obese woman to use HRT, compared with over 90% for a woman with a past MI, 80% for a woman with diabetes or hypertension, and over 70% for a woman who smokes (Figure 8).

Summary and Conclusions

Obese women appear to attain equal levels of CHD prevention from HRT and are less at risk for breast cancer associated with HRT than lean women. However, obese women may be encouraged less strongly to use HRT. We do not know the reasons behind these findings. Perhaps, because fracture prevention is a primary indication for long-term HRT and obese women are at decreased risk of fracture, providers are less inclined to approach the subject of HRT in obese women.

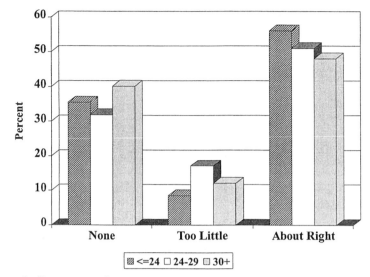

Figure 6. Responses of women aged 50–80 years to the question "How much information has your doctor given you about the possible health benefits of taking hormone pills"? From the EnPower Women's Survey, 1995, Group Health Cooperative, Seattle, Wash.

In middle-aged and older women, the interactions between obesity, endogenous and exogenous hormones, CHD, osteoporosis, and breast cancer risk are complex. These complicated associations should

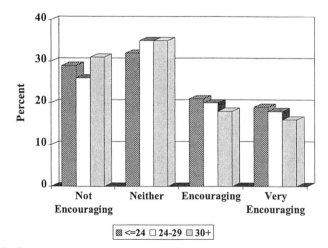

Figure 7. Responses of women aged 50–80 years to the question "To what extent does your doctor encourage you to take hormone pills?" by BMI. From the EnPower Women's Survey, 1995, Group Health Cooperative, Seattle, Wash.

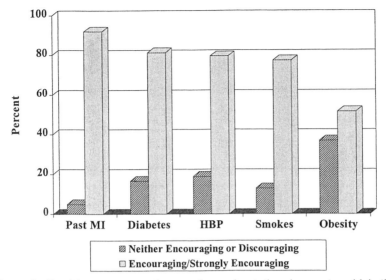

Figure 8. Provider responses to questions about the degree to which the presence of chronic conditions and risk factors affects whether they would encourage or discourage the use of HRT for women over the age of 50 for prevention purposes. EnPower Provider Survey, 1996, Group Health Cooperative, Seattle, Wash.

be considered when counseling women about risk reduction or HRT. Researchers have learned a great deal about these associations, but many questions remain. What factors are associated with the lower rates of HRT in obese women? Do the associations between obesity and CHD, osteoporosis, and breast cancer differ for women with abdominal versus peripheral obesity? Does the influence of HRT on risk for these conditions vary with abdominal versus peripheral obesity? Reanalysis from completed studies could assist in answering many of these important questions for older women.

References

1. Levrant SG, Barnes RB. Pharmacology of estrogen. In: Lobo RA, ed. *Treatment of the Postmenopausal Women: Basic and Clinical Aspects.* New York: Raven Press; 1994:57–68.
2. Judd HL, Shamonki IM, Frumar AM, et al. Origin of serum estradiol in postmenopausal women. *Obstet Gynecol* 1982;59:680–686.
3. Cauley JA, Gutai JP, Kuller LH, et al. The epidemiology of serum sex hormones in postmenopausal women. *Am J Epidemiol.* 1989;129:1120–1131.
4. Siiteri PK. Adipose tissue as a source of hormones. *Am J Clin Nutr* 1987; 45:277–282.

5. Bruschi F, Meschia M, Amicarelli F, et al. Changes in sex hormone-binding globulin plasma concentrations induced by body weight and estrogen status in perimenopausal years. *Menopause* 1997;1:28–31.

6. Thomas HV, Key TJ, Allen DS, et al. Re: Reversal of relation between body mass and endogenous estrogen concentrations with menopausal status. *J Natl Cancer Inst* 1997;89:396–398.

7. Kirschner MA, Samojlik E, Drejka M, et al. Androgen-estrogen metabolism in women with upper body versus lower body obesity. *J Clin Endocrinol Metab* 1990;70:473–479.

8. Matthews KA, Meilahn E, Kuller LH, et al. Menopause and risk factors for coronary heart disease. *N Engl J Med* 1989;321:641–646.

9. Lindquist O, Bengtsson C, Lapidus L. Relationships between the menopause and risk factors for ischaemic heart disease. *Acta Obstet Gynecol Scand Suppl* 1985;130:43–47.

10. Wing RR, Matthews KA, Kuller LH, et al. Weight gain at the time of menopause. *Arch Intern Med* 1991;151:97–102.

11. Colombel A, Charbonnel B. Weight gain and cardiovascular risk factors in the post-menopausal women. *Hum Reprod* 1997;12:134–145.

12. Despres JP, Moorjani S, Lupien PJ, et al. Regional distribution of body fat, plasma lipoproteins, and cardiovascular disease. *Arteriosclerosis* 1990;10: 497–511.

13. Aloia JF, Vaswani A, Russo L, et al. The influence of menopause and hormonal replacement therapy on body cell mass and body fat mass. *Am J Obstet Gynecol* 1995;172:896–900.

14. The Writing Group for the PEPI Trial. Effects of estrogen or estrogen/progestin regimens on heart disease risk factors in postmenopausal women. The Postmenopausal Estrogen/Progestin Interventions (PEPI) Trial. *JAMA* 1995;273:199–208.

15. Khoo SK, Coglan MJ, Wright GR, et al. Hormone therapy in women in the menopause transition. Randomised, double-blind, placebo-controlled trial of effects on body weight, blood pressure, lipoprotein levels, antithrombin III activity, and the endometrium. *Med J Aust* 1998;168:216–220.

16. Kritz-Silverstein D, Barrett-Connor E. Long-term postmenopausal hormone use, obesity, and fat distribution in older women. *JAMA* 1996;275: 46–49.

17. Haarbo J, Marslew U, Gotfredsen A, et al. Postmenopausal hormone replacement therapy prevents central distribution of body fat after menopause. *Metabolism* 1991;40:1323–1326.

18. Grodstein F, Stampfer MJ, Manson JE, et al. Postmenopausal estrogen and progestin use and the risk of cardiovascular disease. *N Engl J Med* 1996; 335:453–461.

19. Stampfer MJ, Willett WC, Colditz GA, et al. A prospective study of postmenopausal estrogen therapy and coronary heart disease. *N Engl J Med* 1985;313:1044–1049.

20. Folsom AR, Mink PJ, Sellers TA, et al. Hormonal replacement therapy and morbidity and mortality in a prospective study of postmenopausal women. *Am J Public Health* 1995;85:1128–1132.

21. Wolf PH, Madans JH, Finucane FF, et al. Reduction of cardiovascular disease-related mortality among postmenopausal women who use hormones: Evidence from a national cohort. *Am J Obstet Gynecol* 1991;164:489–494.

22. Wilson PW, Garrison RJ, Castelli WP. Postmenopausal estrogen use, cigarette smoking, and cardiovascular morbidity in women over 50. The Framingham Study. *N Engl J Med* 1985;313:1038–1043.
23. Manolio TA, Furberg CD, Shemanski L, et al. Associations of postmenopausal estrogen use with cardiovascular disease and its risk factors in older women. The CHS Collaborative Research Group. *Circulation* 1993; 88:2163–2171.
24. Rosenberg L, Palmer JR, Shapiro S. A case-control study of myocardial infarction in relation to use of estrogen supplements. *Am J Epidemiol* 1993;137:54–63.
25. Rodriguez LAG, Pfaff GM, Schumacher MC, et al. Replacement estrogen use and body mass index. *Epidemiology* 1990;1:219–223.
26. Bush TL, Barrett-Connor E, Cowan LD, et al. Cardiovascular mortality and noncontraceptive use of estrogen in women: Results from the Lipid Research Clinics Program Follow-up Study. *Circulation* 1987;75:1102–1109.
27. Barrett-Connor E. Postmenopausal estrogen and prevention bias. *Ann Intern Med* 1991;115:455–456.
28. Derby CA, Hume AL, McPhillips JB, et al. Prior and current health characteristics of postmenopausal estrogen replacement therapy users compared with nonusers. *Am J Obstet Gynecol* 1995;173:544–550.
29. Noppa H, Bengtsson C, Wedel H, et al. Obesity in relation to morbidity and mortality from cardiovascular disease. *Am J Epidemiol* 1980;111:682–692.
30. Harris TB, Ballard-Barbasch R, Madans J, et al. Overweight, weight loss, and risk of coronary heart disease in older women. *The NHANES I Epidemiologic Follow-up Study Am J Epidemiol.* 1993;137:1318–1327.
31. Manson JE, Colditz GA, Stampfer MJ, et al. A prospective study of obesity and risk of coronary heart disease in women. *N Engl J Med* 1990;322:882–889.
32. Willett WC, Manson JE, Stampfer MJ, et al. Weight, weight change, and coronary heart disease in women. Risk within the 'normal' weight range. *JAMA* 1995;273:461–465.
33. Jensen G, Nyboe J, Appleyard M, et al. Risk factors for acute myocardial infarction in Copenhagen, II: Smoking, alcohol intake, physical activity, obesity, oral contraception, diabetes, lipids, and blood pressure. *Eur Heart J* 1991;12:298–308.
34. Hubert HB, Feinleib M, McNamara PM, et al. Obesity as an independent risk factor for cardiovascular disease: A 26-year follow-up of participants in the Framingham Heart Study. *Circulation* 1983;67:968–977.
35. Newton KM, LaCroix AZ. Association of body mass index with reinfarction and survival after first myocardial infarction in women. *J Womens Health* 1996;5:433–444.
36. Lapidus L, Bengtsson C. Regional obesity as a health hazard in women: A prospective study. *Acta Med Scand Suppl* 1988;723:53–59.
37. Collaborative group on hormonal factors in breast cancer. Breast cancer and hormone replacement therapy: Collaborative reanalysis of data from 51 epidemiological studies of 52,705 women with breast cancer and 108,411 women without breast cancer. *Lancet* 1997;350:1047–1059.
38. Ensrud KE, Lipschutz RC, Cauley JA, et al. Body size and hip fracture risk in older women: A prospective study. Study of Osteoporotic Fractures Research Group. *Am J Med* 1997;103:274–280.

39. Cauley JA, Seeley DG, Ensrud K, et al. Estrogen replacement therapy and fractures in older women. Study of Osteoporotic Fractures Research Group. *Ann Intern Med* 1995;122:9–16.
40. Cummings SR, Kelsey JL, Nevitt MC, et al. Epidemiology of osteoporosis and osteoporotic fractures. *Epidemiol Rev* 1985;7:178–208.
41. Cummings SR, Nevitt MC, Browner WS, et al. Risk factors for hip fracture in white women. Study of Osteoporotic Fractures Research Group. *N Engl J Med* 1995;332:767–773.
42. Ensrud KE, Cauley J, Lipschutz R, et al. Weight change and fractures in older women. Study of Osteoporotic Fractures Research Group. *Arch Intern Med* 1997;157:857–863.
43. Grady D, Rubin SM, Petitti DB, et al. Hormone therapy to prevent disease and prolong life in postmenopausal women. *Ann Intern Med* 1992;117:1016–1037.
44. Psaty BM, Heckbert SR, Atkins D, et al. The risk of myocardial infarction associated with the combined use of estrogens and progestins in postmenopausal women. *Arch Intern Med* 1994;154:1333–1339.
45. Anonymous. Hormone replacement therapy. ACOG technical bulletin number 166—April 1992. *Int J Gynaecol Obstet* 1993;41:194–202.
46. Kiel DP, Felson DT, Anderson JJ, et al. Hip fracture and the use of estrogens in postmenopausal women. The Framingham Study. *N Engl J Med* 1987;317:1169–1174.
47. Newton KM, LaCroix AZ, Leveille SG, et al. Women's beliefs and decisions about hormone replacement therapy. *J Womens Health* 1997;6:459–465.
48. Henderson BE, Paganini-Hill A, Ross RK. Decreased mortality in users of estrogen replacement therapy. *Arch Intern Med* 1991;151:75–78.

Late-Breaking Advances in the Biological Understanding of Obesity and Its Sequelae

Robert H. Eckel, MD

Introduction

After years of relative neglect, the science of obesity and body weight regulation has reached at least some level of acceptance. This in part relates to the cloning and/or identification of genes that were not known previously and cause obesity in rodents and/or humans.[1–3] In addition, the increasing appreciation of the importance of obesity to the etiology of a number of common maladies of our age that relate to obesity including heart disease,[4] hypertension,[5] diabetes mellitus,[6] and cancer[7] among others demands attention.

At present, an explosion of research in obesity and body weight regulation is taking place at the very basic, clinical, and population levels. To elaborate on any or all of these broad areas of obesity-related investigation in an attempt to cover the late-breaking advances in the biological understanding of obesity and its sequela would be not only challenging but inappropriate for this chapter. However, the selection of a single recently published paper that represents each of three areas of obesity-related research is the approach chosen. The three areas to be covered include the following: (1) basic science of weight regulation, (2) clinical science of weight regulation, and (3) obesity-related sequela. A brief discussion of weight regulation will precede the papers to be discussed. In closing, some comments that reflect the increasing interest of the National Institutes of Health (NIH) in promoting additional understanding of obesity seem timely.

From: Fletcher GF, Grundy SM, Hayman LL (eds). *Obesity: Impact on Cardiovascular Disease.* Armonk, NY: Futura Publishing Co., Inc.; © 1999.

Weight regulation is a balance between energy intake and energy expenditure. Imbalance in this relationship predicts either weight loss or weight gain. Over years, a slight increase in energy intake relative to energy expenditure results in weight gain. Although most often appropriate for growth and development, after full stature has been achieved excessive energy balance almost always results in an expansion of adipose tissue mass.

Energy expenditure is composed of basal metabolic rate (BMR), physical activity, and the thermogenic effect of food. In general, BMR accounts for 60%–70%, physical activity 20%–30%, and the thermic effect of food 5%–10% of energy expenditure. In humans, BMR is best predicted by lean body mass[8] and genetics,[9] whereas the thermic effect of food relates mostly to the size and macronutrient content of the meal.[10] Physical activity is a mixture of planned exercise and daily movement. As weight increases, lean body mass also increases as does BMR. Thus, a greater number of calories are needed to maintain an expanded body mass than were needed prior to weight gain.[11]

Body weight maintenance relates to a feedback mechanism between the periphery, that is, adipose tissue mass (perhaps certain components of lean body mass also), and the central nervous system. For overweight [body mass index (BMI) 25.0–29.9 kg/m^2] and obese (BMI > 30.0 kg/m^2) subjects, this regulation in general occurs at a higher level of energy intake. The control of energy intake is complex, involving numerous peptidergic and aminergic pathways.[12] In general, the hypothalamus is the central processing area for chemical information where most of the control of energy intake occurs through inhibitory rather than stimulatory pathways. Recently, a newly discovered stimulatory system has been identified following the pursuit of ligands for orphan G-protein coupled cell surface receptors (GPCRs). This orexin/orexin receptor system now will be described.

Basic Science of Weight Regulation

GPCRs are found on a wide variety of cell types and respond to photons, amines, lipids, peptides, and proteases. To evaluate the function of orphan GPCRs, Sakurai et al,[13] pursued high-resolution high-pressure liquid chromatography fractions of tissue extracts for GPCR activity in more than 50 stably transfected orphan GPCR-expressing cell lines. Heterotrimeric G-protein activation was monitored by orphan receptor HFGAN72 evoked calcium release in transfected human embryonic kidney (HEK293) cells. This receptor initially was identified as an expressed sequence tag from human brain. Several extracts (orexins) were identified, which elicited a response. Specificity of orexin-induced signal transduction was identified by the absence of evoked calcium responses in cells expressing an unrelated orphan receptor. Following purification of proteins from the extracts to homogeneity, two peptides were discovered, a major peptide orexin A (a 33 amino acid sequence of 3562 d), and a minor peptide orexin B (a 28 amino acid sequence of 2937-d peptide with 46% sequence homology with orexin A). These two orexins are the result of proteolytic cleavage of a single precursor protein, prepro-orexin. Using highly degenerative primers and reverse transcription–polymerase chain reaction (RT-PCR) of rat brain mRNA, two full-length complementary DNAs (cDNAs) were obtained. Using orexin and orexin receptor riboprobes, orexin was found in the brain and testis whereas orexin receptors were found in the brain only. In fact, prepro-orexin was localized in the hypothalamus (mostly in the lateral hypothalamus), an area of the brain important in the control of energy intake.

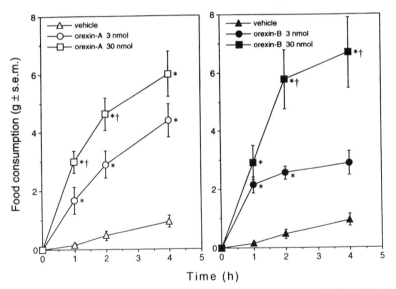

Time (h)

Figure 1. Stimulation of food consumption by intracerebroventricular injection of orexin A and B in freely fed rats. Designated amounts of synthetic human orexin A (**left**) or B (**right**) were administered in a 5-μL bolus through a catheter placed in the left ventricle in early light phase. Cumulative food consumption was plotted over the period of 4 hours after injection. * Significant difference from vehicle controls [$P < 0.05$, $n = 8$–10, analysis of variance (ANOVA) followed by Student—Newman–Keuls test]. † Significant difference between 3-nmol and 30-nmol injections ($P < 0.05$, $n = 8$–10, ANOVA followed by Student–Newman–Keuls test). Similar results were obtained in at least four independent sets of experiments. The same vehicle control curve was replotted in both panels. Reproduced with permission from Reference 13.

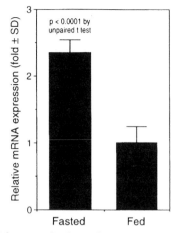

Figure 2. Densitometric quantitation of Northern blot results presented in Figure 7(**A**) of Sakurai et al.[13] The ratio of prepro-orexin and β-actin mRNA signals was determined in each lane, and these normalized values were then compared between the fasted and the fed groups. The mean value for normalized prepro-orixin mRNA expression in the fed group was arbitrarily designated as unity. Reproduced with permission from Reference 13.

To determine the potential role of orexins in energy intake, orexin A and orexin B were injected into the third ventricle of rats and food intake was determined. As shown in Figure 1, injected at 3 and 30 nmol, both peptides increased food consumption above that seen in vehicle-injected controls.[13] At 30 nmol, orexin B increased food consumption by nearly 10-fold. If orexins were to be important in the regulation of energy intake, changes in orexin gene expression might be expected to occur with fasting/feeding. Following a prolonged fast (48 hours), prepro-orexin mRNA increased twofold above fed levels, an effect superior in magnitude to that seen for another major peptide regulator of food intake, neuropeptide Y (Figure 2).[13]

At present, orexins are only the second class of neurotransmitters in the lateral hypothalamus that impact feeding. Melanin concentrating hormone (MCH) also is produced in the lateral hypothalamus and appears to be regulated similarly to orexin by fasting and feeding.[14,15] The hypocretins are secretinlike molecules also produced by the lateral hypothalamus but their role in energy balance has yet to be delineated.[16] The potential contribution of orexins to energy intake has been portrayed nicely by Flier and Maratos-Flier (Figure 3).[17] However, numerous experiments remain, including those that examine relationships of orexins to other peptides and amines that control energy intake, determining if the cells of origin of the orexins are identical to

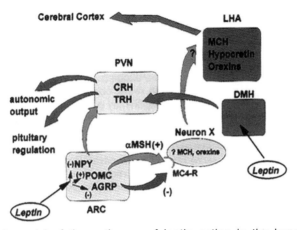

Figure 3. A model of the pathways of leptin action in the hypothalamus. Through direct actions on cell bodies in the arcuate nucleus (ARC), leptin positively regulates pro-opiomelanocortin (POMC) α-melanocyte stimulating hormone (α-MSH) and negatively regulates neuropeptide-Y (NPY) and agouti gene related protein (AGRP). α-MSH neurons project to MD4 receptor-expressing neurons of as-yet-uncertain chemical identity. AGRP-expressing neurons antagonize the α-MSH signal on these neurons. Directly or indirectly, this signal influences neurons in the lateral hypothalamus (LHA) that then influence hunger/satiety by mechanisms that may include long cortical projections involving melanin concentrating hormone (MCH) neurons. NPY projects to the paraventricular nucleus (PVN), which contains neurons expressing corticotropin releasing hormone (CRH) and TRH and other neuropeptides. The PVN influences anterior and posterior pituitary functions; it also directly innervates autonomic preganglionic neurons, both sympathetic and parasympathetic. The dorsomedial hypothalmus (DMH) has neurons that are responsive to leptin and project to the PVN. Reproduced with permission from Reference 17.

those that synthesize MCH and importantly discovering if orexins have any role in the regulation of energy expenditure.

Clinical Investigation

The ongoing controversy about what predicts weight gain has been addressed recently in overfeeding experiments in humans. In past studies, forced overfeeding has resulted in variable amounts of weight gain, an effect with both genetic and environmental influence.[18,19] An explanation of what aspect of energy balance relates to the amount of weight gain has been unclear because until recently the methodology has not been available to address mechanisms. Since the development of doubly labeled water,[20] reasonably accurate assess-

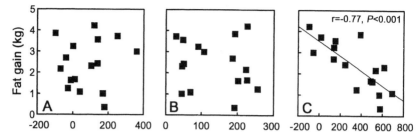

Figure 4. The relation of the change in (**A**) basak netabolic rate, (**B**) postprandial thermogenesis, and (**C**) activity thermogenesis with fat gain after overfeeding. Exercise levels and the thermic efficiency of exercise were unchanged with overfeeding, so that changes in activity thermogenesis represent changes in non-exercise activity thermogenesis (NEAT). Reproduced with permission from Reference 21 and references therein.

ments of energy expenditure can be made to determine what percentage of the excess energy is stored versus dissipated through increased energy expenditure. By assessing BMR and postprandial thermogenesis separately by indirect calorimetry, the amount of energy expended in the form of physical activity can be determined.

A recent study by Levine et al[21] examined the impact of the ingestion of 1000 kcal in excess per day for 8 weeks during maintenance of volitional activity at the level present prior to overfeeding. In 16 participants, the average weight gain was 4.7 kg with a range from 1.4 to 7.2 kg. Although there was no association of the amount of weight gain with the changes in BMR or postprandial thermogenesis, the inverse relationship between the level of nonexercise activity thermogenesis (NEAT) and weight gain was impressive (Figure 4). This form of energy expenditure relates to the activities of daily living that are other than planned exercise including standing, walking, and fidgeting among others.

The accompanying editorial and figure (Figure 5) by Ravussin and Danforth[22] look at the extremes of energy storage during overfeeding by dividing the groups into "easy gainers" and "hard gainers." Presumably, easy gainers have a propensity for fat storage, minimally increasing NEAT in response to overfeeding. Hard gainers resist fat accumulation during overfeeding by increasing NEAT. Whether the short-term effect of caloric overingestion on fat storage predicts the response to subtler overfeeding long term is unclear. Moreover, because volitional activity was maintained in this study, the conscious choice of exercise may be induced sufficiently in some to prevent fat storage. Clearly, physical inactivity during overfeeding predicts weight gain; however, recent unpublished data by Eckel et al[23] suggest that the macronutrient content of the diet also may be important.

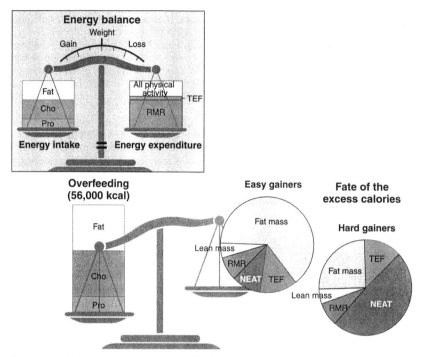

Figure 5. Watching your weight. (**Top**) When energy intake exceeds energy expenditure, weight is gained, with most of the extra energy stored as body fat and smaller amounts as lean tissue (protein and glycogen). When energy expenditure exceeds intake, weight is lost, with most of the loss of energy as body fat and smaller amounts of lean tissue. Physical activity can be divided into the energy used for conscious activities (mostly volitional) and for NEAT. (**Bottom**) In response to overfeeding, an average 39% of the excess calories were stored in the body as fat and 4% as lean tissue (protein and glycogen). The remaining excess calories were dissipated by thermogenic mechanisms. Most of the increase in physical activity was accounted for by an increase in NEAT because volitional activity was kept constant. The variability in the gain of fat was inversely related to the subjects' ability to increase NEAT, resting metabolic rate (RMR), and the thermal effect of food energy (TEF). Reproduced with permission from Reference 22.

When subjects were made inactive for 24 hours on a high-fat diet, fat storage was promoted whereas a similar period on a high-carbohydrate diet was associated with a variable amount of fat gain, but on the average no fat gain.

The importance of this chapter is to challenge health care professionals to encourage the increasingly overfed and inactive public to ward off fat gain during periods of overeating. This can be accomplished in a number of ways, but just moving more is an easy place to start. Both the time and the cost of this change in behavior appears to

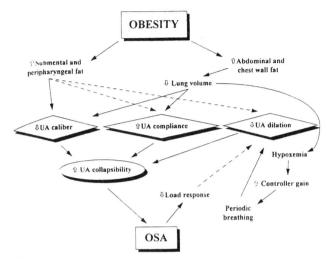

Figure 6. The pathophysiologic role of obesity in obstructive sleep apnea. Reproduced with permission from Reference 26.

be acceptable for most. However, perhaps this type of activity is less conscious and favors the thrifty gene hypothesis[24] of weight regulation in an environment where food is available and physical activity is not needed for most.

Obesity-Related Sequelae

Obstructive sleep apnea is a common and potentially serious complication of obesity that is appreciated insufficiently and diagnosed by primary care physicians and specialists.[25] Potential cardiopulmonary complications include congestive heart failure, cor pulmonale, pulmonary hypertension, systemic hypertension, cardiac arrthymias, and sudden death. A schematic presentation of how obesity and obstructive sleep apnea relate is portrayed in the figure of Storable and Rosen (Figure 6).[26] Factors that predict the presence and/or severity of the defect relate not only to the amount of adipose tissue in the submental and peripharyngeal region, but the distribution of fat in the chest and abdomen. Here, lung volume can be influenced negatively. Of additional importance is the size of the airway, which in part is inherited, and may not relate directly to the amount of adjacent fat. Through interactions between alterations in airway structure, function, balance between ventilatory drive and load, and obesity-induced hypoxemia, obstructive sleep apnea may result.

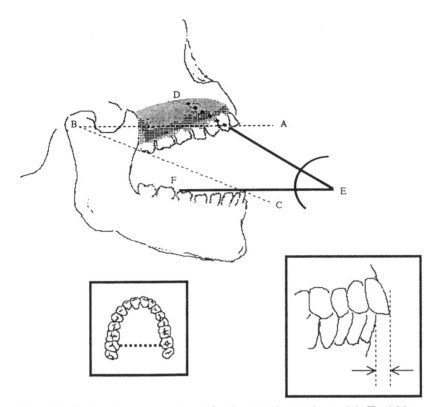

Figure 7. Oral cavity measurements for the morphometric model. (**Top**) Measurement of the palatal height by two separate calipers, labeled ABD and DEF. Angle ABC is a 20° angle between the maxillary and mandibular incisor tips with the vertex (B) of an externally placed caliper at the mandibular condyle. Angle DEF represents a caliper placed inside the oral cavity. The vertical distance DF is equal to P (palatal height) in millimeters. (**Bottom left**) Measurement from the mesial surfaces of the crowns of the second molars to obtain either Mx (maxillary intermolar distance) or Mn (mandibular intermolar distance) in millimeters. (**Bottom right**) Measurement of overjet (OJ) or the horizontal overlap of the crowns of the maxillary and mandibular right central incisors in millimeters. Reproduced with permission from Reference 27.

To assess the propensity of an individual to be at risk for obstructive sleep apnea, accurate and predictive assessments are needed, which can be applied in the ambulatory setting. If effective, such a tool could not only serve to identify patients with obstructive sleep apnea, but save the expense of unnecessary radiological, oximetric and formal sleep studies. The morphometric model recently described by Kushida et al[27] may prove useful to this end. Using measurements of BMI, neck circumference, and the oral cavity (Figure 7), a mathematical model (Figure 8) can be created for the patient. Using polysomnography to

The morphometric model is as follows:

$$\boxed{P + (Mx - Mn) + 3 \times OJ} + 3 \times [\text{Max } (BMI - 25, 0)] \times (NC \div BMI)$$

where P is palatal height (in millimeters), or the distance from the dorsum of the tongue at the median lingual sulcus to the highest point of the palate, measured with the tongue in a relaxed position and the maxillary and mandibular incisor tips subtending an angle of 20 degrees from the mandibular condyle; Mx is the maxillary intermolar distance (in millimeters) between the mesial surfaces of the crowns of the maxillary second molars; Mn is the mandibular intermolar distance (in millimeters) between the mesial surfaces of the crowns of the mandibular second molars; OJ is the overjet (in millimeters), or the horizontal overlap of the crowns of the maxillary and mandibular right central incisors; BMI (24) is the body mass index (kg/m^2; ideal BMI $\leq$ 25); and NC is neck circumference (in centimeters) measured at the level of the cricothyroid membrane.

Figure 8. Reproduced with permission from Reference 27.

determine the number of abnormal respiratory events during sleep in 300 subjects, the model had a sensitivity of 97.6%, specificity of 100%, a positive predicative value of 100% with a negative predictive value of 88.5% (Table 1). Even in the absence of symptoms of obstructive sleep apnea, this rapid and accurate measurement could identify those at risk even at lesser degrees of obesity development. The application of this model as a screening tool is premature but hopefully further research will prove to validate a technique, which will either encourage or discourage the use of polysomnography for confirmation.

Trans-NIH Initiative

On April 27, 1998 Dr. Harold Varmus, Director of the NIH, called a meeting of NIH directors where obesity is supported, representatives of the extramural research community, and one liaison from the American Obesity Association to discuss the development of a trans-NIH initiative to address scientifically the increasing girth of America. Four areas of emphasis for NIH action in obesity research were identified. These included genetics of human obesity, prevention of obesity, interdisciplinary interactions/research consortia to strengthen basic/clinical research, and training.

Table 1 (Ref. 27)

Two-by-Two Contingency Tables for Patients with and without the Obstructive Sleep Apnea Syndrome*

Variable	Patients with OSAS	Patients without OSAS	Total patients	Sensitivity (95% CI)	Specificity (95% CI)	Positive predictive value (95% CI)	Negative predictive value (95% CI)
	n				%		
Morphometric model value ≥70	248	0	248	97.6 (95–98.9)	100 (92–100)	100 (98.5–100)	88.5 (77–96)
Morphometric model value <70	6	46	52				
Total	254	46	300				
BMI >25 kg/m²	235	12	247	92.5 (89.3–95.8)	73.9 (61.2–86.6)	95.1 (92.5–97.8)	64.1 (51.2–77.1)
BMI ≤25 kg/m²	19	34	53				
Total	254	46	300				
Neck circumference ≥40 cm	154	3	157	60.6 (54.6–66.6)	93.4 (86.3–100)	98.1 (95.9–100)	30.1 (22.6–37.6)
Neck circumference <40 cm	100	43	143				
Total	254	46	300				

* OSAS = obstructive sleep apnea syndrome; CI = confidence interval; BMI = body mass index.

In the area of genetics, the following four areas of emphasis were defined:

1. Develop core resources to make the latest genomic technologies widely accessible
2. Foster coordination between groups working with human populations
3. Develop a coordinated population resource for obesity genetics
4. Expand minority population research

For obesity prevention, the following four areas also were identified:

1. Develop small grants in obesity prevention research
2. Develop new methods to facilitate obesity prevention studies
3. Expand trans-NIH research efforts directed to understanding the biology of behavior, sustained behavioral change, and motivated behavior
4. Integrate treatment and prevention programs in high-risk families

In the area of interdisciplinary interactions/research consortia to strengthen basic/clinical research, the following were recommended:

1. Foster interdisciplinary interactions and research consortia through existing mechanisms, for example, PO1s, SCORs, U19s
2. Foster interactions with industry in obesity research

For training, the following two recommendations were made:

1. Foster interdisciplinary research, for example, basic scientists in behavioral research and behavioral scientists in basic research
2. Develop skills in new technologies applicable to obesity research

Overall, if and when implemented, these recommendations should do much to further the understanding of obesity as a chronic disorder and hopefully provide steps that will lead to effective prevention and therapeutics.

Conclusions and Questions

Obesity in America and increasingly around the world is epidemic. When will it stop? The public wants simple solutions but none at the present are available. Prevention must be emphasized, but is this capable of being accomplished, and is lifestyle alone enough? Scientific progress in a number of areas is occurring. How therapeutically applicable will this knowledge be?

The NIH appears increasingly to be positioned to respond. Will they and if so how? Industry is already proactive, and new drugs will likely result from the application of basic science knowledge they and academia gather. Will drugs be developed that are both safe and effective and if so, will combination therapy be necessary to prevent and/or treat this metabolic disorder?

References

1. Chua SC Jr. Monogenic models of obesity. *Behav Genet* 1997;27:277–284.
2. Perusse L, Chagnon YC, Weisnagel J, et al. The human obesity gene map: The 1998 update. *Int J Obesity* 1999;7:111–129.
3. Ristow M, Muller-Wieland D, Pfeiffer A, et al. Obesity associated with a mutation in a genetic regulator of adipocyte differentiation. *N Engl J Med* 1998;339:953–959.
4. Eckel RH. Obesity and heart disease: A statement for healthcare professionals from the Nutrition Committee, American Heart Association. *Circulation* 1997;96:3248–3250.
5. Reisin E, Messerli FH. Obesity-related hypertension: Mechanisms, cardiovascular risks, and heridity. *Curr Opin Neph Hyperten* 1996;4:67–71.
6. Maggio CA, Pi-Sunyer FX. The prevention and treatment of obesity. Application to type 2 diabetes. *Diabetes Care* 1997;20:1744–1766.
7. Anonymous. Nutritional aspects of the development of cancer. Report of the Working Group on Diet and Cancer of the Committee on Medical Aspects of Food and Nutrition Policy. *Rep Health Soc Subj (Lond)* 1998;48: i–xiv,1–274.
8. Gallagher D, Belmonte D, Deurenberg P, et al. Organ-tissue mass measurement allows modeling of REE and metabolically active tissue mass. *Am J Physiol* 1998;275:E249–E258.
9. Bogardus C, Lillioja S, Ravussin E, et al. Familial dependence of the resting metabolic rate. *N Engl J Med* 1986;315:96–100.
10. Jequier E, Acheson K, Schutz Y. Assessment of energy expenditure and fuel utilization in man. *Annu Rev Nutr* 1987;7:187–208.
11. Lichtman SW, Pisarska K, Berman ER, et al. Discrepancy between self-reported and actual caloric intake and exercise in obese subjects. *N Engl J Med* 1992;327:1893–1898.
12. Thorburn AW, Proietto J. Neuropeptides, the hypothalamus and obesity: Insights into the central control of body weight. *Pathology* 1998;30:229–236.
13. Sakurai T, Amemiya A, Ishii M, et al. Orexins and orexin receptors: A family of hypothalamic neuropeptides and G protein-coupled receptors that regulate feeding behavior. *Cell* 1998;92:573–585.

14. Bittencourt JC, Presse F, Arias C, et al. The melanin-concentrating hormone system of the rat brain: An immuno- and hybridization histochemical characterization. *J Comp Neurol* 1992;319:218–245.
15. Qu D, Ludwig DS, Gammeltoft S, et al. A role for melanin-concentrating hormone in the central regulation of feeding behaviour. *Nature* 1996;380: 243–247.
16. de Lecea L, Kilduff TS, Peyron C, et al. The hypocretins: Hypothalamus-specific peptides with neuroexcitatory activity. *Proc Natl Acad Sci U S A* 1998;95:322–327.
17. Flier JS, Maratos-Flier E. Obesity and the hypothalamus: Novel peptides for new pathways. *Cell* 1998;92:437–440.
18. Sims EA, Danforth E Jr, Horton ES, et al. Endocrine and metabolic effects of experimental obesity in man. *Recent Prog Horm Res* 1973;29:457–496.
19. Bouchard C, Tremblay A, Despres JP, et al. The response to long-term overfeeding in identical twins. *N Engl J Med* 1990;322:1477–1482.
20. Coward WA, Roberts SB, Cole TJ. Theoretical and practical considerations in the doubly-labelled water (2H2(18)O) method for the measurement of carbon dioxide production rate in man. *Eur J Clin Nutr* 1988;42:207–212.
21. Levine JA, Eberhardt NL, Jensen MD. Role of nonexercise activity thermogenesis in resistance to fat gain in humans. *Science* 1999;283:212–214.
22. Ravussin E, Danforth E Jr. Beyond sloth: Physical activity and weight gain. *Science* 1999;283:184–185.
23. Shepart TY, Jensen DR, Sharp TA, et al. Dietary macronutrient composition affects fuel substrate utilization and balance differently in normal and obese subjects. *Int J Obesity* 1998;22:575.
24. Neel J. Diabetes mellitus: A "thrifty" genotype rendered detrimental by "progress"? *Am J Human Genet* 1962;14:353–361.
25. Vgontzas AN, Tan TL, Bixler EO, et al. Sleep apnea and sleep disruption in obese patients. *Arch Intern Med* 1994;154:1705–1711.
26. Strobel RJ, Rosen RC. Obesity and weight loss in obstructive sleep apnea: A critical review. *Sleep* 1996;19:104–115.
27. Kushida CA, Efron B, Guilleminault C. A predictive morphometric model for the obstructive sleep apnea syndrome. *Ann Intern Med* 1997;127:581–587.

Part 3

Assessment, Interventions, Treatment, and Outcomes

Chapter 13

Body Composition Assessment: Epidemiological, Clinical, and Research Tools

Mary Ellen Sweeney, MD

Introduction

The incidence of obesity has increased over the past 10 years at an alarming rate. One-third of adults are considered obese and the incidence in children is similar.[1] Obesity has been associated with an increased incidence of diabetes, coronary artery disease (CAD), abnormal blood lipids, and hypertension. In general terms, obesity implies a body weight that is greater than 20% above ideal for age and gender. However, many of the sequela attributed to obesity may be found in patients whose weight lies within the normal range.[2] Evidence such as this has led researchers to investigate the extent to which components of excess body weight, that is, fat-free mass (FFM), fat, and percent body fat, contribute to the development of disease. The distribution of body fat, that is, subcutaneous versus visceral or intra-abdominal adiposity, may be an even greater indicator of risk.[3] Body composition assessment has evolved significantly over the past two decades with the development of complex and highly accurate methodologies. Great strides have been made from the earliest methodology, which utilized analytical chemical methods to determine the composition of human cadavers.[4] Yet, work such as this serves as the basis for today's body composition assessment techniques.

The most common techniques currently being utilized for body composition assessment can be divided into epidemiological, clinical, and research tools (Table 1). Epidemiological techniques are those that can be applied easily and uniformly to large populations. These meth-

From: Fletcher GF, Grundy SM, Hayman LL (eds). *Obesity: Impact on Cardiovascular Disease.* Armonk, NY: Futura Publishing Co., Inc.; © 1999.

Table 1

Body Composition Assessment Tools

Epidemiological	Clinical	Research
Body weight	Skin folds	Hydrostatic weighing
Weight-stature	Bioelectrical impedance	Computerized tomography
Circumference	Dual energy absorptiometry	Magnetic resonance imaging
	Air plethysmography	Neutron activation analysis
		Total body potassium
		Deuterium-labeled water

ods generally are categorized as doubly indirect methods of analysis when using the groupings proposed by Deurenberg and Schutz.[4] They divided body composition methods into three main groups: direct, such as carcass analysis; indirect, such as densitometry; or doubly indirect, such as anthropometric methods, which are based on a statistical relationship between easily measured parameters, such as body weight, and data obtained from direct or indirect methods. Clinical assessment tools include those that are available in the medical setting, either in the outpatient clinic or at a hospital or medical center. These include both indirect and doubly indirect methods. Research assessment tools generally are available only in university or research centers. These methods are more complicated to administer and usually require specialized equipment. These include both direct and indirect methods. During the past decade, there has been an emphasis on the development of body composition assessment equipment that can be utilized in the sports and wellness arenas. Companies seek to provide devices that are inexpensive, portable, and do not require extensive training to operate. Bioelectrical impedance analyzers (BIAs) are a good example of this type of device. In addition, over the past 10 years, radiological equipment, originally developed for medical purposes, has been adapted for use in body composition assessment. Examples of these include dual-photon absorptiometry, computerized tomography (CT), and nuclear magnetic resonance imaging (MRI).

Epidemiological Assessment Methods

Anthropometry is the use of body weight, height, skin fold, and circumference measures to predict percent body fat. The accuracy of the resulting value increases when multiple measures are combined, such as height and weight or height, weight, and skin folds, etc. The most common "gross" measure of body fat is body weight. Individuals who are overweight generally are overfat. Determination of the degree of overweight is done by comparing actual body weight to the ideal weight for height and sex. Ideal body weight (IBW) is calculated using height-weight tables, such as the Metropolitan Life Insurance Tables.[5] Percent IBW is determined by body weight/ideal weight × 100 = % IBW. Obesity is categorized as greater than 120% of IBW. Data from the Framingham Heart Study showed that increased body weight after age 25 increased the risk of CAD for both men and women.[6] Each standard deviation increment in relative weight is associated with a 15% and 22% increase in cardiovascular events in men and women, respectively.[7] Although weight is highly correlated with both body fat and percent body fat,[8] the addition of height to form a weight-to-stature ratio improves the validity of the measure. Different ratios can be used such as weight/height, weight/height^2 and weight/height^3; however, body mass index (BMI) [weight (kg)/height (m^2)], has been the most widely utilized and validated measure. When used in combination with age, BMI can predict percent body fat with a standard error of the estimate of 3.4%.[9,10] BMI has been shown to correlate independently and positively with cardiovascular disease (CVD).[2,11] Using the data from 13 242 participants in the First National Health and Nutrition Examination Survey (NHANES I) Epidemiological Follow-up Study, estimates of BMI at which minimum mortality occurs was determined to be 27.1 for black men, 24.8 for white men, 26.8 for black women, and 24.3 for white women.[12] However, the use of BMI to describe body fat is limited by its inability to differentiate between muscle weight and fat weight. It also does not account for the distribution pattern of fat, which is thought to be more highly correlated to the development of CAD, diabetes, and hypertension.

Circumference measures can be done at numerous body locations. These measures can provide information about subcutaneous fat, visceral fat, and muscle tone. They can be used in virtually all populations, from children to morbidly obese adults. Sites used for measurements include upper arm, chest, abdomen, waist, hips, midthigh, and calf. Body circumferences are correlated with total body fat and percent body fat, but the correlation coefficients are smaller than between skin fold thickness and total body fat and percent body fat.[13]

The waist-to-hip ratio (WHR), calculated by measuring the smallest (waist) and largest (hip) truncal diameters has been shown to be a good indicator of fat distribution and is positively correlated to an increased risk of diabetes,[14,15] hypertension,[15] and coronary artery disease.[16,17] A normal WHR is generally thought to be less than 0.80 for women and less than 0.95 for men. WHR has also been found to be a better predictor of stroke risk than BMI. In a study of 28 684 US male health professionals, men in the highest quintile of WHR (WHR > 0.95) had a 2.3 times greater risk of stroke than did men in the lowest quintile.[18] It has been shown that 90% of the variance in the waist circumference can be attributed to the levels of total body fat, subcutaneous fat, and deep abdominal fat, whereas these same variables explain only 50% of the variance in the WHR.[19] Therefore, the waist circumference appears to be the single most important variable in CAD risk estimation. Body weight, percentage of body fat, BMI, and WHR are all gross determinants of body fat. These parameters are easy to measure using a scale and a tape measure and thus, they are well suited to large epidemiological studies. All of these techniques may be performed in the clinical setting.

Clinical Assessment Methods

Clinical assessment methods are those methods that usually are performed in a medical or professional setting by trained personnel. Measurement of skin fold thickness using calipers applied to folds of skin at various sites has been shown to be a good estimate of subcutaneous body fat. Seven sites are chosen that include chest, axilla, triceps, subscapula, abdomen, suprailium, and thigh. The sum of these sites then is correlated to body density standards as determined by underwater weighing. The percentage of body fat then is estimated. For men, the sum of chest, abdomen, and thigh skin folds and for women the sum of triceps, suprailium, and thigh have been found to be highly correlated with the sum of seven.[20] Though skin fold measurements can be used to estimate body fat in large population studies within an error of +3% and can be adapted easily to the clinical setting, they have been found to underestimate the amount of body fat when compared with underwater weighing and total body water by deuterium dilution in obese patients.[21]

The bioelectrical impedance (BIA) technique for body composition assessment is used widely in both research and sports and fitness communities. It is contained in an easily portable unit and can be performed by nonmedical personnel. It is based on the introduction of a small alternating electrical current into the body at the toes and fingers via source electrodes. The detecting electrodes measure the voltage drop caused by this circuit at the same anatomical landmarks. This technique is based on the principle that cells have electrical characteristics that form capacitors. The supporting or relatively noncellular environment is the transport mass and is resistive only. Thus, the impedance in the human body can be modeled by a combination of capacitance and resistance elements measured in series or in parallel. A thorough discussion of principles of BIA can be found in the proceedings from the National Institutes of Health Technology Assessment Conference.[22] Under stable conditions, the conductivity of a body segment or region is directly proportional to the amount of electrolyte-rich fluid present. Fat is anhydrous and under stable conditions, all body water and fluids are bound to the fat-free body mass component. Therefore, BIA estimates FFM, and body fat is calculated as the difference between body weight and FFM.[22] Conditions that can lead to an error in BIA measurements include inaccurate measurement of height and/or weight, the length of time the subject is recumbent before the measurement is performed, adduction or crossing of limbs, consumption of food or fluids less than 8 hours before measurements are taken, moderate to strenuous exercise within hours of BIA, and disease-associated fluid alterations.[23]

Dual energy X-ray absorptiometry (DXA) is a relatively new method for body composition assessment. Originally, it was developed as a technique for assessing bone mineral density and subsequently validated as a tool to assess total body composition.[24] The DXA X-ray source produces a polychromatic photon spectrum with two energy peaks. Exponential attenuation of the photons occurs as they pass across the subject. Detectors on the other side of the subject record the diminished photon intensity for each of the energies. Then, the attenuation characteristics in each pixel are used to estimate the components of fat, FFM, and bone mineral density[25] (see Figure 1). Many studies have examined DXA for accuracy and reproducibility in body composition assessment. The results are highly reproducible with coefficients of variation of 1% for total body mineral, 0.8% for fat, and 2% for fat-free soft tissue.[26] With the advent of effective drug treatments for osteoporosis, DXA is available in most hospitals and many office practices. It is fairly rapid and patient friendly but does require a trained technician to administer the test.

Air displacement plethysmography was developed on the same principles as hydrostatic weighing except body volume is determined by air and not water displacement. Patients are first weighed in the air and then step into a small chamber, dressed in a swimsuit and bathing cap. Thoracic gas volume is measured while the patient is in the chamber. Air volume displacement is measured and body volume is calculated. Percent body fat then is calculated using the Siri formula.[27] The test takes approximately 3–5 minutes to perform and the analysis is totally automated. Patients are not required to submerge themselves in a tank of water and breath holding is not done, which makes this technology easier to perform in special populations such as children, the elderly, and the frail. When compared with hydrostatic weighing

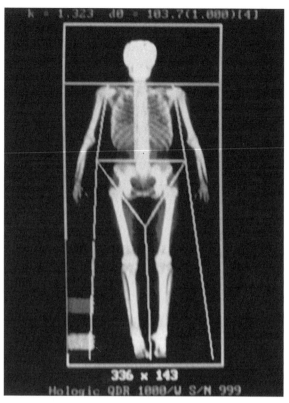

Figure 1. Example of a body composition assessment scan using dual-photon X-ray absorptiometry.

in a group of 68 adults with varying degrees of obesity, air plethysmography was shown to be highly reliable and valid.[28]

Research Assessment Tools

Research-associated body composition assessment tools include those that generally are performed only in university or research centers. Hydrostatic or underwater weighing has long been considered the gold standard for body composition. Although it is used widely around the world, its use generally is restricted to universities, body composition assessment laboratories, and large corporations with a strong philosophy of wellness and prevention. It is based on Archimedes principle that a solid is heavier than a fluid, and if a solid is placed in the fluid it will sink to the bottom. The solid, when weighed in the fluid, will be lighter than its true weight by the weight of the fluid displaced. In other words, the object placed in the fluid will be buoyed up by a counterforce, which will equal the weight that it displaces. The density of bone and muscle is greater than that of water, but the density of fat at 0.9 is less than that of water. Therefore, a person with a greater proportion of muscle will weigh more in water and will have a greater body density compared with a fatter person. The following equation is utilized: $Db = Wa/((Wa - Ww)/Dw)û (RV + 100$ mL) where Db = body density; Wa = body weight out of water; Ww = body weight in the water; Dw = density of water; and RV = residual volume.[29] The 100 mL is the estimated air volume in the gastrointestinal tract and RV is residual volume left in the lungs after maximum expiration. Multiple trials are done by placing the subject in a tank of water, seated on a chair suspended from a scale or load cell. Subjects must maximally exhale, submerge their head under water, and hold perfectly still while the weight is computed. Percent body fat then is calculated using the body density.[27] Although highly accurate and reproducible, the test itself may be difficult to perform in the very obese, the elderly, and the very young.

Although CT scanning and MRI are available in most hospitals and medical centers, their use as body composition assessment tools

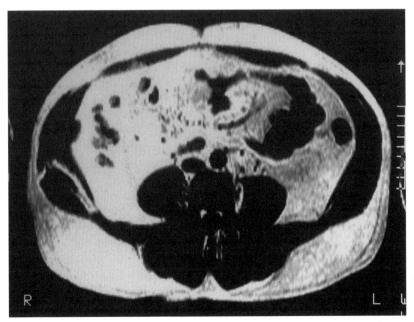

Figure 2. Magentic resonance imaging (MRI) scan at the level the fourth lumbar vertebra in a male patient with a high predominance of visceral adiposity.

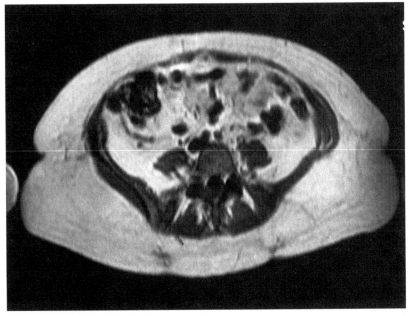

Figure 3. MRI scan at the level of the fourth lumbar vertebra in a male patient with a high predominance of subcutaneous adiposity.

still is limited to the research setting. The main advantage of these methods is that they provide a three-dimentional representation of body fat distribution (see Figures 2 and 3). Not only can subcutaneous adiposity be determined, but also visceral or intra-abdominal adipose tissue can be imaged, quantitated, and compared with other measures. Elegant studies have been done correlating body fat with serial CT scans throughout the trunk and extremities.[30] A single CT or MRI scan done at the level of the umbilicus or the fourth lumbar vertebra can be used to extrapolate the amount of total body subcutaneous and visceral fat.[31] When followed by serial CT scans, patients who have lost weight have demonstrated changes in the ratio of their visceral to subcutaneous fat.[32] Measurement of visceral obesity may be important particularly when assessing the risk of diseases such as hypertension, diabetes, and CAD. It has been shown that excess visceral fat is associated with alterations in glucose homeostasis and lipoprotein metabolism.[33,34] The relationship between obesity and CAD is complex and probably mediated by a multitude of factors such as cholesterol, triglycerides (TGs), free fatty acids, insulin, and blood pressure.[3]

Total body water can be used as an estimate of FFM, using total body potassium and doubly labeled water. These procedures can be performed in a large range of populations, including children. In the doubly labeled water method, the subject drinks a known quantity of an isotope, usually deuterium, which is not metabolized and is known to mix freely with body fluids. After an equilibration period, the concentration of the isotope in a body fluid can be used to estimate total body water. The determination of total body potassium using naturally occurring 40K assumes a constant amount of potassium in the FFM.[35] Total body potassium is calculated using a gamma counter and body composition is calculated using standardized equations.

In vivo neutron activation (IVNA) involves the controlled application of neutron irradiation to induce the release of gamma rays from tissue nuclei. These gamma rays have specific, detectable energies that can quantify elements such as carbon, hydrogen, nitrogen, oxygen, sodium, calcium, phosphorus, and chloride.[25] Two types of neutron-nuclear interactions are utilized in IVNA, the inelastic scattering of fast neutrons, which are optimal for tissue penetration and favor some forms of neutron-nuclear interactions, and the radiative capture of thermal neutrons by elemental nuclei. Neutron activation systems are costly and require highly trained scientists to maintain and operate the centers. However, these facilities provide valuable references and standards by which other body composition techniques can be measured.

Summary

The science of body composition assessment has advanced significantly over the past half of the century producing highly accurate clinical and research methodologies. Complex elemental and molecular analysis systems have provided the reference base for a broad range of techniques in the epidemiological and clinical arenas. In the future, improved methods of direct analysis will provide the groundwork for the development of body composition assessment methods that are more compact, fully automated, and patient friendly.

References

1. Kuczmarski RJ, Flegal KM, Campbell SM, et al. Increasing prevalence of overweight among US adults. The National Health and Nutrition Examination Surveys, 1960 to 1991. *JAMA* 1994;272:205–211.
2. Willett WC, Manson JE, Stampfer MJ, et al. Weight, weight change, and coronary heart disease in women. Risk within the "normal" weight range. *JAMA* 1995;273:461–465.
3. Larsson B. Obesity, fat distribution and cardiovascular disease. *Int J Obes* 1991;15:53–57.
4. Deurenberg P, Schutz Y. Body composition: Overview of methods and future directions of research. *Ann Nutr Metab* 1995;39:325–333.

5. 1983 Metropolitan height and weight tables. *Stat Bull Metrop Life Found* 1983;64:3–9.
6. Hubert HB, Feinleib M, McNamara PM, et al. Obesity as an independent risk factor for cardiovascular disease: A 26-year follow-up of participants in the Framingham Heart Study. *Circulation* 1983;67:968–977.
7. Kannel WB, D'Agostino RB, Cobb JL. Effect of weight on cardiovascular disease. *Am J Clin Nutr* 1996;63:419S–422S.
8. Roche AF, Chumlea WC. New approaches in the clinical assessment of adipose tissue. In: Bjorntorp P, Brodoff BN, eds. *Obesity*. Philadelphia, Pa: J. B. Lippincott Co., 1992:55–66.
9. Norgan NG, Ferro-Luzzi A. Weight-height indices as estimators of fatness in men. *Hum Nutr Clin Nutr* 1982;36:363–372.
10. Revicki DA, Israel RG. Relationship between body mass indices and measures of body adiposity. *Am J Public Health* 1986;76:992–994.
11. Gartside PS, Wang P, Glueck CJ. Prospective assessment of coronary heart disease risk factors: The NHANES I Epidemiologic Follow-Up Study (NHEFS) 16-Year Follow-Up. *J Am Coll Nutr* 1998;17:263–269.
12. Durazo-Arvizu RA, McGee DL, Cooper RS, et al. Mortality and optimal body mass index in a sample of the US population. *Am J Epidemiol* 1998; 147:739–749.
13. Tran ZV, Weltman A. Predicting body composition of men from girth measurements. *Hum Biol* 1988;60:167–175.
14. Hartz AJ, Rupley DC Jr, Kalkhoff RD, et al. Relationship of obesity to diabetes: Influence of obesity level and body fat distribution. *Prev Med* 1983;12:351–357.
15. Kalkhoff RK, Hartz AH, Rupley D, et al. Relationship of body fat distribution to blood pressure, carbohydrate tolerance, and plasma lipids in healthy obese women. *J Lab Clin Med* 1983;102:621–627.
16. Larsson B, Svardsudd K, Welin L, et al. Abdominal adipose tissue distribution, obesity, and risk of cardiovascular disease and death: 13 year follow up of participants in the study of men born in 1913. *Br Med J (Clin Res Ed)* 1984;288:1401–1404.
17. Hartz A, Grubb B, Wild R, et al. The association of waist hip ratio and angiographically determined coronary artery disease. *Int J Obes* 1990;14: 657–665.
18. Walker SP, Rimm EB, Ascherio A, et al. Body size and fat distribution as predictors of stroke among US men. *Am J Epidemiol* 1996;144:1143–1150.
19. Despres JP. Lipoprotein metabolism in visceral obesity. *Int J Obes* 1991;15: 45–52.
20. Jackson AS, Pollock ML. Practical assessment of body composition. *Phys Sportsmed* 1995;13:76–89.
21. Gray DS, Bray GA, Bauer M, et al. Skinfold thickness measurements in obese subjects. *Am J Clin Nutr* 1990;51:571–577.
22. Foster KR, Lukaski HC. Whole-body impedance: What does it measure? *Am J Clin Nutr* 1996;64:388S–396S.
23. Kushner RF, Gudivaka R, Schoeller DA. Clinical characteristics influencing bioelectrical impedance analysis measurements. *Am J Clin Nutr* 1996;64: 423S–427S.
24. Mazess RB, Barden HS, Bisek JP, et al. Dual-energy x-ray absorptiometry for total-body and regional bone-mineral and soft-tissue composition. *Am J Clin Nutr* 1990;51:1106–1112.

25. Heymsfield SB, Wang Z, Baumgartner RN, et al. Human body composition: Advances in models and methods. *Annu Rev Nutr* 1997;17:527–558.
26. Modlesky CM, Lewis RD, Yetman KA, et al. Comparison of body composition and bone mineral measurements from two DXA instruments in young men. *Am J Clin Nutr* 1996;64:669–676.
27. Siri WE. Body composition from fluid spaces and density: Analysis of methods. In: Brozek J, Henschel A, eds. *Techniques for Measuring Body Composition*. Washington, DC: NAS/NRC, 1961:223–224.
28. McCrory MA, Gomez TD, Bernauer EM, et al. Evaluation of a new air displacement plethysmograph for measuring human body composition. *Med Sci Sports Exerc* 1995;27:1686–1691.
29. Brozek JF, Grande F, Anderson JT. Densitometric analysis of body composition: Revision and some quantitative assumptions. *Ann NY Acad Sci* 100:113–140.
30. Sjostrom L. A computer-tomography based multicompartment body composition technique and anthropometric predictions of lean body mass, total and subcutaneous adipose tissue. *Int J Obes* 1991;15:19–30.
31. Tokunaga K, Matsuzawa Y, Ishikawa K, et al. A novel technique for the determination of body fat by computed tomography. *Int J Obes* 1983;7:437–445.
32. Sweeney ME, Nelso RC, Almon ML, et al. Changes in intraabdominal and subcutaneous adipose tissue with different levels of caloric restriction and exercise. Annual Meeting of the American Heart Association, 1994:101. Abstract.
33. Peiris AN, Sothmann MS, Hennes MI, et al. Relative contribution of obesity and body fat distribution to alterations in glucose insulin homeostasis: Predictive values of selected indices in premenopausal women. *Am J Clin Nutr* 1989;49:758–764.
34. Peiris AN, Sothmann MS, Hoffmann RG, et al. Adiposity, fat distribution, and cardiovascular risk. *Ann Intern Med* 1989;110:867–872.
35. Forbes GB. *Human Body Composition*. New York: Springer-Verlag; 1995.

Chapter 14

Dietary Strategies: Issues of Diet Composition

Sachiko T. St. Jeor, PhD, RD, and Judith M. Ashley, PhD, RD

Introduction

The ideal macronutrient composition of the diet for weight loss and weight maintenance still is being debated highly. Although consensus was seemingly established around the efficacy and desirability of the low-fat (LF) diet, the growing worldwide epidemic of obesity, and differences in dietary patterns have caused considerable concern and interest.[1] A serious reexamination of dietary factors, which may have significant contributory roles, not only in the increasing incidence of obesity but also in the prevention of weight gain and health promotion, currently is occurring. Inherent advantages of different diets, such as the Mediterranean diet (rich in monounsaturated fatty acids), Asian diets (rich in vegetable proteins), European diets (including alcohol and saturated fat), and the emerging American diet (lower in fat) are being compared. Confusion of health professionals regarding which diet to recommend also is exhibited by confused consumers trying to find which diet or nutrients they should consume. Of importance is the fact that 35% to 40% of Americans take dietary supplements.[2] Additionally, the weight-loss industry claims over $100 billion per year for its economic costs, which includes at least $33 billion for diet foods and drinks.[3,4] Although it is doubtful that there will ever be a clear answer to the exact diet composition or macronutrient ratio that is best for the prevention and treatment of obesity, the following are the objectives of this discussion: (1) to outline current dietary intake patterns and theories regarding macronutrient variations; (2) to dis-

From: Fletcher GF, Grundy SM, Hayman LL (eds). *Obesity: Impact on Cardiovascular Disease.* Armonk, NY: Futura Publishing Co., Inc.; © 1999.

cuss treatment options and their implications; and (3) to evaluate desired outcomes, especially with regard to cardiovascular disease (CVD) risk factors.

Obesity and Dietary Intake Patterns

The current intake of Americans reflects a decline in total fat intake from 36% to 34% of total energy (kcal) but a concomitant rise from 100 to 300 kcal consumed over the 10 years comparing the Second National Health and Nutrition Examination Survey (NHANES II) (1976–1980) to NHANES III (1988).[4] Thus, despite the apparent success of the "LF" message and consequent consumption of foods and diets lower in fat, the average weight in US adults has increased, in part because of this increase in overall energy intake. Approximately one in three adults were classified as overweight, with a mean increase in weight of 3.6 kg or approximately 8 lbs during one 10-year period.[5] This includes over 20% of men and 25% of women in America[1] who are now classified as truly obese with a body mass index (BMI) ≥ 30.[6] Thus, the challenge in diet composition is not only for the treatment of obesity (weight loss) but also for prevention of weight gain or regain (weight maintenance).

Low-Fat (Higher Carbohydrate) Diets

The average American diet for adults 20 years and older has been described as containing approximately 34% kcal from total fat, 49% kcal from carbohydrates, 15% to16% kcal from protein, and 2% to 3% kcal from alcohol.[4] Comparatively, current dietary recommendations made by the 1995 US Dietary Guidelines,[7] American Heart Association (AHA)[8] and the National Cholesterol Education Program[9] include lower fat intakes to <30% kcal of fat. The World Health Organization Study Group[10] recommends that dietary intakes of fat should not fall below 15% kcal fat, which has been defined as a "very LF diet"[11] to ensure adequacy and safety in provision of essential fatty acids. The comparative total fat in grams are listed below for kilocalorie percent intakes at 1200, 2000, and 3000 kcal/d and compared with regard to how carbohydrate intake levels vary in these diets in Figure 1.

	Average diet (34% kcal fat)	Lower fat diet (30% kcal fat)	Very low fat diet (15% kcal fat)
1200 kcal/d	49 g	40 g	20 g*
2000 kcal/d	82 g	67 g	33 g
3000 kcal/d	123 g	100 g	50 g

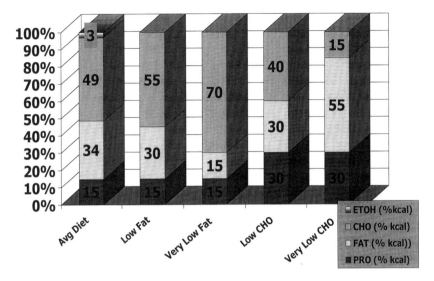

Figure 1. Macronutrient composition of the diet.

If protein intake remains constant at approximately 15% kcal, the difference in total energy per day will be made up by variations of carbohydrate intake from 49% to 70% kcal. Consideration for nutrient adequacy (especially protein) should be made with LF diets, which also are low in total kilocalories. The adequacy of the essential fatty acid, linoleic acid, generally is not a concern in these diets because it is provided in sufficient quantity at 1%–2% of total kilocalories to prevent clinical and biochemical evidence of deficiency.[12] Importantly, LF diets are associated with healthier eating patterns, according to data reported in the USDA's 1995 Continuing Survey of Food Intakes, with increases in fruit, grains, and skim milk and concomitant decreases in saturated fat with total fat.[13] Thus, by definition, a very LF diet (15% kcal) also is a very high carbohydrate diet (70% kcal). However, there is still debate whether LF diets should be defined in kilocalorie percents or total fat because total kilocalories vary.

Low-Carbohydrate (Higher Fat) Diets

For purposes of this discussion, the very low carbohydrate diet will be defined as those that contain ≤100 g total carbohydrate per day, which is the minimum needed by the body to maintain blood glucose levels, provide fuel to the brain, and prevent ketosis. This approximates 40% kcal at a 1000-kcal intake, 33% kcal at 1200 kcal, 20% kcal at 2000 kcal, and 13%

at 3000 kcal. To account for the total macronutrient intake, diets low in carbohydrate become very high fat (HF) diets (ranging from 45% to 70% kcal) and higher protein diets (ranging in fat from 20% to 40% kcal/d). At the lower levels of caloric intake, the low levels of carbohydrate, which may be imposed to minimize food selection and lower caloric intakes, are achieved because foods pure in fat and protein without carbohydrate also limit intake, palatability, and desirability. Alternatively, at extremes of higher energy intake with lower carbohydrate levels imposed, diets must be extremely high in fat and protein as they become the major source of energy. However, the overall macronutrient ratios stay somewhat the same. Figure 1 shows predicted macronutrient ratio comparisons for very low carbohydrate diets at 40% and 15% kcal. As illustrated, a low-carbohydrate diet at 40% kcal likely can consist of 30% kcal as protein and 30% kcal as fat and a very low carbohydrate diet at 15% kcal likely can consist of 30% kcal as protein and 55% kcal as fat. The level of carbohydrate that is recommended, even for low-calorie diets for weight reduction, is 55% kcal with emphasis on provisions from complex carbohydrate sources.[14] The comparative total carbohydrate (CHO) in grams are listed below for percentage of kilocalorie intakes at 1200, 2000, and 3000 kcal/d.

	Average diet (55% kcal CHO)	Low CHO diet (40% kcal CHO)	Very low CHO diet (15% kcal CHO)
1200 kcal/d	165 g	120 g	45 g*
2000 kcal/d	275 g	200 g	75 g*
3000 kcal/d	412 g	300 g	112 g

Thus, diets that are very low in carbohydrate (15%) by definition also are very high in fat and protein and usually do not provide the recommended minimum of 100 g of carbohydrate daily (these are indicated by an asterisk in above list). From a practical viewpoint, the major concerns with low-carbohydrate diets are their ability to maintain nutrient adequacy, long-term palatability, and consequent effects on overall health because of their avoidance or limitation of certain food groups. Overall, caloric intake usually is limited due to the nature of allowed foods that are high in protein and/or fat without added carbohydrates to compliment intake or provide a variety of foods. Because these diets often become very restrictive, care should be taken to maximize the nutrient value of the diet, such as including mono-unsaturated rather than saturated fat sources. Additionally, serious considerations should be given to vitamin and mineral supplements when dairy foods, enriched grains, fruits, and/or vegetables are restricted severely or omitted. It is important to consider that carbohydrates are ubiquitous in plain, basic foods and add up rapidly (1 slice bread ~ 25 g CHO, 1 cup milk ~ 12 g CHO, ½ cup potatoes or rice ~

15 g CHO, and 1/2 cup fruit or 1 cup vegetable ~ 10 to 15 g CHO). Thus, very low carbohydrate diets are prone to dietary imbalance and inadequacy. Low-carbohydrate diets vary in level of carbohydrate provided and may be self-limiting because of restrictions imposed by the quantity and type of foods allowed.

High-Protein Diets

The majority of dietary advice has focused around fats and carbohydrates in the diet because of their obvious impact on heart disease, cancer, and obesity. However, because of the essential nature of protein and its complexity, this has led to its popularity with numerous popular diet fads. However, the fact is that most Americans eat too much protein. The average protein intake for Americans reportedly is 12%–16% of total energy intake (approximately 88 to 92 g/d in males and 63–66 g/d in females).[4] This exceeds the protein requirement for most individuals, which is approximately 0.8 g/kg per day of reference protein of high biological value from animal sources such as albumen from egg whites and casein from milk.[12] Special conditions when extra protein is needed include those of accelerated growth, pregnancy and lactation, and disease states when patients are depleted nutritionally or have increased requirements.

High-protein diets have been popular because of special attributes that are associated with metabolism, structure, and/or role in the diet. Recent emphasis has been on beneficial aspects associated with glucose control, insulin regulation, muscle building, regulation, or increases in metabolism. Regardless of anecdotal data, the intake of extra protein alone will not build more muscle, provide more growth, or stimulate weight loss. Extra protein is not utilized efficiently by the body and provides a burden for its degradation rather than contributing overall to its beneficial effects. Further, protein is the most expensive source of calories. Although high-protein intakes afford little immediate risk to healthy individuals who have normal kidney and liver function, the long-term burden on the body to metabolize excess protein and nutrients has been of concern in the development of other diseases for the susceptible individual. Because of the nature of the dietary protein supply, high-protein diets usually are associated with higher intakes of saturated fat. Additionally, if food selection is limited by definition of the diet emphasizing only protein intake, nutrient deficiencies are likely to occur. Thus, a high-protein diet provides no benefit beyond meeting the recommended requirement for the essential amino acids and protein. Alone, it is not associated with health, weight loss, or muscle building.

The percentage of kilocalories from protein at various levels of total energy intake are outlined below. It is evident that as the total energy intake increases, the protein (% kcal) should decrease and the total amount of protein in grams, rather than the percentage of kilocalories, should be emphasized. Alternatively, as the total energy intake in the diet decreases, the percentage of kilocalories or total amount in grams and the quality of protein (complete, high-biological value sources) should increase in order to assure protein adequacy and provision of the essential amino acids. The average adult female needs >50 g and the average adult male needs >60 g high-quality protein. A reasonable range of protein in the diet is >50 to 100 g of protein intake per day.

	Low protein diet (<10% kcal)	Average diet (15% kcal)	High protein diet (20% kcal)	Very high protein diet (30% kcal)
1200 kcal	30 g*	45 g*	60 g	90 g
2000 kcal	50 g*	75 g	100 g†	150 g†
3000 kcal	75 g	112 g†	150 g†	225 g†

Thus, *low-calorie diets (indicated by the asterisk in the above list) used for weight reduction should be evaluated carefully for protein content. Also, +higher protein diets should be evaluated simultaneously for associated levels of saturated fat, cost, and necessity. High-protein diets that generally are advocated at the expense of severely limiting other foods become monotonous, self-limiting because of their long-term acceptability, and do not provide all of the needed nutrients. They can affect health adversely if prolonged and nutrient imbalances are permitted to occur. The overall benefits of high-protein diets are minimal.

Energy Deficit Diets for Weight Loss and Energy Balance Diets for Weight Maintenance

During weight reduction, it appears that the greatest impact of diet is from its total energy deficit and the diet composition has little effect on the rate or magnitude of weight loss over the short term.[15–17] However, for long-term weight maintenance, the total energy requirement may be affected by many factors and diet composition is focused on prevention of weight gain or obesity and maintenance of health.

Energy intake is highly variable and if energy deficits for weight loss or energy balance for long-term weight maintenance are to be achieved, questions regarding the effects of diet composition on the three major components of energy expenditure (EE) [resting energy expenditure (REE), energy cost of physical activity, and thermogenesis] must be considered. Studies have demonstrated that changes in body composition, especially fat-free mass (FFM), affect the major component of EE or REE.[18,19] During weight maintenance, there is little or no change in REE unless there are major changes in FFM. Thus, HF diets that may promote major changes in adiposity (even without changes in total weight) may contribute to small increases in REE by changes in FFM.[20,21] However, maintenance of a reduced (−10%) or elevated (+10%) body weight over usual weight, in both obese and nonobese subjects, have demonstrated compensatory changes of +16% increase and −15% decrease, respectively, in total 24 hour EE, mainly caused by changes in FFM.[21] The implications of these findings suggest that major caloric adjustments are needed (±15% of 2500 kcal = 375 kcal/d) and when ignored, these small differences or imbalance over the long term may be one of the chief reasons why many individuals are unable to maintain weight losses and gain weight.[21] An important concept in the regulation of body weight is that very small differences over longer time periods make a significant difference as illustrated below.

Intake:
- +50 kcal/d = 350 kcal/wk
- +350 kcal/wk = 3500 kcal/10 wk = 1 lb
- +3500 kcal/10 wk = +5 lb/y

Output:
- −100 kcal/d = 700 kcal/wk
- −700 kcal/wk = 3500 kcal/5 wk
- −3500 kcal/5 wk = −10 lb/y

Assuming that ±3500 kcal approximates a weight change of approximately 1 lb (indicated by the asterisk in the above list), a small difference of 375 kcal/d caused by this change could result in as much as 2625 kcal/wk or a weight change of approximately ¾ lb or 39 lb/y. Exaggerating this comparison further in terms of food intake and EE, 2–3 bites less of food (~ −100 kcal) plus a mile walk (~ −100 kcal) or equivalent increase in physical activity (30 min/d), could make up only part of this difference. The projected 200 kcal/d or 1400 kcal/wk would approximate a weight change of approximately 20 to 26 lb/y.

Weight Change Equivalents:
  1 lb of water = 0 kcal
  1 lb of pure protein (75% hydrated) ≈ 450 kcal
  1 lb of pure fat (15% hydrated) ≈ 3700 kcal
  3500 kcal/lb assumes mostly fat loss, which is highly variable,
      but preferred.
  −500 kcal/d ≈ −3500 kcal/wk ≈ −1 lb/wk

The effects of diet composition on energy expended through increased physical activity is highly individualized, complex, and in need of further study. High-carbohydrate diets generally have been promoted for periods of prolonged and/or exacerbated bouts of increased physical activity or exercise to maximize glycogen stores and serve as readily available glucose. Because the REE remains relatively constant from day to day, the amount of energy expended in physical activity is the component that is most sensitive to adjusting EE to total energy intake despite differences in overall dietary composition.[20]

With regard to energy metabolism, the independent effects of the different macronutrients overall pose interesting questions. Although the overall caloric effects of carbohydrates energetically are more expensive, those from fat are utilized more efficiently with the tendency to facilitate lipogenesis.[18,22] This caloric savings through the overall thermic effect of food (TEF) is regulated largely, but usually unquantitated and seemingly small. However, it can definitely make a difference in overall caloric balance and adiposity over the longer term. Thus, it appears evident that both total kilocalories or energy provided and the macronutrient composition of the diet play major roles in the regulation of weight and promotion/maintenance of health. Furthermore, although there is evidence that energy needs are fairly stable over long periods of time,[23] alterations in metabolic efficiency of ±10%–15% occur with under- or overfeeding and changes in body weight,[21,24] interindividual differences in energy intake, diet composition and EE affect energy balance,[25] and nutritional adaptation may be different for obese versus normal-weight individuals.[23]

Table 1, adapted from Hill et al,[15] demonstrates the potential effects that diet composition can have on the overall TEF in kilocalories per day. It is evident that the TEF is lowered when overall food intake is reduced (1200 versus 2500 kcal intake). However, on an LF diet, the total kilocalories is 30 kcal/d more because of the overall differences in carbohydrate from the HF diet. Thus, this illustrates the important

Table 1

Diet Composition and Thermic Effect of Food (kcal/d)

LF = 20%F, 60%C, 20%P HF = 40%F, 40%C, 20%P	2500 kcal/d		1200 kcal/d	
	LF	HF	LF	HF
Carbohydrate 8% TEF	120	80	58	38
Fat 2% TEF	90	20	5	10
Protein 20% TEF	100	100	48	48
Total	230	200	111	96

Adapted with permission from Reference 15.

point that on the low-calorie diets during weight loss, this difference is not significant and becomes significant only during extended periods of time (several months) when small differences can make a difference, as discussed previously.

Treatment Options and Implications

Weight Loss

The dietary prescription starts with an estimation of total energy needs in kilocalories per day. As discussed, during periods of active weight loss, the deficit in total kilocalories per day is most important. The rationale is that active weight-loss phases are associated necessarily with large energy deficits over relatively short periods of time. However, of importance is that the weight-reduction diet be balanced in nutrients to meet daily needs and provide the option of eating a variety of foods to meet these nutrient requirements. Diets below 1200 kcal/d are at risk for providing all the needed nutrients and a well-formulated multivitamin and mineral supplement should be considered.[26] An excellent guide is that which follows the Food Guide Pyramid using the lower allowance for each food group and is presented in Table 2[26,27]; it is an LF diet with adequate protein and carbohydrates.

Adherence to a weight-loss diet may be affected by its caloric level, macronutrient composition, recommended dietary patterns and foods, and departure from usual intake. The caloric deficit must be assessed carefully, because some individuals may not need or tolerate the lower calorie diets. The rate and magnitude of weight loss is determined by the overall compliance and duration of the weight-reduction diet itself. Thus, the diet composition representing more normal and usual eating patterns of the individual is critically important, because fads and monotonous diets usually are shorter in duration.

Weight Maintenance

The important factor in weight maintenance is energy balance over the long term. Wide variations in food intake and overall energy balance occur day to day; yet most adults maintain stable body compositions and weight during long periods, often by restricting food on certain days so they can "overeat" on others.[28] Diet composition, thus, varies widely and the question regarding contributions of the three macronutrients to energy balance and promotion of fat deposition is of critical interest. The regulation of protein, carbohydrate, and fat balances is related to their oxidation and stores in the body. Figure 2 (adapted from Swinburn and Ravussin[29]) outlines the effects of nutrient intake of alcohol as well as these three macronutrients with regard to overall nutrient stores and oxidative autoregulation potential. The intake of alcohol, which contributes approximately 2%–3% of kilocalories for the average adult, receives little attention as it is associated with increasing energy intake and usually minimized or avoided in low-calorie diets. Because it is metabolized efficiently, it has little effect beyond its contribution to the energy pool on nutrient stores. Because obesity reflects high-nutrient stores, dietary factors that promote fat stores or adiposity are of concern. The autoregulation of carbohydrate and protein are efficient and body stores of both glycogen and protein are limited. However, fat stores are not limited and their capacity to increase with increasing excess energy is evident. Further, because fat intake does not stimulate fat oxidation a positive fat balance results.[29] Obesity is promoted by a positive fat balance, which is promoted by an HF diet or HF-to-carbohydrate ratio[29–31] independent of total energy intake in susceptible individuals.[32–35] Thus, maintenance of fat balance requires that such factors as negative energy balance or exercise must

---

Table 2

Modification of the Food Guide Pyramid for a 1200-kcal Diet

Food group	Number of servings for a 1200-kcal[*,†]
Bread group	6[‡]
Vegetable group	3
Fruit group	2
Milk group	2[§]
Meat group (ounces)	4[‖]

Adapted with permission from Reference 27.

* Not recommended for pregnant or lactating women, children (depending on age), or those who have special dietary needs. At or below this low level of kilocalorie intake, it may not be possible to obtain recommended amounts of all nutrients from foods; therefore, it is important to make careful food choices, and the need for dietary supplements should be evaluated.

† This plan allows up to 1 teaspoon (4 g) of added sugar and 5 g of added fat.

‡ For maximum nutritional value, make whole-grain, high-fiber choices.

§ Choose skim milk products. The discretionary 5 g of added fat can be used here to select low- or reduced-fat dairy products. With the increase in recommendations for calcium intake, if 3 servings from this group are encouraged, the 80–100 kcal additional to be provided should be accommodated.

‖ Select lean meat and use cooking methods that do not require added fat.

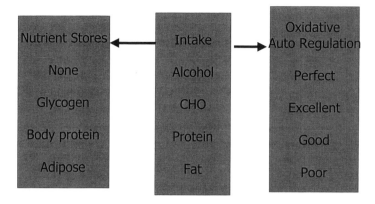

Figure 2. Effect of nutrient intake on storage and oxidative autoregulation.

compensate for the fat consumed in the diet.[15] For weight maintenance, the diet prescription must be for energy balance and fat balance.
Diets lower in fat are preferred and the upper level of <30% kcal of fat
is recommended strongly as the starting point.[6-9]

Health Maintenance

The overall energy load of the diet is of major interest as obesity
is being recognized as a disease and major contributor to the cause of
other chronic diseases in the world.[36] However, the ideal macronutrient composition of the diet becomes the center of interest for health
maintenance and disease prevention over the long term. The contribution of HF intakes to fat storage (adiposity) and the promotion of the
obese state have been discussed. Thus, the undesirability of HF intake
overall is underscored especially when strong associations of LF intake
also are linked to reduced CVD risk. However, although LF diets
have been associated with decreases in total cholesterol and low-
density lipoprotein (LDL) cholesterol, they also have been associated
with important increases in triglycerides (TG) and decreases in high-
density lipoprotein (HDL) cholesterol.[11,37,38] Thus, strong controversy
emerged regarding whether higher fat diets rich in monounsaturated
fats should be promoted because they also have been found to lower
total cholesterol, do not lower HDL cholesterol, and lower TGs, as
well.[38,39] The link between dietary fat and certain cancers and the
associations with saturated and trans fat and increases in CVD have
further underscored the importance of the LF diet. Importantly, lower
fat diets (<30%) seem the best compromise because these intakes are

associated with decreases in saturated and trans fats; increases in fruits, vegetables, and fiber; and improvements in overall nutrient content.[11,40] When modified in type of fat (increasing monunsaturated fats), the diet effects can be maximized.

Treatment Outcomes

The ideal macronutrient composition of the diet associated with the best treatment outcomes is believed to be one that promotes weight maintenance without promoting adiposity. Thus, the diet should be geared toward energy balance without excess calories from any source, especially fat. The AHA recently has recognized obesity as an independent risk factor for CVD.[41] The treatment of obesity with reduction of fat to <30% kcal has been promoted by major organizations and currently appears to be the best recommendation in balance. This by definition is a lower fat diet (with approximately 15% protein and 55% carbohydrate), which will promote dietary balance, a variety of foods, and healthy intake patterns that can be maintained over the longer term. Thus, the prevention as well as treatment of obesity becomes of central importance and the long-term compliance to dietary interventions becomes the key. Emphasis on reduction of saturated fat and individualized approaches to increase motivation along with new and innovative approaches to renew interest in overall healthier eating patterns and more active lifestyles for EE are needed.

References

1. *Obesity: Preventing and Managing the Global Epidemic.* Geneva: World Health Organization, 1998.
2. Federation of American Societies for Experimental Biology. Third Report on Nutrition Monitoring in the United States: Executive Summary. Washington, DC: US Government Printing Office; 1995.
3. Wolf AM, Colditz GA. Current estimates of the economic cost of obesity in the United States. *Obes Res* 1998;6:97–106.
4. McDowell MA, Briefel RR, Alaimo K, et al. Energy and macronutrient intakes of persons ages 2 months and over in the United States: Third National Health and Nutrition Examination Survey, Phase I, 1998–1991. October 24 ed., Washington, DC: US Government Printing Office, 1994.
5. Kuczmarski RJ, Flegal KM, Campbell SM, et al. Increasing prevalence of overweight among US adults. The National Health and Nutrition Examination Surveys, 1960 to 1991. *JAMA* 1994;272:205–211.
6. Anonymous. Clinical guidelines on the identification, evaluation, and treatment of overweight and obesity in adults: The evidence report. National Institutes of Health. *Obes Res* 1998;6:51S–209S.

7. US Department of Agriculture and US Department of Health and Human Services. *Nutrition and Your Health: Dietary Guidelines for Americans.* 4th ed., Washington, DC: US Government Printing Office, 1995.

8. Krauss RM, Deckelbaum RJ, Ernst N, et al. Dietary guidelines for healthy American adults. A statement for health professionals from the Nutrition Committee, American Heart Association. *Circulation* 1996;94:1795–1800.

9. Anonymous. Summary of the second report of the National Cholesterol Education Program (NCEP) Expert Panel on Detection, Evaluation, and Treatment of High Blood Cholesterol in Adults (Adult Treatment Panel II). *JAMA* 1993;269:3015–3023.

10. Anonymous. Diet, nutrition, and the prevention of chronic diseases. Report of a WHO Study Group. *WHOrgan Tech Rep Ser* 1990;797:1–204.

11. Lichtenstein AH, Van Horn L. Very low fat diets. *Circulation* 1998;98: 935–939.

12. Food and Nutrition Board. *Recommended Dietary Allowances.* 10th ed. Washington, DC: National Academy Press; 1989.

13. Lichtenstein AH, Kennedy E, Barrier P, et al. Dietary fat consumption and health. *Nutr Rev* 1998;56:S3–S19. Discussion S19–S28.

14. Dwyer JT, Lu D. Popular diets for weight loss: From nutritionally hazardous to healthful. In: Stunkard AJ, Wadden, eds. *Obesity: Theory and Therapy.* 2nd ed. New York, NY: Raven Press, 1993:231–252.

15. Hill JO, Drougas H, Peters JC. Obesity treatment: Can diet composition play a role? *Ann Intern Med* 1993;119:694–697.

16. Golay A, Allaz AF, Morel Y, et al. Similar weight loss with low- or high-carbohydrate diets. *Am J Clin Nutr* 1996;63:174–178.

17. Hill JO, Peters JC, Reed GW, et al. Nutrient balance in humans: Effects of diet composition. *Am J Clin Nutr* 1991;54:10–17.

18. Leibel RL, Hirsch J, Appel BE, et al. Energy intake required to maintain body weight is not affected by wide variation in diet composition. *Am J Clin Nutr* 1992;55:350–355.

19. Mifflin MD, St Jeor ST, Hill LA, et al. A new predictive equation for resting energy expenditure in healthy individuals. *Am J Clin Nutr* 1990;51:241–247.

20. Hill JO, Drougas H, Peters JC. Physical activity and moderate obesity. In: Bouchard C, Shephard R, Stephens T, eds. Physical Activity, Fitness, and Health. Toronto: Human Kinetics Publishers; 1993.

21. Leibel RL, Rosenbaum M, Hirsch J. Changes in energy expenditure resulting from altered body weight. *N Engl J Med* 1995;332:621–628.

22. Dattilo AM. Dietary fat and its relationship to body weight. *Nutr Today* 1992:13–19.

23. Hirsch J, Hudgins LC, Leibel RL, et al. Diet composition and energy balance in humans. *Am J Clin Nutr* 1998;67:551S–555S.

24. James WP, McNeill G, Ralph A. Metabolism and nutritional adaptation to altered intakes of energy substrates. *Am J Clin Nutr* 1990;51:264–269.

25. Waterlow JC. Nutritional adaptation in man: General introduction and concepts. *Am J Clin Nutr* 1990;51:259–263.

26. Committee to Develop Criteria for Evaluating the Outcomes of Approaches to Prevent and Treat Obesity. *Weighing the Options. Criteria for Evaluating Weight-Management Programs.* Washington, DC: National Academy Press; 1995.

27. US Department of Agriculture. *USDA's Food Guide Pyramid.* Washington, DC: Home and Garden Bulletin No. 202 ed.; 1992.

28. Flatt JP. What do we most need to learn about food intake regulation? *Obes Res* 1998;6:307–310.
29. Swinburn B, Ravussin E. Energy balance or fat balance? *Am J Clin Nutr* 1993;57:766S–770S. Discussion 770S–771S.
30. Astrup A, Raben A. Obesity: An inherited metabolic deficiency in the control of macronutrient balance? *Eur J Clin Nutr* 1992;46:611–620.
31. Westerterp-Plantenga MS, MJ IJ, Wijckmans-Duijsens NE. The role of macronutrient selection in determining patterns of food intake in obese and non-obese women. *Eur J Clin Nutr* 1996;50:580–591.
32. Romieu I, Willett WC, Stampfer MJ, et al. Energy intake and other determinants of relative weight. *Am J Clin Nutr* 1988;47:406–412.
33. Astrup A, Buemann B, Western P, et al. Obesity as an adaptation to a high-fat diet: Evidence from a cross-sectional study. *Am J Clin Nutr* 1994; 59:350–355.
34. Ravussin E, Tataranni PA. Dietary fat and human obesity. *J Am Diet Assoc* 1997;97:S42–S46.
35. Tucker LA, Kano MJ. Dietary fat and body fat: A multivariate study of 205 adult females. *Am J Clin Nutr* 1992;56:616–622.
36. Grundy SM. Multifactorial causation of obesity: Implications for prevention. *Am J Clin Nutr* 1998;67:563S–572S.
37. Connor WE, Connor SL. Should a low-fat, high-carbohydrate diet be recommended for everyone? The case for a low-fat, high-carbohydrate diet. *N Engl J Med* 1997;337:562–563. Discussion 566–567.
38. Katan MB, Grundy SM, Willett WC. Should a low-fat, high-carbohydrate diet be recommended for everyone? Beyond low-fat diets. *N Engl J Med* 1997;337:563–6. Discussion 566–7.
39. Grundy SM. What is the desirable ratio of saturated, polyunsaturated, and monounsaturated fatty acids in the diet? *Am J Clin Nutr* 1997;66:988S–990S.
40. Dougherty RM, Fong AK, Iacono JM. Nutrient content of the diet when the fat is reduced. *Am J Clin Nutr* 1988;48:970–979.
41. Eckel RH. Obesity and heart disease: A statement for healthcare professionals from the Nutrition Committee, American Heart Association. *Circulation* 1997;96:3248–3250. Figure 1. Macronutrient composition of the diet.

Chapter 15

Energy Expenditure and Obesity

James O. Hill, PhD,
and Adamandia D. Kriketos, PhD

Introduction

The fact that body weight is influenced by an interaction of genetic and environmental factors[1] must be considered when examining the role of energy expenditure (EE) in the etiology of obesity. In Figure 1, we have illustrated the change in the body mass index (BMI; kg/m^2) distribution that has occurred in the United States over the past 4 decades. As the environment has become more obesity promoting, the BMI distribution has changed. Both the average BMI and the spread in the BMI distribution have increased in response to the changing environment. In this chapter we will consider the role of EE in contributing to differences between body weights of different individuals within the same environment and between the same individual in different environments.

The Nature of Body Weight Regulation

Stability of body weight requires an equality between energy intake and EE.[2] The traditional view of energy balance is shown in Figure 2. Adjustments in energy intake and/or EE in response to daily variations in food intake or physical activity would serve to maintain a constant body weight and body composition over time. According to this view, obesity would arise because of a failure of this regulatory system.[3]

From: Fletcher GF, Grundy SM, Hayman LL (eds). *Obesity: Impact on Cardiovascular Disease.* Armonk, NY: Futura Publishing Co., Inc.; © 1999.

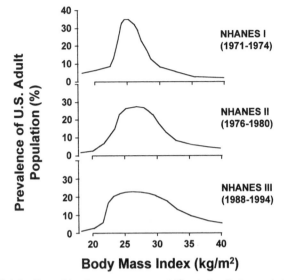

Body Mass Index (kg/m²)

Figure 1. Distribution of body mass among US adults. Data are taken from the National Health and Nutrition Examination Surveys conducted from 1971 to 1994.

An alternative view of an energy regulatory system assumes that the body's ability to adjust energy intake and EE to defend a constant body weight is limited. When faced with a challenge to the system (eg, increased energy intake or decreased physical activity) that exceeds the adaptive capacity of intake and expenditure, body mass changes. The change in body mass is not the result of defective regulation, but

Obesity results from an "error" in regulating energy balance

$$E_{in} = E_{out}$$

or

$$E_{in} = RMR + TEF + EE_{ACT}$$

Figure 2. The traditional view of energy balance. Energy balance occurs when energy intake (E_{in}) is equal to energy expenditure (E_{out}). The E_{out} is equivalent to the sum of resting metabolic rate (RMR), the thermic effect of food (TEF), and the energy expended during physical activity (EE_{act}). Obesity would be the result of a regulatory error.

represents an important component of the regulatory system, which helps restore energy balance. This occurs through a change in resting metabolic rate (RMR) (associated with the altered body mass) and perhaps through signals to alter energy intake.

More specifically, obesity is a problem of fat balance, because while the body has a good ability to adjust oxidation rates of protein and carbohydrate to alterations in the intake of each, it does not have this ability for fat.[2,4–7] This means that following a perturbation that produces positive or negative energy balance, protein and carbohydrate balances are achieved quickly and, thus, imbalances in energy become imbalances in fat.[2,4–7] This produces changes in the body fat mass, which serve to increase or decrease fat oxidation to reachieve fat balance and energy balance.[7] The body fat mass stabilizes at the point where fat oxidation has been increased or decreased sufficiently to restore fat balance. Figure 3 illustrates that body fat mass is an integral part of the energy balance regulatory system.

Components of Energy Expenditure

Daily EE can be considered as having multiple components.[8] For purposes of this discussion, we will consider the following components of daily EE: RMR, the thermic effect of food (TEF) and the EE in physical activity (EEact). RMR is determined largely by the amount of body mass, with fat-free mass (FFM) having a much higher rate of EE than fat mass. The TEF is determined largely by the amount and composition of energy consumed. EEact is influenced primarily by the

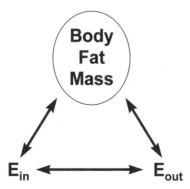

Figure 3. An alternative view of an energy regulatory system. This model depicts that changes in the body fat mass are not simply the result of regulatory errors, but that body fat mass is an integral component of the regulatory system. An increase in body fat mass, for example, is necessary under some circumstances to achieve energy and fat balance.

amount and type of physical activity performed. The term obligatory thermogenesis often is used to designate the rate of EE that arises as a function of the size of body size. This is estimated as the sum of RMR and TEF (there may be a small part of TEF that is not obligatory, but this is controversial). Alternatively, facultative thermogenesis is considered as the component of EE that varies because of factors other than body size (eg, energy expended as a function of amount of physical activity).

How Does the Environment Affect Body Weight Regulation: Role of Energy Expenditure

There are many examples of how body weight is affected by the environment. One of the most compelling is a comparison of Pima Indians living on reservations in Arizona to Pima Indians, that are genetically similar, living as subsistence farmers in Mexico.[9] Figure 4 shows that the BMI of the former group is substantially greater than the BMI of the latter group. A second example is migration of subjects from obesity-retardant environments to obesity-promoting environments. Curb and Marcus[10] have shown that BMI increases when Japanese individuals move to the United States. Finally, the increase in the prevalence of obesity in the United States from the 1970s to the 1990s is another example of how changes in the environment can influence the average BMI of the population.[11]

How does the environment affect energy balance and body weight regulation? The environment can have substantial effects on energy

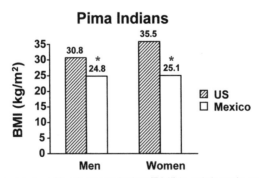

Figure 4. Comparison of body mass index (BMI) in adult male and female Pima Indians living on a reservation in Arizona (filled boxes) and in a farming community in Mexico (open boxes). The Mexican Pima Indians in each gender group have a significantly lower (P < 0.0001) BMI than their Arizona-living counterparts. Adapted with permission from Reference 9.

intake and physical activity. The current environment in the United States, for example, is characterized by an abundant supply of cheap, high-fat/high-energy density foods and by low levels of physical activity.[12] This environment promotes positive energy balance, because the body does not have a good ability to adjust energy intake downward to match reduced EE.[12] It is difficult to accept that the increase in obesity that has occurred over the past 2 decades in the United States is caused by widespread defects in energy balance regulation. It is more plausible that the effects of the environment on energy intake and physical activity for most people exceed the capacity to adjust energy intake and EE to keep body weight at a non-overweight level.

Human physiology developed in an environment where avoiding depletion of body energy stores was likely a high priority, and where avoiding accumulation of body energy stores was a selective advantage. It makes sense that we would have evolved stronger physiological systems to oppose loss of body energy than to oppose accumulation of body energy. This is illustrated in Figure 5. Acute alterations in energy intake in either direction appear to produce rather weak ad-

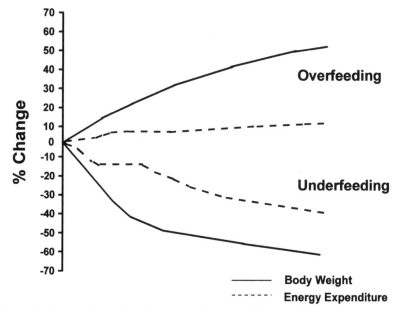

Figure 5. Acute alterations in energy intakes, either under- or overfeeding, produce weak adjustments of energy expenditure (EE). More prolonged alterations in energy intakes, in either direction, lead in more substantial changes in body weight. These changes appear to be greater for food restriction than for overfeeding.

justments of EE, which may be somewhat higher for under- than overfeeding. Jebb et al[13] found that over 12 days, EE was decreased by 10.5% in subjects underfed by 1/3 and increased by 8.9% in subjects overfed by 1/3. Others[14–16] found similar increases in EE with overfeeding. The changes in EE were insufficient to prevent subjects from being in considerable energy imbalance. However, with sustained food restriction and loss of body energy, the decline in EE appears to be greater than can be explained by loss of body mass.[17] With overfeeding, there does not appear to be an increase in EE beyond that which would be associated with increased body mass. Because there appears to be a better protection against loss of body weight than against gain of body mass, an increase in obligatory EE is not likely to be a major factor in preventing obesity.

Differences in Body Weight Regulation between Individuals in a Common Environment

The next question we will ask is whether differences in EE play a primary role in determining which individuals will become obese within a given environment.

Resting Metabolic Rate

RMR is the largest component of 24-hour EE and has been studied extensively as a factor in the development of obesity. FFM is the major determinant of RMR, but fat mass also can contribute to variance in RMR.[18] These factors can explain 60%–80% of variance in RMR, leaving some unexplained variance. Some unexplained variance may be caused by genetic factors, because RMR expressed per kilogram FFM shows fewer variations within families than between families.[19]

Although RMR is greater in obese individuals than lean individuals, this is caused by higher FFM in the former group.[20] There is general agreement that obese individuals do not have a systematically higher RMR than lean individuals when the known determinants of RMR are considered.[20]

However, it has been suggested that a low RMR may cause obesity and the process of becoming obese then normalizes RMR. Ravussin et al[21] provided support for this hypothesis in studies of Pima Indians. Ravussin and his colleagues showed in a longitudinal study of Pima Indians that low rates of EE, adjusted for FFM, fat mass, age, and gender, were significant predictors of weight gain.[21] The adjusted 24-hour EE was related inversely to the amount or rate of change in body weight. After a weight gain, the new adjusted RMR increased to a value similar to that in persons who did not gain weight. Similarly, Roberts et al[22] reported that a low rate of EE predicted weight gain in infants. However, other studies have not found RMR to be a predictor of either weight gain or weight loss in adults[23,24] or a predictor of weight gain in children.[25,26]

Another way to test the hypothesis is to examine reduced-obese subjects. In such subjects, weight loss may unmask the low RMR that led to obesity. Although this literature is somewhat controversial, a large number of studies have failed to show a reduced RMR in reduced-obese subjects.[27-34] Perhaps the strongest data come from the National Weight Control Registry, a registry of successful weight-reduced subjects, each of whom has maintained at least a 30-lb weight loss for at least 1 year.[35] Thompson et al[36] showed a normal RMR in 40 successful weight-reduced subjects compared with a never-reduced control group.

Finally, although a low RMR has been documented in African American subjects,[37-40] it is not clear that this low RMR is a major cause of obesity. First, the low RMR is present in African American men and women[40] as compared with Caucasians, but the prevalence of obesity between African Americans and Caucasians is only higher in women. Second, the low RMR is seen in subjects across a range of BMI from very lean to obese, with no evidence that developing obesity normalizes RMR.

Thermic Effect of Food

TEF is defined as the increase in RMR following the ingestion of a meal and includes energy costs of digestion, absorption, and metabolism of ingested food.[41] Meal size, meal composition, the nature of the previous diet, insulin resistance, physical activity, aging, and body composition can all influence TEF.[41,42] Although this component of 24-hour EE accounts for a relatively small proportion of total EE (6%–10%), it has been suggested that differences in TEF could play a role in the development and/or maintenance of obesity.[43]

The role of TEF in energy balance in man remains controversial. For example, D'Alessio et al[44] cite 15 papers reporting a reduced TEF in obese subjects as compared with lean subjects and 12 papers reporting no difference in the TEF between the two groups. There are no data that have examined whether a low TEF may be factor in obesity development and then may be normalized with development of obesity.

In a study comparing the TEF in obese versus lean individuals, the extent of the difference in TEF is equivalent to a 1%–2% proportion of 24-hour EE, that is, approximately equal to a half sandwich.[30]

Energy Expended in Physical Activity

The total amount of EE during physical activity (EEact) is determined by the amount of physical activity multiplied by the cost of that activity, (ie, the efficiency with which it is performed). Although the cost of activity is dependent on the amount of body mass being moved, this component is highly variable because of individual differences in amount of physical activity performed. EEact may represent 15%–50% of 24-hour EE in active subjects.[45,46] This range may be reduced in sedentary subjects but likely remains high. For example, Ravussin et al[18] reported an interindividual variation in EEact of 138–685 kcal/d in Pima Indians studied for a day in a whole-room calorimeter.

Negative relationships between measures of physical activity (usually self-reports) and indices of obesity (usually BMI) are seen in most data sets obtained from the general US population.[47,48] The relationship appears to be similar in men and women, and across all ages.[49–54] Further, there is evidence for a similar relationship in African Americans[52] and Hispanics.[53]

In several data sets, body weight gain over time has been shown to be correlated negatively with baseline level of physical activity and with changes in level of physical activity.[50,55,56]

There does not appear to be any data to suggest that an increased efficiency of physical activity plays a role in the etiology of obesity. An obese individual has an increased work efficiency because of their greater FFM; however, following weight reduction, the efficiency of physical activity is decreased, which is explained by the decline in body mass.[57]

Variation in Components of Energy Expenditure

In Table 1, we have estimated the extent of the between-subject variation in each component of EE. These estimations are based on between-subject variation reported in the scientific literature and assume that subjects have a daily energy requirement of 3000 kcal. The greatest between-subject variation was in EEact, and this would seem the most likely place where differences in EE could lead to differences in susceptibility to obesity. However, it is possible that the variation in

Table 1

Potential Between-Subject Differences in Energy Expenditure

Component	Assumptions*	Extent of differences between subjects
RMR	1. 20%–40% unexplained variation in RMR; 2. Individuals vary in this unexplained variation by 10%	60–120 kcal/d
TEF	1. TEF = 10% of total energy intake 2. Individuals differ by 1%–2%	30–60 kcal/d
EEact	1. EEact ranges from 15% to 50% of total EE	450–1500 kcal/d

* Assumes all subjects would have energy requirements of 3000 kcal/d for weight maintenance.

RMR and TEF also could contribute to differences between subjects in the level of body weight maintained within a given environment.

Summary

Changes in body fat mass are an integral part of the regulatory system involved in maintenance of energy balance. When an individual is in an environment with abundant food and low levels of physical activity, there is an increased likelihood of sustained or periodic positive energy balance. This is because food intake does not appear to be matched precisely to the low levels of EE and because there is only a weak ability to increase obligatory EE in response to positive energy. Under these circumstances, increases in body fat mass result from positive fat and energy balance and can serve to increase fat oxidation and total EE to restore energy and macronutrient balance.

Within a given environment, individuals differ widely in body weight and body composition. This likely is caused by individual differences in how the environment affects food intake and to individual differences in some components of EE. The greatest individual variation in EE is seen in the EEact. EEact has been shown to correlate negatively with BMI and with change in BMI. There is less individual variation in RMR and TEF. Although there is some suggestion that differences in RMR may predict obesity, the majority of data suggest differences in RMR are not a strong predictor of body weight change. There are no data to suggest that a low TEF is predictive of obesity.

The notion that obesity arises from an abnormally low rate of EE has not been supported by the majority of data collected in human subjects. The component of EE most associated with differences in obesity is the EEact. This is the most modifiable component of EE, and efforts to increase physical activity could be extremely helpful in preventing obesity.

References

1. Hill JO, Pagliassotti MJ, Peters JC. Non genetic determinants of obesity and body fat topography. In: Bouchard C, ed. *The Genetics of Obesity*. Boca Raton: CRC Press, Inc.; 1994:35–48.
2. Flatt JP. Importance of nutrient balance in body weight regulation. *Diabetes Metab Rev* 1988;4:571–581.
3. Schwartz MW, Seeley RJ. The new biology of body weight regulation. *J Am Diet Assoc* 1997;97:54–58. Quiz 59–60.
4. Bennett C, Reed GW, Peters JC, et al. Short-term effects of dietary-fat ingestion on energy expenditure and nutrient balance. *Am J Clin Nutr* 1992;55:1071–1077.
5. Schutz Y, Flatt JP, Jequier E. Failure of dietary fat intake to promote fat oxidation: A factor favoring the development of obesity [see comments]. *Am J Clin Nutr* 1989;50:307–314.
6. Flatt JP, Ravussin E, Acheson KJ, et al. Effects of dietary fat on postprandial substrate oxidation and on carbohydrate and fat balances. *J Clin Invest* 1985;76:1019–1024.
7. Astrup A, Buemann B, Western P, et al. Obesity as an adaptation to a high-fat diet: Evidence from a cross-sectional study. *Am J Clin Nutr* 1994; 59:350–355.
8. Ravussin E, Rising R. Daily energy expenditure in humans: Measurements in a respiratory change and by doubly labeled water. In: Kinney JM, Tucker HN, eds. *Energy Metabolism: Tissue Determinants and Cellular Corollaries*. New York: Raven Press, Ltd.; 1992:81–96.
9. Ravussin E, Valencia ME, Esparza J, et al. Effects of a traditional lifestyle on obesity in Pima Indians. *Diabetes Care* 1994;17:1067–1074.
10. Curb JD, Marcus EB. Body fat and obesity in Japanese Americans. *Am J Clin Nutr* 1991;53:1552S–1555S.
11. Kuczmarski RJ, Flegal KM, Campbell SM, et al. Increasing prevalence of overweight among US adults. The National Health and Nutrition Examination Surveys, 1960 to 1991. *JAMA* 1994;272:205–211.
12. Hill JO, Peters JC. Environmental contributions to the obesity epidemic. *Science* 1998;280:1371–1374.
13. Jebb SA, Prentice AM, Goldberg GR, et al. Changes in macronutrient balance during over- and underfeeding assessed by 12-d continuous whole-body calorimetry. *Am J Clin Nutr* 1996;64:259–266.
14. Horton TJ, Drougas H, Brachey A, et al. Fat and carbohydrate overfeeding in humans: Different effects on energy storage. *Am J Clin Nutr* 1995;62: 19–29.
15. Roberts SB, Fuss P, Heyman MB, et al. Effects of age on energy expenditure and substrate oxidation during experimental underfeeding in healthy men. *J Gerontol A Biol Sci Med Sci* 1996;51:B158–B166.

16. Bouchard C, Tremblay A. Genetic influences on the response of body fat and fat distribution to positive and negative energy balances in human identical twins. *J Nutr* 1997;127:943S–947S.

17. Keys A, Henschel A, Michelson O, et al. *The Biology of Human Starvation.* Minneapolis, Minn: University of Minnesota Press; 1950.

18. Ravussin E, Lillioja S, Anderson TE, et al. Determinants of 24-hour energy expenditure in man. Methods and results using a respiratory chamber. *J Clin Invest* 1986;78:1568–1578.

19. Bogardus C, Lillioja S, Ravussin E, et al. Familial dependence of the resting metabolic rate. *N Engl J Med* 1986;315:96–100.

20. Owen OE. Resting metabolic requirements of men and women. *Mayo Clin Proc* 1988;63:503–510.

21. Ravussin E, Lillioja S, Knowler WC, et al. Reduced rate of energy expenditure as a risk factor for body-weight gain. *N Engl J Med* 1988;318:467–472.

22. Roberts SB, Savage J, Coward WA, et al. Energy expenditure and intake in infants born to lean and overweight mothers. *N Engl J Med* 1988;318:461–466.

23. Seidell JC, Muller DC, Sorkin JD, et al. Fasting respiratory exchange ratio and resting metabolic rate as predictors of weight gain: The Baltimore Longitudinal Study on Aging. *Int J Obes Relat Metab Disord* 1992;16:667–674.

24. Kreitzman SN, Coxon AY, Johnson PG, et al. Dependence of weight loss during very-low-calorie diets on total energy expenditure rather than on resting metabolic rate, which is associated with fat-free mass. *Am J Clin Nutr* 1992;56:258S–261S.

25. Goran MI, Shewchuk R, Gower BA, et al. Longitudinal changes in fatness in white children: No effect of childhood energy expenditure. *Am J Clin Nutr* 1998;67:309–316.

26. Stunkard A, Berkowitz R, Stallings V, et al. Growth and development on infants born to obese and lean mothers. *Obes Res* 1997;5:1–36.

27. Burstein R, Prentice AM, Goldberg GR, et al. Metabolic fuel utilisation in obese women before and after weight loss. *Int J Obes Relat Metab Disord* 1996;20:253–259.

28. Amatruda JM, Statt MC, Welle SL. Total and resting energy expenditure in obese women reduced to ideal body weight. *J Clin Invest* 1993;92:1236–1242.

29. de Groot LC, van Es AJ, van Raaij JM, et al. Energy metabolism of overweight women 1 mo and 1 y after an 8-wk slimming period. *Am J Clin Nutr* 1990;51:578–583.

30. Nelson KM, Weinsier RL, James LD, et al. Effect of weight reduction on resting energy expenditure, substrate utilization, and the thermic effect of food in moderately obese women. *Am J Clin Nutr* 1992;55:924–933.

31. Weinsier RL, Nelson KM, Hensrud DD, et al. Metabolic predictors of obesity. Contribution of resting energy expenditure, thermic effect of food, and fuel utilization to four-year weight gain of post-obese and never-obese women. *J Clin Invest* 1995;95:980–985.

32. Weigle DS, Sande KJ, Iverius PH, et al. Weight loss leads to a marked decrease in nonresting energy expenditure in ambulatory human subjects. *Metabolism* 1988;37:930–936.

33. Larson DE, Ferraro RT, Robertson DS, et al. Energy metabolism in weight-stable postobese individuals. *Am J Clin Nutr* 1995;62:735–739.

34. James WP, Lean ME, McNeill G. Dietary recommendations after weight loss: How to avoid relapse of obesity. *Am J Clin Nutr* 1987;45:1135–1141.

35. Klem ML, Wing RR, McGuire MT, et al. A descriptive study of individuals successful at long-term maintenance of substantial weight loss. *Am J Clin Nutr* 1997;66:239–46.

36. Thompson HR, Grunwald GK, Seagle HM, et al. Resting energy expenditure in reduced-obese subjects in the National Weight Control Registry. *Obes Res* 1997;5:IV-38.

37. Carpenter WH, Fonong T, Toth MJ, et al. Total daily energy expenditure in free-living older African-Americans and Caucasians. *Am J Physiol* 1998;274: E96–E101.

38. Albu J, Shur M, Curi M, et al. Resting metabolic rate in obese, premenopausal black women. *Am J Clin Nutr* 1997;66:531–538.

39. Foster GD, Wadden TA, Vogt RA. Resting energy expenditure in obese African American and Caucasian women. *Obes Res* 1997;5:1–8.

40. Hill JO, Sharp T, Sidney S, et al. Differences in resting metabolic rate between Caucasian and African-American young adults in the CARDIA study. *Obes Res* 1997;1997:IV-18.

41. Reed GW, Hill JO. Measuring the thermic effect of food. *Am J Clin Nutr* 1996;63:164–169.

42. de Jonge L, Bray GA. The thermic effect of food and obesity: A critical review. *Obes Res* 1997;5:622–631.

43. Schutz Y, Bessard T, Jequier E. Diet-induced thermogenesis measured over a whole day in obese and nonobese women. *Am J Clin Nutr* 1984;40:542–552.

44. D'Alessio DA, Kavle EC, Mozzoli MA, et al. Thermic effect of food in lean and obese men. *J Clin Invest* 1988;81:1781–1789.

45. Livingstone MB, Strain JJ, Prentice AM, et al. Potential contribution of leisure activity to the energy expenditure patterns of sedentary populations. *Br J Nutr* 1991;65:145–155.

46. Dauncey MJ. Activity and energy expenditure. *Can J Physiol Pharmacol* 1990;68:17–27.

47. Crespo CJ, Keteyian SJ, Heath GW, et al. Leisure-time physical activity among US adults. Results from the Third National Health and Nutrition Examination Survey. *Arch Intern Med* 1996;156:93–98.

48. DiPietro L, Williamson DF, Caspersen CJ, et al. The descriptive epidemiology of selected physical activities and body weight among adults trying to lose weight: The Behavioral Risk Factor Surveillance System Survey, 1989. *Int J Obes Relat Metab Disord* 1993;17:69–76.

49. Anderssen N, Jacobs DR Jr, Sidney S, et al. Change and secular trends in physical activity patterns in young adults: A seven-year longitudinal follow-up in the Coronary Artery Risk Development in Young Adults Study (CARDIA). *Am J Epidemiol* 1996;143:351–362.

50. Williamson DF, Madans J, Anda RF, et al. Recreational physical activity and ten-year weight change in a US national cohort. *Int J Obes Relat Metab Disord* 1993;17:279–286.

51. Kok FJ, Matroos AW, Hautvast JG, et al. Correlates of body mass index in 1926 Dutch men and women. *Hum Nutr Clin Nutr* 1982;36:155–165.

52. Washburn RA, Kline G, Lackland DT, et al. Leisure time physical activity: Are there black/white differences? *Prev Med* 1992;21:127–135.

53. Winkleby MA, Fortmann SP, Rockhill B. Health-related risk factors in a sample of Hispanics and whites matched on sociodemographic characteristics. The Stanford Five-City Project. *Am J Epidemiol* 1993;137:1365–1375.
54. Haffner S, Gonzalez Villalpando C, Hazuda HP, et al. Prevalence of hypertension in Mexico City and San Antonio, Texas. *Circulation* 1994;90: 1542–1549.
55. Owens JF, Matthews KA, Wing RR, et al. Can physical activity mitigate the effects of aging in middle-aged women? *Circulation* 1992;85:1265–1270.
56. French SA, Jeffery RW, Forster JL, et al. Predictors of weight change over two years among a population of working adults: the Healthy Worker Project. *Int J Obes Relat Metab Disord* 1994;18:145–154.
57. Hill JO, Saris WHM. Energy expenditure and physical activity. In: Bray G, Bouchard C, James WPT, eds. *Handbook of Obesity*. New York, NY: Marcel Dekker, Inc.; 1997:457–474.

Chapter 16

Physical Activity in the Management of Obesity: Issues and Implementation

Marcia L. Stefanick, PhD

Introduction

The Third National Health and Nutrition Examination Survey (NHANES III), conducted from 1988–1994, showed a marked increase in the prevalence of obesity in the United States since the NHANES II (1976–1980). Specifically, the percent of the US population that is obese, that is, having a body mass index (BMI) $\geq 30 \ kg/m^2$, increased from 14.5% to 22.5% between surveys.[1] With 54.5% of US adults aged 20 years or older being overweight or obese, the National Heart Lung and Blood Institute's Obesity Education Initiative and National Institute of Diabetes and Digestive and Kidney Diseases convened the Expert Panel on the Identification, Evaluation, and Treatment of Overweight and Obesity in Adults.[2]

An important question raised by the Expert Panel was "What treatments are effective?" After evaluating the literature to determine the most appropriate treatment strategies that would constitute evidence-based clinical guidelines, the Panel recommended physical activity "as part of a comprehensive weight-loss therapy and weight control program, because it: modestly contributes to weight loss in overweight and obese adults, may decrease abdominal fat, increases cardiorespiratory fitness, and may help with maintenance of weight loss."[2] The Panel recommended the exercise prescription developed by the Centers for Disease Control and Prevention and the American College of Sports Medicine in 1995[3] and embraced by the National Institutes of Health (NIH) Consensus Development Panel on Physical

From: Fletcher GF, Grundy SM, Hayman LL (eds). *Obesity: Impact on Cardiovascular Disease.* Armonk, NY: Futura Publishing Co., Inc.; © 1999.

Activity and Cardiovascular Health.[4] Specifically, the Panel recommended that moderate levels of physical activity be encouraged for 30 to 45 minutes, 3 days a week, initially, with a long-term goal of accumulating at least 30 minutes or more of moderate-intensity physical activity on most and preferably all days of the week.[2] This chapter will review the literature that pertains to these recommendations.

The review will be restricted primarily to randomized, controlled clinical trials of exercise in initially sedentary or overweight or obese individuals, with or without dietary interventions, with some attention to type of "dose" of exercise, that is, frequency and duration of exercise, length of training period, and treatment regimens. This approach is intended to provide clinicians and health educators with reasonable expectations for the exercise recommendations they are being encouraged to prescribe for the management of obesity in overweight patients and the general public.

In this context, it is worth recognizing that relationships found in epidemiological studies between obesity and a sedentary lifestyle, both of which are highly prevalent in the population, or observations of lower-body weights in individuals who engage in higher levels of physical activity, do not provide evidence that overweight individuals will lose weight by exercising at a level that may be associated with leanness in the general population.[5] Recognizing that 1 kg of body fat supplies enough energy to support approximately 100 km of walking or jogging and that it is fat mass loss, which should be the goal of any weight-loss program, must be understood that weight loss by exercise alone would be a slow and gradual process. Furthermore, it is imperative that caloric intake is not increased in response to the increase in energy expenditure; therefore, attention to diet is important.

Randomized, Controlled Trials
of Aerobic Exercise Only

In evaluation of randomized, controlled trials of the effect of physical activity on weight loss, abdominal fat, and cardiorespiratory fitness, the Expert Panel focused on 13 published articles.[6–18] Three of these articles[7–9] presented different data from the first Stanford Weight Control Project (SWCP-I),[7–9] in which weight loss by exercise, with no change in diet, was the intervention goal, as opposed to an outcome variable and two of them should not be regarded as separate trials.[8,9] Two of the other trials seem to have been misclassified, in that the "control" group in one actually was instructed to consume a low-fat, ad libitum–carbohydrate diet and lost 5.8 kg[10] and another had neither an exercise-only group nor a control group because all groups were placed on a 5000 kJ diet.[12] Finally, as the Panel acknowledged, one of the articles was a follow-up study[15] of a controlled trial of three different exercise regimens[13]; and the control group was no longer part of the study.[15]

Table 1 presents the basic study design (randomized intervention groups), key subject recruitment criteria, length of training period, initial obesity status, and weight changes for the eight remaining trials, which were deemed acceptable by the Expert Panel. A small study[19] and four larger trials[20–23] have been added, which seem in accordance with the minimum criteria outlined by the Expert Panel, that is, of at least 4 months duration and not relying on self-reported weights.[2] An additional small, but elegant, 12-week metabolic ward study appears, which included both a weight maintenance and a weight-loss exercise group, as well as a diet-induced weight-loss group and control.[24] Although it is likely that there are many other small studies in the literature that report weight changes in exercise only versus control groups, particularly in the sports medicine literature, the 15 trials in this table include a broad range of men and women, at different levels of normal weight, overweight, and obesity and several exercise interventions. However, none of them focus on minority groups, for whom data are extremely limited.

It is interesting to note that several of the earlier trials reported baseline weight, without height, and did not report BMI, thereby making it difficult to know the weight status of the participants. Furthermore, many of these studies reported significant weight changes within groups, that is, baseline versus posttreatment weights, but do not specify whether there were significant differences between groups, thereby making poor use of the control group.

The first two trials in Table 1 were designed to determine whether aerobic exercise increases high-density lipoprotein cholesterol (HDLC) in middle-aged men who were not selected to be overweight.[20,22] In the Finnish trial,[20] men aged 40–45 years were assigned to exercise ($N = 50$) or control ($N = 50$). Exercisers were given an individualized training program that consisted of walking, jogging, swimming, skiing, or cycling and included 3 weekly sessions during the first 8 weeks, at a target heart rate of resting heart rate $+ 0.40 \times$ [maximum heart rate (HRmax) $-$ resting heart rate], with HRmax extrapolated from values assessed during a submaximal exercise test on a bicycle ergometer. After this period, exercisers were expected to do a minimum of one unsupervised training session on alternate days, at a higher intensity of resting heart rate $+ 0.66 \times$ (HRmax $-$ resting heart rate), and one supervised session a month, and to meet with study exercise physiologists regularly. Controls were asked to maintain previous exercise habits. Both exercisers and controls were instructed to reduce dietary

Table 1

Randomized Trials with Aerobic Exercise Only versus Control Groups

Study	Interventions: treatment groups	N post (randomized) sex; basic (key) inclusion criteria	Training period duration	Initial BMI (or weight in kg)	Weight (kg) (or BMI) change	Differences among groups (weight changes)
Huttunen et al.[20]	1: Aerobic exercise 2: Control	90 (100) men; middle-aged	4 months	1: (78.4) 2: (79.9)	1: −0.9 2: −0.6	NS
Wood et al.[21]	1: Aerobic exercise 2: Control	78 (81) men; sedentary	9–12 months	1: (76.4) 2: (78.0)	1: −1.9 2: +0.6	P = 0.002
Sopko et al.[24]	1: Aerobic exercise (weight loss) 2: Aerobic exercise with no weight change 3: Hypocaloric diet (weight loss) 4: Control (weight maintenance)	21 (40) men: 110% standard body weight, sedentary	12 weeks	1: (81.2) 2: (99.3) 3: (100.3) 4: (82.5) 2 and 3 vs. 4 P < 0.05	1: −6.2 2: −0.5 3: −6.0 4: −0.5	Not reported. Pre vs post, 1: P < 0.001 3: P < 0.001
Ronnemaa et al.[6]	1: Aerobic exercise 2: Control	25 (30) men (33%) + women with NIDDM	4 months	1: (85.2) 2: (82.8)	1: −2.0 2: +0.5	Not reported 1: pre vs post P < 0.05
Wood et al.[8]	1: Aerobic exercise (weight loss) 2: Hypocaloric diet (weight loss) 3: Control (weight maintenance)	131 (155) men; 120%–160% ideal weight; sedentary	9–12 months	1: (94.1) 2: (93.0) 3: (95.4)	1: −4.0 2: −7.2 3: +0.6	1 and 2 vs. 3 P < 0.001 1 vs. 2 < 0.01

Study	Groups	Sample	Duration	Baseline	Change	Significance
Verity and Ismail[11]	1: Aerobic exercise 2: Control	10 (10) women, postmenopausal with NIDDM, >120% ideal weight; sedentary	4 months	1: 27.3 2: 33.4 NS	1: −4.1 2: −2.9	NS
King et al.[13]	1: Aerobic exercise—higher intensity, group-based 2: Aerobic exercise—higher intensity, home-based 3: Aerobic exercise—lower intensity, home-based 4: Control	167 (197) men; 160 (131), women, postmenopausal, not on HRT; sedentary	9–12 months	1: 27.4 2: 28.0 3: 27.1 4: 27.0 1: 26.3 2: 27.1 3: 25.7 4: 27.1	1: (−0.2) 2: (−0.2) 3: (−0.9) 4: (+0.1) 1: (+0.4) 2: (+0.1) 3: (−0.6) 4: (0.0)	No group differences, in either sex
Duncan et al.[22]	1: Aerobic walking (8.0 km/h) 2: Brisk walking (6.4 km/h) 3: Strolling (4.8 km/h) 4: Control	59 (102) women, premenopausal; sedentary	24 weeks	1: (60.3) 2: (64.2) 3: (62.0) 4: (66.5)	1: +1.1 2: +0.1 3: +0.8 4: +3.7	2 vs. 4, $P < 0.05$ No other differences

continues

Table 1 Continued

Study	Interventions: treatment groups	Training period duration	N post (randomized) sex; basic (key) inclusion criteria	Initial BMI (or weight in kg)	Weight (kg) (or BMI) change	Differences among groups (weight changes)
Hellenius et al.[14]	1: Aerobic exercise 2: Low-fat diet 3: Aerobic exercise + low-fat diet 4: Control	6 months	157 (158) men; mildly elevated TC	1: 26.1 2: 25.3 3: 25.2 4: 24.5	1: (−0.3) 2: (−0.3) 3: (−0.6) 4: (+0.3)	1 and 2 vs. 4 $P < 0.01$; 3 vs. 4 $P < 0.001$
Katzel et al.[16]	1: Aerobic exercise with no weight change (low-fat diet) 2: Hypocaloric, low-fat diet 3: Control	9 months	111 (170) men; 120%–160% ideal weight, sedentary	1: 30.4 2: 30.8 3: 29.5	1: −0.5 2: −9.5 3: +0.2	None reported Pre vs. post, 2: $P < 0.05$
Ready et al.[19]	1: Aerobic exercise (walking) 2: Control	6 months	25 (40) women, postmenopausal; high TC; sedentary	1: 29.4 2: 32.1	1: −1.9 2: −0.6	$P < 0.05$
Anderssen et al.[17]	1: Aerobic exercise 2: Hypocaloric (low-fat) diet 3: Aerobic exercise + hypocaloric diet 4: Control	1 year	209 men + women	1: 2: 3: 4:	1: −0.9 2: −4.0 3: −5.6 4: +1.1	1 vs. 4 $P < 0.05$ 2 vs. 3 NS

Study	Interventions	Duration	Subjects	Baseline	Change	Significance
Pritchard et al.[23]	1: Aerobic exercise (weight loss) 2: Hypocaloric low-fat diet 3: Control (weight maintenance)	12 months	58 (66) men; overweight	1: 29.2 2: 29.0 3: 28.6	1: −2.6 2: −6.3 3: +0.9	1 and 2 vs. 3 $P < 0.05$ Pre vs. post, 1: $P < 0.05$ 2: $P < 0.001$
Stefanick et al.[18]	1: Aerobic exercise 2: Low-fat diet 3: Aerobic exercise + low-fat diet 4: Control	9–12 months	190 (197) men, 177 (180) women postmenopausal; with low HDL-C + elevated LDL-C	All men BMI: 27.0 (weight 84.2) All women BMI: 26.3 (weight: 69.6)	1: −0.6 2: −2.8 3: −4.2 4: +0.5 1: −0.4 2: −2.7 3: −3.1 4: +0.8	1 vs. 4 NS 1 vs. 2 $P < 0.05$ 1 vs. 3 $P < 0.001$ 2 and 3 vs. 4 $P < 0.001$ 1 vs. 4 NS 1 vs. 2 $P < 0.05$ 1 vs. 3 $P < 0.01$ 2 and 3 vs. 4 $P < 0.001$

BMI = body mass index; NS = not significant; NIDDM = non-insulin-dependent diabetes mellitus; HRT = hormone replacement therapy; TC = total cholesterol; HDL-C = high-density lipoprotein cholesterol; LDL-C = low-density lipoprotein cholesterol.

saturated fats and simple carbohydrates and alcohol; however, there was no dietary assessment. Neither group was encouraged to lose weight. Maximal oxygen uptake was increased significantly in exercisers and decreased in controls, and changes differed between groups ($P < 0.001$). A small but significant reduction in body weight was evident in both exercises (-0.9 kg) and controls (-0.6 kg), but weight changes were not significantly different between groups.

In the Stanford Exercise Study,[21] sedentary men, aged 30–55, who spanned a range of BMI (mean 24.8 kg/m^2) were assigned randomly for 1 year to control ($N = 33$) or aerobic exercise ($N = 48$), consisting of approximately 45 minutes of supervised walking or jogging three times per week, with a choice on any given day of doing approximately 8 km at a 10–12 km/h pace, 5 km at 8–9 km/h, or 3 km at 6–7 km/h. No instruction on diet was provided to either group, both of which completed 3-day food records at several points. At 1 year, exercisers had increased mean maximum aerobic capacity, VO$_{2max}$ (9.0 mL/kg per minute; $P < 0.0001$), compared with controls, but did not change caloric intake or percent of calories from any given food source. Compared with controls, exercisers lost significant weight (2.5 kg; $P < 0.001$) and reduced percent body fat, as assessed by hydrostatic weighing (3.8%; $P < 0.0001$). Secondary analyses, which separated exercisers into four "treatment-dose" groups (based on weekly jogging/walking distance: 0–6.2, 6.3–12.6, 12.7–20.6, and 20.8+ km), showed that distance correlated significantly with body fat changes ($r = -0.49$; $P = 0.002$).

Sopko et al, designed a study to "tease apart" the relationships of diet- and exercise-induced weight loss to lipid changes.[24] Men, aged 19–44 who were slightly overweight (110% of standard weight) were assigned randomly to control weight loss by caloric restriction; weight loss by exercise; and exercise with weight maintenance. Meals were prepared in a metabolic kitchen for all groups and were fixed at 40% of calories from fat. Caloric intake was adjusted to maintain weight every 3 days according to group assignment. Exercisers engaged in supervised treadmill walking with an energy expenditure of 700 kcal per session, five times a week, to total 3500 kcal per week, at a pace of 5.6–6.4 km/h for most subjects. Significant weight was lost by men assigned to weight loss by exercise (-6.2 kg), but not to control (-0.5 kg) or exercise with weight maintenance (-0.5 kg), clearly demonstrating the role of caloric intake in determining the effectiveness of exercise on weight loss.

Ronnemaa et al[6] randomized 20 male and 10 female non–insulin-dependent diabetes mellitus (NIDDM) type II patients, aged 45–60, to control or exercise, consisting of 5–7 weekly 45-minute (or longer) periods of walking, jogging, or skiing at a recommended pulse rate equal to resting pulse rate $+$ 0.6 $\times$ (maximum pulse rate $-$ resting pulse rate), which corresponds approximately to 70% of VO_{2max}. No dietary advice was provided to patients. The mean increase in VO_{2max} in the exercise group was 9.7%, with no change in controls. Exercisers lost 2.0 kg while controls increased weight by 0.5 kg; however, it was not reported whether or not there was a significant difference between groups.

Verity and Ismail[11] also assigned postmenopausal women with NIDDM to control or exercise. Women in the exercise group attended an adult fitness program that met three times per week and included stretching, progressive calisthenics, and walking at a pace requiring 65%–80% of predicted cardiac preserve, with an expenditure of 240–300 kcal per session. Both exercisers and controls lost weight (-4.1 kg and -2.1 kg, respectively), but the differences between groups was not significant.

The SWCP-I[7] was designed to determine differential effects of diet-induced and exercise-induced weight loss on cardiovascular risk factors. Sedentary, moderately overweight (20%–50% above ideal body weight) men, aged 35–59, were randomized to control; weight loss by caloric restriction, without changing diet composition or activity level; or weight loss by increased aerobic exercise, consisting of approximately 45 minutes of supervised walking or jogging three times per week, with no dietary changes. Caloric reduction, assessed by 7-day food records, was significant ($P < 0.01$) in dieters versus controls at 7 months (approximately 335 kcal/d) and 1-year (approximately 240 kcal/d), while caloric intake did not differ between exercisers and controls at either time point. At 1 year, VO_{2max} had increased in exercisers, compared with controls (6.5 mL/kg per minute, $P < 0.001$), and dieters (4.1 mL/kg per minute; $P < 0.001$). Compared with controls, total and fat weight losses were significicnatly greater ($P < 0.001$) in both dieters (7.8 and 6.2 kg, respectively) and exercisers (4.6 and 4.4 kg); while lean mass loss was greater only in dieters (2.1 kg), who also lost more lean weight than exercisers (1.4 kg; $P < 0.01$). Fat weight loss did not differ between dieters and exercisers.

Ready et al[19] randomized postmenopausal women with mildly elevated serum cholesterol (5.9 to 8.0 mmol/L) to walking ($N = 24$) or control ($N = 16$) for 6 months. Walkers were asked to walk for 60 mins/d, 5 d/wk at an initial intensity of 60% HRmax reserve. Walkers attended supervised sessions twice a week for the first 2 weeks and once a week thereafter. Average walking speed increased from 5.5 to 6.0 km/h. The estimated weekly energy expenditure was 6367 kJ. The 6-month program resulted in an increase in VO_{2max} of 11% in walkers, which was significant versus controls ($P < 0.01$). Analysis of 3-day food frequency records indicated that there were no significant changes in energy intake or diet composition throughout the program. Walkers lost a small but significant amount of weight (-1.3 kg) and fat mass (-1.7 kg) compared with controls ($P < 0.05$ kg).

King et al[13] conducted a much larger study of 160 postmenopausal women and 197 men, aged 50–65, the Stanford-Sunnyvale Health Improvement Program (SSHIP) Trial, which compared group-based and home-based programs of higher intensity (73%–88% peak heart rate, as assessed by a maximal graded exercise treadmill test) versus lower intensity (60%–73%). Women and men assigned to group-based, higher intensity exercise were encouraged to attend an exercise program consisting primarily of walking and jogging three times a week during which they were expected to have at least 40 minutes of higher intensity exercise. Participants assigned to home-based exercise were expected to do either high-intensity exercise three times per week or lower intensity exercise five times per week depending on assignment. All three exercise conditions significantly ($P < 0.03$) improved VO_{2max}, averaging approximately 5% increase, compared with controls; however, there were no significant weight or body composition changes in either gender.

Duncan et al[22] also randomized women to control or three different exercise intensities: aerobic walking (8.0 km/h), brisk walking (6.4 km/h), or strolling (4.8 km/h), with each group walking a distance of 2.4 km, 5 days per week initially, and increasing this to 4.8 km by the 7th week, which was maintained through the remainder of the 24-week trial. The VO_{2max} was increased in all three exercise conditions compared with controls, but there was a linear dose-response gradient across exercise conditions, with aerobic walkers experiencing the greatest increase in VO_{2max}. In contrast, weight changes did not differ among exercise groups and only was different between brisk walkers and controls, with the difference developing because of weight gain in controls.

Hellenius et al[14] randomized men aged 35–60 years, who were at slightly elevated cardiovascular risk, to exercise only; a National Cholesterol Education Program (NCEP) step I diet only (total fat $\leq 30\%$ and saturated fat $\leq 10\%$ of calories, dietary cholesterol ≤ 300 mg/d); the combination of exercise and diet; or control for 6 months. Men in the exercise groups were advised to increase exercise gradually until they could do regular aerobic-type exercise (walking, jogging, etc.) two to three times a week at an intensity of 60%–80% of maximal heart rate and lasting 30–45 minutes. Men assigned to diet followed the diet with the goal of reducing calories to bring about weight loss, if appropriate. BMI decreased significantly in exercise only and exercise + diet groups and diet-only group versus control, with the decrease being most apparent in the combined group. Waist circumference also decreased in all three intervention groups versus control, with the combination group being most effective.

To specifically compare the effects of weight loss (achieved without a change in activity level) to aerobic exercise (not accompanied by weight loss), Katzel and colleagues[16] randomly assigned 170 sedentary, obese (120%–160% of ideal body weight) men, aged 46–80, for 1 year to control; weight loss by a hypocaloric, reduced-fat diet, similar to the NCEP step I diet; or aerobic exercise with weight maintenance. Therefore, effort was made to prevent weight loss by exercise. The exercise consisted of 45 minutes of treadmill and cycle ergonometer workouts, three times per week. Prior to baseline testing, all three groups were instructed for 3 months on an isoenergetic reduced-fat diet and men in both the aerobic exercise and control groups were encouraged to continue this diet, without losing weight, throughout the trial. Of those who completed the trial, dieters lost approximately 9.5 kg, 75% of which was fat mass, and did not change VO_{2max}; whereas exercisers did not change average weight, although percent body fat was decreased 0.8% (< 0.005) but did increase VO_{2max} (approximately 7.0 mL/kg of fat-free mass (FFM) per minute; ie, 17% above baseline) compared with the other two groups ($p < 0.001$).

To compare effects on body composition of weight loss through diet with weight loss through exercise, using dual x-ray absorptiometry (DEXA), Pritchard et al[23] randomized overweight men to 12 months of aerobic exercise ($N = 21$); low-fat, hypocaloric (-500 kcal/d) diet ($N = 18$); or control ($N = 19$). Exercisers selected their own aerobic exercise regimen, with a minimum participation set at three sessions of 30 min/wk at 65%–75% of HRmax. Of the 21 exercisers, 11 walked, 4 jogged (2 alternated jogging with swimming), 3 attended a gymnasium (45 minutes of aerobic workout, 15 minute resistance, anaerobic), and 3 rode an exercise bike. Greater weight loss occurred in dieters (6.4 kg) than in those with aerobic exercise alone (2.6 kg); DEXA scans revealed that 40% of dieters' weight loss was lean tissue; while more than 80% of weight loss by exercisers was fat.

The diet and exercise for elevated risk (DEER) Trial[18] investigated the effects of a NCEP step II diet and aerobic exercise in normotensive, euglycemic men and postmenopausal women who had HDLC levels below the sex-specific mean of the population (≤ 44 mg/dL, men; ≤ 59 mg/dL, women) combined with moderately elevated low-density lipoprotein cholesterol (LDLC) (125–189 mg/dL, men; 125–209 mg/dL, women). Men, aged 30–64 and ≤ 34 kg/m^2, and postmenopausal women, aged 45–64 and ≤ 32 kg/m^2, were assigned for 1 year to control ($N = 47$ men and 46 women); aerobic exercise, with 45 minutes of walking, jogging, or comparable activity, at 60%–80% of HRmax at least three times per week ($N = 50$ men and 44 women); NCEP step II diet with recommendations to adjust caloric intake to reach or maintain desirable body weight (N = 49 men and 47 women); or step II NCEP diet + aerobic exercise (N = 51 men and 43 women). Mean dietary goals were achieved by both diet and diet + exercise in men and women, as assessed by five unannounced 24-hour recalls at baseline and 1 year. Dietary fat and cholesterol changes were significant versus control and exercise only in both sexes. Aerobic capacity (mL/kg per minute) was increased significantly, compared with controls, in exercise (2.7) and diet + exercise (5.5) men and in exercise (3.4) and diet + exercise (4.7) women and was similarly increased in exercisers and dieting exercisers.

Although DEER participants were not selected to be overweight, the mean baseline BMI was 27.0 kg/m^2 in men and 26.3 kg/m^2 in women. At 1 year, total fat and weight losses were significant compared with controls in dieters and dieting exercisers in both sexes, but did not differ between diet only and diet + exercise in either sex. In men, dieters lost a mean of 3.3 kg (2.1 kg fat weight) and dieting exercisers lost 4.7 kg (3.5 kg fat weight) compared with controls, while weight loss in exercisers (1.2 kg, 1.0 kg fat weight) was not significant. Closer scrutiny of the caloric data revealed increases in both exercise-only women and men in the order of approximately 100 kcal/d, which were not significant compared with other groups, but which certainly would counteract the 700–900 kcal/wk energy expenditure achieved by most exercisers. Lean mass loss did not differ between dieters or dieting exercisers and control men, but was significantly greater in both dieting groups compared with exercise only (1.3 kg) for both. In DEER women, dieters lost a mean of 3.5 kg and dieting exercisers lost 3.9 kg compared with controls; while weight loss in exercisers (1.2 kg) was not significant. Lean mass losses were minimal and did not differ between groups.

In summary, the randomized controlled trials reviewed here generally show only modest (or no) weight loss with aerobic exercise programs that meet the recommended exercise prescription, even though these consistently result in improved cardiorespiratory fitness. Caloric intake clearly determines whether exercise will produce weight loss or maintenance and should be monitored.

Weight-Loss Trials of Aerobic Exercise Plus Diet versus Diet Only

The Expert Panel stated that a combination of reduced calorie diet and increased physical activity produces greater weight loss than diet alone or exercise alone, based on results from 12 studies,[10,14,17,18,25–32] which appear in Table 2, with the exception of one article, which actually is a follow-up study[32] of a trial that does appear on this table.[33] The reader also is referred to a review by King and Tribble,[34] which presents at least 15 studies that are not described in this review. Table 2 includes seven additional trials that seem to meet the criteria of the Expert Panel.[35-41] The participants in these trials generally are more obese than those described in the studies that appear in Table 1.

Wing et al[25] assigned women and men with NIDDM to a hypocaloric diet alone and combined with exercise in which participants walked a 3-mile route three times a week with study therapists and exercised once a week on their own. Calorie restriction was calculated to produce 1 kg/wk weight loss. The addition of exercise resulted in greater weight loss than diet alone (-9.3 kg vs. -5.6 kg; $P < 0.01$) in a 10-week period.

Hammer et al[10] randomized premenopausal obese women to either exercise or no exercise combined with either a low-fat, ad libitum–carbohydrate diet or a calorie-restricted low-fat, high-carbohydrate diet. Exercise consisted of brisk walking and/or jogging 5 d/wk on an indoor track. The distance was increased by 0.8 km/wk until 4.8 km was achieved by the 5th or 6th week and maintained for the remaining 10 weeks. Work intensity was $\geq 60\%$ HRmax (HRmax) (determined during a VO_{2max} treadmill test) in week 1 and then was increased to 70%–85% HRmax. There were no significant effects of exercise, whereas women assigned to calorie restriction lost more weight than the ad libitum group.

Hill, et al.[35] tested whether a constant 1200-kcal diet differed from a diet that alternated from very low calorie (600 and 900 kcal) to 1200 and 1500 kcal with or without an exercise component involving brisk walking five times per week at a target heart rate of 60%–70%, (determined by a treadmill fitness test). The diet pattern made no difference; however, the women assigned to exercise lost significantly more weight than diet alone.

Bertram et al[12] prescribed a 5000-kJ diet to three randomized treatment groups of women: control; diet combined with special lectures; and exercise in the form of three sessions per week consisting of stretching, 30 minutes of walking or jogging at an intensity calculated to maintain heart rate at 70% of predicted maximum, and strengthening exercises. All groups lost significant weight, but there was no greater weight loss in the exercise group than the other groups.

Donnelly et al[36] assigned women to one of four groups for 90 days: endurance exercise (EE), weight training (WT), combination of EE and WT, and no exercise, with all four groups receiving a liquid-formula very low calorie diet containing 2184 kJ/d. Both EE and WT were conducted 4 d/wk. EE consisted of various modes of exercise,

Table 2

Randomized Trials with Aerobic Exercise + Diet versus Diet Only Groups

Study	Interventions: treatment groups	N post (randomized) sex; basic (key) inclusion criteria	Training period duration	Initial BMI (or weight in kg)	Weight (kg) [or BMI] change	Differences among groups (weight changes)
Wing et al.[25]	1: AE + hypocaloric diet 2: Hypocaloric diet	21 women + 9 men >20% ideal wt, 30–65 yrs old, with type II diabetes	10 weeks + 1 year follow-up	1: 37.5 2: 37.9	1: −9.3 2: −5.6	1 vs. 2 $P < 0.01$
Hammer et al.[10]	1: AE + hypocaloric diet 2: Hypocaloric diet 3: AE + control diet 4: Control low-fat, ad libitum diet	26 (36) women, premenopausal	16 weeks	1: 32.2 2: 32.2 3: 30.6 4: 37.0	1: −12.9 2: −9.5 3: −6.7 4: −5.8	1 vs. 2 NS 3 vs. 4 NS 1 + 3 vs. 2 + 4 NS
Hill et al.[35]	1: AE + constant 1200 kcal/d diet 2: Constant 1200 kcal/d diet 3: AE + alternating (600, 900, 1200, 1500 kcal/d) diet 4: Alternating diet	32 (40), women; 130%–160% ideal body weight	12 weeks	1: 30 2: 31 3: 31 4: 31	1 + 3: −8.6 2 + 4: −6.5 1 + 2: −7.9 3 + 4: −7.7	1 + 3 vs. 2 + 4 $P < 0.05$ 1 + 2 vs. 3 + 4 NS
Bertram et al.[12]	Hypocaloric (5000 kJ) diet + 1: AE + stretch/strengthen 2: Diet lectures 3: Control	36 (45) women, obese	1 year	1: 34.6 2: 34.3 3: 34.8	1: −7.0 2: −9.3 3: −8.1	No differences. Pre vs. Post, $P < 0.01$ for all

Study	Intervention	Sample	Duration	Results	Statistics
Donnelly et al.[36]	Hypocaloric (liquid) diet 1: AE (endurance) 2: No exercise 3: Weight training 4: Endurance exercise + weight training (Women could self-select group)	69 women	90 days	1: 37.5 2: 38.2 3: 38.2 4: 38.3	1: −21.4 2: −20.4 3: −20.9 4: −22.9	No group differences.
Wood et al.[26]	1: AE + hypocaloric, low-fat diet 2: Hypocaloric, low-fat diet 3: Control	119 (132) men; BMI = 28–34, 112 (132) women, premenopausal; BMI = 24–30; sedentary	1 year	All men BMI: 30.7 (weight 98.4) All women BMI: 27.9 (weight 75.0)	1: −8.7 2: −5.1 3: +1.7 1: −5.1 2: −4.1 3: +1.3	1 vs. 2 $P < 0.01$ 1 and 2 vs. 3 $P < 0.001$ 1 vs. 2 NS 1 and 2 vs. 3 $P < 0.001$
Sweeny et al.[37]	Hypocaloric diet – severe, 40% + moderate, 70% (combined) 1: AE (walking) 2: No exercise 3: AE + circuit weight training	30 (47) women, premenopausal; 135–185% ideal body weight	6 months	1: 34.9 2: 33.4 3: 37.1	1: −15 2: −13 3: −11 based on graph	No group differences.

continues

Table 2 Continued

Study	Interventions: treatment groups	N post (randomized) sex; basic (key) inclusion criteria	Training period duration	Initial BMI (or weight in kg)	Weight (kg) [or BMI] change	Differences among groups (weight changes)
Svendsen et al.[27]	1: Aerobic + anaerobic exercise + hypocaloric (formula) diet 2: Hypocaloric (formula) diet 3: Control	118 (121) women, postmenopausal; BMI ≥25 kg/m²	12 weeks	1: (78.1) 2: (78.1) 3: (76.6)	1: −10.3 2: −9.5 3: +0.5	1 vs. 2 NS 1 and 2 vs. 3 $P < 0.001$
Hellenius et al.[14]	1: AE + low-fat diet 2: Low-fat diet 3: AE 4: Control	157 (158) men; mildly elevated TC	6 months	1: 25.2 2: 25.3 3: 26.1 4: 24.5	1: (−0.6) 2: (−0.3) 3: (−0.3) 4: (+0.3)	1 vs. 2 NS 1 vs. 3 NS 1 vs. 4, $P < 0.001$
Singh et al.[38]	1: AE + prudent diet + fruits and vegetables 2: Prudent diet only	457 (463) Asian men (90%) + women with CHD risk	24 weeks	1: 24.6 2: 24.1	1: −6.6 2: −0.3	1 vs. 2, $P < 0.01$
Dengel et al.[39]	1: AE + hypocaloric low-fat diet 2: Hypocaloric, low-fat diet 3: Control	66 (148) men; 120%–160% wt, sedentary >45 years of age	10 months	1: 30.3 2: 30.1 3: 29.5	1: −8.1 2: −9.3 3: +0.4	1 vs. 2 NS 1 and 2 vs. 3, $P < 0.05$
Blonk et al.[28]	1: AE + behavior + diet 2: Hypocaloric diet	53 (20 + 40) men + women; BMI >27, with type II diabetes	24 months	1: 31.3 2: 32.8	1: −3.5 2: −2.1	NS

Study	Intervention	Duration	Baseline	Change	Results
Marks et al.[29]	1: AE (cycling) + diet 2: RT + diet 3: AE + RT + diet 4: Hypocaloric, low-fat diet 5: Control	80 women, premenopausal; 120%–150% ideal body weight	20 weeks	1: 28.7 2: 30.4 3: 31.3 4: 30.1 5: 29.4	1: −4.5 2: −3.5 3: −5.4 4: −3.7 5: +1.5	1, 2, 3 and 4 vs. 5 $P < 0.05$ No other group differences
Andersen et al.[30]	Hypocaloric (liquid) diet + 1: AE 2: ST 3: AE + ST 4: No Exercise	53 (66) women, obese	48 weeks	All (mean) 36.2	1: −13.4 2: −17.9 3: −15.3 4: −12.9	No group differences.
Anderssen et al.[17]	1: AE + hypocaloric low-fat diet 2: Hypocaloric, low-fat diet 3: AE 4: Control	209 men + women	1 year	1: 2: 3: 4:	1: −5.6 2: −4.0 3: −0.9 4: +1.1	1 vs. 2 NS 2 vs. 3 NS 1 vs. 4 $P < 0.05$
Fox et al.[40]	1: Aerobic + resistance exercise (200 kcal/d E expenditure) + hypocaloric (−500 kcal/d) diet 2: Hypocaloric diet (−500 kcal/d) 3: Hypocaloric diet (−700 kcal/d)	40 (46), women, postmenopausal; 120%–140% ideal weight; ≥60 years of age	24 weeks	1: 30.6 2: 29.8 3: 30.4	1: −7.1 2: −6.6 3: −5.8	No group differences.

continues

Table 2 Continued

Study	Interventions: treatment groups	N post (randomized) sex; basic (key) inclusion criteria	Training period duration	Initial BMI (or weight in kg)	Weight (kg) [or BMI] change	Differences among groups (weight changes)
Gordon et al.[31]	1: AE + low-fat diet 2: Low-fat diet 3: AE	48 (17 + 38) men + women, 21–65 years, with 130–179 mm Hg SBP and/or 85–109 mm Hg DBP	12 weeks	1: (92.7) 2: (100.5) 3: (101.9)	1: −7.1 2: −5.8 3: −1.0	1 vs. 2 NS 1 and 2 vs. 3 $P < 0.001$
Wadden et al.[33]	Very low caloric diet + 1: AE 2: ST 3: AE + ST 4: No exercise	120 (128), women; obese	48 weeks	1: 37.3 2: 36.5 3: 35.3 4: 36.4	1: −13.7 2: −17.2 3: −15.2 4: −14.4	No group differences.
Stefanick et al.[18]	1: AE + low-fat diet 2: Low-fat diet 3: AE 4: Control	190 (197) men, 177 (180) women postmenopausal; with low HDL-C + elevated LDL-C	9–12 months	All men BMI: 27.0 (weight: 84.2) All women BMI: 26.3 (weight: 69.6)	1: −4.2 2: −2.8 3: −0.6 4: +0.5 1: −3.1 2: −2.7 3: −0.4 4: +0.8	1 and 2 vs. 4 $P < 0.001$ 1 vs. 3 $P < 0.001$ 2 vs. 3 $P < 0.05$ 1 and 2 vs. 4 $P < 0.001$ 1 vs. 3 $P < 0.01$ 2 vs. 3 $P < 0.05$

AE = aerobic exercise; CHD = coronary heart disease; RT = resistance training; ST = strength training; SBP = systolic blood pressure; DBP = diastolic blood pressure; see Table 1 for other definitions.

including treadmill walking, stationary bicycling, rowing, etc., at an intensity set at 13 rated perceived exertion initially and replaced with 70% heart rate reserve. Strength training (ST) was performed on universal gym equipment and progressed from two sets to eight repetitions at 80% 1 repetition maximum (RM). Changes in body weight, percent body fat, fat weight, and FFM did not differ between groups, all of whom lost over 20 kg.

The second Stanford Weight Control Project (SWCP-II)[26] initially studied sedentary, moderately overweight premenopausal women (BMI = 24–30 kg/m^2) and men (BMI = 28–34 kg/m^2), aged 25–49. SWCP-II assigned women and men to 1-year treatments: control; a hypocaloric NCEP step I diet; or the hypocaloric NCEP step I diet plus aerobic exercise consisting of approximately 45 minutes of supervised walking or jogging, three times per week. Dietary changes, assessed by 7-day food records, were nearly identical in the two diet groups for men and women. Aerobic capacity (mL/kg per minute) improved significantly ($P < 0.001$) in diet + exercise men, compared with control (8.8) and diet-only (7.0) men and in diet + exercise women versus control (6.4) and diet-only (5.0) women. Weight loss was significant ($P < 0.001$) in both diet men (6.8 kg) and diet + exercise men (10.4 kg), compared with controls, as was fat weight loss (5.5 and 9.0 kg respectively), with greater fat loss in dieting exercisers versus dieters ($P < 0.001$). Lean mass loss also was significant ($P < 0.05$) in diet (1.3 kg) and diet + exercise men (1.4 kg) versus control but did not differ between dieters and dieting exercisers.

In SWCP-II women, weight loss was significant ($P < 0.001$) in both dieters (5.4 kg) and dieting exercisers (6.4 kg) compared with controls, as was fat weight loss (4.5 and 6.0 kg respectively), with no significant differences between weight-loss groups. This may suggest a sex difference or may have occurred because of a lower return rate in diet women versus diet + exercise ($P = 0.6$). Lean mass loss did not differ between groups.

Sweeney et al[37] assigned obese women to either moderate or severe dietary restrictions and to aerobic exercise, primarily brisk walking, 3 d/wk or aerobic exercise plus circuit WT, or no exercise for 6 months. Neither exercise program resulted in greater weight loss than diet alone.

Svendsen et al[27] assigned 121 overweight (self-reported BMI ≥ 25 kg/m^2) postmenopausal women, aged 45–54 years, to control, a hypocaloric formula diet, or the diet plus three sessions per week of 1–1.5 hours of aerobic exercise (bicycling, stair climbing, and treadmill running) and resistance training. Aerobic capacity (mL/kg per minute) increased in the dieting exercisers, compared with controls (5.1) and dieters (4.6). Total weight loss was significant in both diet-only (10.0

kg) and diet + exercise (10.8 kg) women, compared with controls and did not differ between groups; however, the dieting exercisers lost significantly ($P < 0.001$) more fat weight (1.8 kg) than diet only. The latter lost 1.2 kg lean weight, while dieting exercisers lost none ($P < 0.05$ vs. dieters).

The Hellenius et al[14] study was described in the previous section. BMI changes in the aerobic exercise + diet men (-0.6) did not differ significantly from either diet only (-0.3) or exercise only (-0.3). Both D + E and E groups reduced BMI significantly versus control ($+0.03$), whereas diet only was not significant. The D + E group also reduced waist significantly versus both control and diet only but not versus exercise only.

The Oslo Diet and Exercise Study [17] also was discussed in the previous section. The ODES data were presented by diastolic blood pressure tertiles (<84, $84-91$, >91 mm Hg) for each treatment group, rather than by treatment assignment, requiring some interpretation of the statistical outcomes. Weight loss was presented by treatment group versus control but not by individual treatment or control groups. There appeared to be no difference in weight loss for diet-only versus diet plus exercise groups, and both appeared to be significant compared with control.

The Diet and Moderate Exercise Trial[38] randomly assigned 419 men and 44 women from a South Asian population, who had one or more coronary heart disease (CHD) risk factors, to one of two groups for 24 weeks: (1) group A, American Heart Association (AHA) step I (reduced-fat) diet + fruits and vegetables + exercise, consisting of brisk walking 3–4 km/d or spot running, 10–15 min/day ($N = 231$); or (2) group B, AHA step I diet only ($N = 232$). At 24 weeks, after 20 weeks of exercise in addition to the dietary regimen, group A had lost 6.5 kg (9.8% reduction from baseline), while group B had lost only 0.3 kg ($P < 0.01$ versus A).

Dengel et al[39] assigned obese men over 45 years of age to control or a hypocaloric, low-fat diet with or without aerobic exercise consisting of stationary cycling and walking and jogging outdoors and on a treadmill three times per week for 10 months. Both diet-only and diet with exercise groups lost significant weight versus control; however, the addition of exercise did not increase weight loss.

Blonk et al[28] randomized obese women with type II diabetes to a conventional program of diet counseling or a comprehensive program, which added exercise and behavioral modification in a long-term study (24 months). The comprehensive plan resulted in greater weight loss by 6 months but not by 24 months.

Marks et al[29] randomized premenopausal women to control; a hypocaloric, low-fat diet; the diet combined with aerobic exercise on a life cycle, a computerized stationary cycle, with training at 70%–85% of attained HRmax; the diet combined with resistance training utilizing life circuit; and the diet plus both life cycle and life circuit training. All four diet intervention groups lost weight compared with control, but there were no differences between diet-only and exercise groups or among exercise groups.

Andersen[30] randomized obese women to a hypocaloric (liquid) diet with no exercise; a step aerobics exercise program; a resistance training program; and a combined step aerobics and resistance exercise program for 48 weeks. All groups lost substantial weight, but there was no difference between the diet only group and any of the exercise groups or among exercise groups.

Fox et al[40] randomized postmenopausal women over 60 years of age to either a −500-kcal/d or −700-kcal/d hypocaloric diet, using the AHA exchange system, or to a −500-kcal/d diet combined with a 3-d/wk 1-hour walking program + 2-d/wk light resistance exercise program designed to use 12 major muscles, with the exercise program expected to expend 200 kcal/d. Loss of body weight was significant for all groups at 24 weeks, but did not differ among groups.

Gordon et al[31] randomized women and men with high normal blood pressure or stage 1 or 2 hypertension to a hypocaloric, low-fat diet, aerobic exercise, or diet + aerobic exercise. Exercise consisted of 30–45 minutes of aerobic exercise, primarily walking, on 3–5 d/wk at a heart rate of 60%–85% of maximal value achieved during baseline exercise testing and a perceived exertion rating of 11–13 on the Borg 6–20 scale. In these patients, both diet alone and diet + exercise elicited greater weight reduction than exercise alone, but there was no difference between diet + exercise and diet alone.

Wadden et al[33] randomized obese women to a 48-week study in which all women were prescribed a very low calorie diet and randomized to one of four groups: aerobic exercise, WT, the combination of aerobic exercise and WT, and no exercise. All groups lost substantial weight, but there were no differences among groups.

The DEER Trial was described in the previous section.[18] The combined exercise and diet group lost significantly more weight than exercise-only groups, for both sexes; however, weight loss did not differ between the diet + exercise women (−3.1 kg) and diet-only women (−2.4 kg) or men (−4.2 kg vs. −2.8 kg), although this arose because all pairwise comparisons had a Bonferroni adjustment; that is, $P < 0.05$ was not regarded as significant.

In summary, 11 of these 19 studies showed no benefit of the addition of aerobic exercise to a weight-reducing diet for weight loss, two others suggested no benefit for women but a benefit for men, or at least a strong tendency, and six others showed greater weight loss with the addition of exercise to a hypocaloric diet.

Selected Follow-Up Studies

Table 3 presents a few long-term follow-up studies from randomized, controlled trials of exercise + diet versus diet only. Wing et al[25] published two small trials together with their follow-up studies. The 2-year weight change data for the study with aerobic exercise + diet (−7.9 kg) and diet only (−3.8 kg) were similar to those for the study with aerobic exercise + diet (−7.8 kg) versus a low-intensity, flexibility ("placebo") exercise + diet group (−4.0 kg); however, the differences between groups reached significance in the first study but not the second.

Svendsen et al[41] published a 6-month follow-up to the 12-week study described in the previous section. Both the exercise + diet and the diet-only women gained approximately 2 kg during this period and although weight loss was still significant versus control, it remained not significant between the combined and diet-only women.

Skender et al[42] published a 1-year follow-up to a trial in which obese men and women had been assigned randomly to a Help Your Heart Eating Plan (HYHEP) or to aerobic exercise, primarily walking, for three to five 45-minute periods per week, at an intensity that subjectively felt "vigorous" but not "strenuous," without changing diet, or to exercise + the HYNEP. At 1 year, the exercise-only group (−2.9 kg) had lost less weight than the diet-only (−6.8 kg) or exercise + diet group [−8.9 kg; analysis of variance (ANOVA) $P < 0.09$]; however, both the diet-only and the exercise + diet groups regained weight during the 2nd year, while the exercise-only group maintained its weight loss. Weight change from baseline to year 2 for 86 (of an original 127) women who returned was diet only (+0.9), exercise only (−2.7 kg), and diet + exercise (−2.2 kg).

Wadden et al[32] reported 1-year follow-up data for the study described in the previous section. All groups, regardless of assignment to aerobic exercise, ST, a combination, or no exercise, gained back a substantial portion of the weight they had lost in the initial year and there were no differences among groups.

These few studies do not support the notion that the addition of exercise to diet enhances a diet-only approach. The Skender[42] study is particularly intriguing because it suggests that exercise only may be a better approach for long-term benefits, despite the modest weight loss that is seen initially. It is clear that long-term follow-up studies are needed to evaluate the true value of any given weight-loss strategy, before drawing any conclusions.

Table 3

Follow-up Studies of Trials with Aerobic Exercise + Diet versus Diet Only

Study	Interventions: treatment groups	N post (randomized) sex; basic (key) inclusion criteria	Training period duration	Initial BMI (or weight)	Wt (kg) change in (year 1)	Wt (kg) change by (year 2)
Wing et al.[25]	Hypocaloric diet + 1: Aerobic exercise 2: Control	28 (30) women + men; >20% ideal weight, 30–65 years old, with type II diabetes	10 weeks + 1 year follow-up	1: 37.5 2: 37.9	1: −9.3 2: −5.6	1: −7.9 2: −3.8 1 vs. 2 P < 0.01
Wing et al.[25]	Hypocaloric diet + 1: Aerobic exercise (walking) 2: Low intensity, flexibility exercise	19 (25) women + men; >20% ideal weight, 30–65 years old, with type II diabetes	10 weeks + 1-year follow-up	1: 38.1 2: 37.5	1: −8.5 2: −7.3	1: −7.8 2: −4.0 1 vs. 2 NS
Svendsen et al.[41]	1: Aerobic + anaerobic exercise + hypocaloric (formula) diet 2: Hypocaloric (formula) diet	110 (118) women, postmenopausal; BMI ≥25 kg/m²	12 weeks	1: (78.1) 2: (78.1) 3: (76.6)	1: −10.3 2: −9.5 3: +0.5 1 vs. 2 NS	1: −8.5 2: −7.5 3: +0.5 1 vs. 2 NS
Skender et al.[42]	1: Aerobic exercise + HYHEP Diet 2: Diet (HYHEP) 3: Aerobic exercise	86 (127) men + women, 25–45 years ≥14 kg overweight sedentary year 2: 86 (61)	Year 1: weight loss intervention Year 2: follow-up	1: (100.1) 2: (98.5) 3: (93.7)	1: −8.9 2: −6.8 3: −2.9 ANOVA P < 0.09	1: −2.2 2: +0.9 3: −2.7
Wadden et al.[32]	Hypocaloric diet + 1: Aerobic exercise 2: ST 3: Aerobic exercise + ST 4: No exercise	77 (99), women; obese	Year 1: weight loss intervention; Year 2: follow-up	All BMI = 36.5 (all weight: 95.8)	1: −13.5 2: −17.3 3: −17.3 4: −15.3	1: −8.5 2: −10.1 3: −8.6 4: −6.9 No group differences

HYHEP = Help Your Heart Eating Plan; ANOVA = analysis of variance; see previous tables for other definitions.

Randomized Trials with Aerobic Exercise versus Resistance Exercise or Control

Several of the randomized controlled trials presented in previous sections compare two different exercise types, in particular aerobic exercise, which favors fat burning, and resistance exercise, or ST, which favors retention of lean body mass (5). Table 4 presents studies that have resistance exercise or WT regimens, all of which were conducted in women. The studies by Donnelly et al,[36] Sweeney et al,[37] Marks,[29] Anderson et al,[30] and Wadden[33] are described in previous sections.

Manning et al[43] assigned premenopausal obese women to control or ST, involving three sets of six to eight repetitions with sets 1 and 2 at 60%–70% of one repetition maximum three times a week for 12 weeks. The program did not result in weight change, BMI, or caloric intake, but did improve strength.

Boyden et al[44] randomly assigned premenopausal women to control or supervised resistance exercise for 5 months. Training consisted of 12 exercises to load major muscle groups in the arms, legs, trunk, and lower back, performed at 70% of a maximal single weight lift with three sets of eight repetitions, 3 d/wk, 1 h/d. There were no significant changes in body weight in either group; however, the exercise group had a significant decrease in percentage of body fat and increase in FFM that was not seen in the control group.

Ross and Rissanen[45] prescribed a hypocaloric diet to obese women who were assigned randomly to aerobic exercise or resistance exercise for 16 weeks. Participants could choose the mode of aerobic exercise, which varied between stationary cycling, walking on a motorized treadmill, and stair-stepping on a Stairmaster, and built up to 60-minute sessions 5 d/wk. The resistance WT exercise was done 3 d/wk on seven Nautilus stations. Adipose tissue was studied by magnetic resonance imaging (MRI). Both groups reduced their volume ratio of visceral to subcutaneous fat, but there were no differences between groups.

The studies in Table 4 find no differences between weight loss in women engaged in aerobic exercise versus ST or in resistance training and control.

Randomized Trials Comparing Different Exercise Programs

Table 5 presents a set of behavioral studies of relevance to the role of exercise in managing obesity. Obviously, the mere prescribing of physical activity to overweight or obese individuals will not result in weight loss, regardless of the exercise program. The patient or person must do it. There is an increasing interest in determining an optimal exercise dose and volume (frequency, duration, intensity, etc.) and whether breaking up daily exercise into multiple short periods, rather than employing single long periods, will improve adherence and thus outcomes. The study by King et al,[13] which focused on adherence issues surrounding group- versus home-based exercise, also addressed the question of optimal intensity of exercise. With respect to weight loss, there were no differences among groups, regardless of assignment to lower or higher intensity exercise. The Duncan study[22] also suggested that walking speed has little effect on weight loss.

To investigate the possible benefit of multiple short periods for weight loss, Jakicic et al[46] randomly assigned overweight women, aged 25–50, to a behavioral weight-loss program consisting of a calorie-restricted diet combined with 5 d/wk of either single aerobic exercise periods per day, starting as 20-minute periods (weeks 1–4), increasing to 30-minute periods (weeks 5–8), and to 40-minute periods (weeks 9–20); or multiple 10-minute periods per day, starting as two-periods per day, increasing to three and then four, respectively.[23] Both groups reduced calories and percent of calories from fat significantly. Women performing multiple short periods lost 8.9 kg in the 20-week period, while those exercising in single long periods lost 6.4 kg (not significant). Because the dietary changes (caloric restriction) probably contributed the most to weight loss, it was not possible to determine the independent contribution of the exercise components; however, exercising in multiple short periods was shown to improve adherence to exercise and to result in significantly greater improvement in aerobic capacity, as well as a trend for greater weight loss.

To further study the importance of the exercise setting, Perri et al[47] assigned obese women to either a group-based or home-based 15-month behavioral weight-loss program, which included a moderate intensity walking program (30 min/d, 5 d/wk). At 15 months, participants in the home program demonstrated significantly greater weight losses than those in group programs, presumably because of greater adherence to exercise.

Recently, two studies appeared on lifestyle activity versus structured aerobic exercise. The lifestyle groups were instructed to accumulate 30 minutes of moderate-intensity activity in a way that is adapted uniquely to the individual and may include such daily activities as walking instead of driving, using stairs instead of elevators, etc. In contrast, structured exercise usually is initiated with a prescription of a targeted percent of maximal power to work on or specific workload to achieve within a specific amount of time.

Table 4

Randomized Trials with Aerobic versus Resistance Exercise

Study	Interventions: treatment groups	N post (randomized) sex; basic (key) inclusion criteria	Training period duration	Initial BMI (or weight in kg)	Weight (kg) (or BMI) change	Differences among groups (weight changes)
Donnelly et al.[36]	Very low calorie (liquid) diet + 1: Aerobic EE 2: WT 3: EE + WT 4: No exercise	69 women, obese	90 days	1: 37.5 2: 38.2 3: 38.3 4: 38.2	1: −21.4 2: −20.9 3: −22.9 4: −20.4	No group differences.
Manning et al.[43]	1: ST 2: Control	22 (24) women; obese; sedentary	12 weeks	1: 31.4 2: 32.8	1: +1.4 2: +0.4	NS
Boyden et al.[44]	1: RT 2: Control	103 (88), women, premenopausal	5 months	1: 22.1 2: 22.6	1: +0.4 2: 0.0	NS
Sweeney et al.[37]	Hypocaloric diet— severe + moderate 1: AE (walking) 2: AE + circuit weight training 3: No exercise	30 (47) women, premenopausal; 135–185% ideal body weight	6 months	1: 2: 3:	1: −15 2: −13 3: −11	No group differences.
Ross et al.[45]	Hypocaloric diet + 1: AE 2: Resistance exercise	24 (29), women, premenopausal; BMI >27; WHR >0.85	16 weeks	B1: 34.4 1: 96.0 B2: 31.8 2: 86.1	1: −10.9 2: −10.1	NS

Study	Intervention	Sample	Duration	All (mean)		Group differences
Andersen et al.[30]	Hypocaloric (liquid) diet + 1: AE 2: ST 3: AE + ST 4: No exercise	53 (66) women, obese	48 weeks	36.2	1: −13.4 2: −17.9 3: −15.3 4: −12.9	No group differences.
Marks et al.[29]	1: AE (cycling) + diet 2: RT + diet 3: AE + RT + diet 4: Hypocaloric, low-fat diet 5: Control	80 women, premenopausal; 120–150% ideal body weight	20 weeks	1: 28.7 2: 30.4 3: 31.3 4: 30.1 5: 29.4	1: −4.5 2: −3.5 3: −5.4 4: −3.7 5: +1.5	1, 2, 3, and 4 vs. 5 $P < 0.05$ 1 vs. 2 NS 1 vs. 3 NS 1 and 3 vs. 4 NS
Wadden et al.[33]	Hypocaloric diet + 1: AE 2: ST 3: AE + ST 4: No Exercise	120 (128), women; obese	48 weeks	1: 37.3 2: 36.5 3: 35.3 4: 36.4	1: −13.7 2: −17.2 3: −15.2 4: −14.4	No group differences.

EE = endurance exercise; WT = weight training; WHR = waist-to-hip ratio; see previous tables for other definitions.

Table 5

Randomized Trials of Different Exercise Programs

Study	Interventions: treatment groups	N post (randomized) sex; basic (key) inclusion criteria	Training period duration	Initial BMI (or weight in kg)	Weight (kg) (or BMI) change	Differences among groups (weight changes)
Wing et al.[25]	1: AE (moderate intensity, walking) + hypocaloric diet 2: Low-intensity, flexibility exercise + hypocaloric diet	21 women + 4 men >20% ideal weight, 30–65 yrs old, with type 2 diabetes	10 weeks	1: 38.1 2: 37.5	1: −8.5 2: −7.3	1 vs. 2 NS 1 and 2: pre vs. post, $P < 0.001$
King et al.[13]	1: AE—higher intensity, group-based 2: AE—higher intensity, home-based 3: AE—lower intensity, home-based 4: Control	167 (197) men; 131 (160), women, postmenopausal, not on HRT; sedentary	9–12 months	1: 27.4 2: 28.0 3: 27.1 4: 27.0 1: 26.3 2: 27.1 3: 25.7 4: 27.1	1: (−0.2) 2: (−0.2) 3: (−0.9) 4: (+0.1) 1: (+0.4) 2: (+0.1) 3: (−0.6) 4: (0.0)	No group differences, in either sex

Study	Intervention/Groups	Subjects	Duration	Baseline	Change	Significance
Duncan et al.[22]	1: Aerobic walking (8.0 km/h) 2: Brisk walking (6.4 km/h) 3: Strolling (4.8 km/h) 4: Control	59 (102) women, premenopausal; sedentary	24 weeks	1: (60.3) 2: (64.2) 3: (62.0) 4: (66.5)	1: +1.1 2: +0.1 3: +0.8 4: +3.7	2 vs. 4, $P < 0.05$ No other differences
Jakicic et al.[46]	Hypocaloric, low-fat diet + 1: Long-bout aerobic exercise 2: Short-bout aerobic exercise	52 (56), women; 120%–175% ideal weight sedentary	20 weeks	1: 33.8 2: 34.1	1: −6.5 2: −8.9	NS
Perri et al.[47]	Behavioral (diet) weight loss + 1: Group-based exercise 2: Home-based exercise	41 (49) women; BMI = 27–45; 40–60 years old	15 months	1: 34.0 2: 33.1	1: −7.0 2: −11.7	$P < 0.05$
Dunn et al.[48]	1: Structured AE (3–5 group sessions per week) 2: Lifestyle physical activity (accumulate 30 minute moderate-intensity exercise most days)	190 (235) men + women (50%); 35–60 years old sedentary	24 months	1: 28.0 2: 28.4	1: +0.7 2: −0.1	NS
Andersen et al.[49]	Behavioral (+diet) weight loss + 1: Structured AE 2: Lifestyle physical activity	38 (40), women; ≥15 kg ideal weight	16 weeks	1: 31.4 2: 32.4	1: −8.3 2: −7.9	NS

Dunn et al[48] demonstrated that a lifestyle physical activity intervention was as effective as a structured exercise program in improving physical activity, cardiorespiratory fitness, and blood pressure; however, neither group changed their weight, which is not surprising considering the modest effect on weight loss associated with structured aerobic exercise.

Andersen et al[49] combined these exercise options with a low-fat hypocaloric diet in a 16-week randomized trial. Mean weight losses were 8.3 kg with structured aerobic exercise + diet and 7.9 kg with lifestyle activity + diet. There was no difference between them; however, the aerobic group lost less FFM. During a 1-year follow-up, the aerobic group regained 1.6 kg, while the lifestyle group regained 0.08 kg.

Discussion

This review presents over 40 randomized clinical trials designed to assess the role of physical activity in the management of obesity. In general, neither aerobic exercise nor resistance exercise seem to be powerful enough to cause major weight loss without the addition of caloric restriction; yet the long-term benefits of reducing excess body fat by increasing energy expenditure and preserving lean body mass with resistance exercise, instead of relying on caloric deficit, remain to be explored. Many different kinds of structured exercise programs have been utilized in these studies, but there is no clear evidence that one is better than another or that there is an optimal intensity of exercise for promoting weight loss. In general, it seems that controlling caloric intake and expending as much energy as one can is the best approach. This is unlikely to be embraced with enthusiasm by the population; therefore we must continue to identify key components of improving adherence and developing patience with slow weight loss from exercise.

In the meantime, the evidence that exercise improves other disease risk factors associated with obesity continues to accumulate. It is becoming increasingly clear that engaging in exercise at the recommended 30-min/d dose may provide the overweight and obese individual many benefits, even if it facilitates only modest weight loss and maintenance.

References

1. Flegal KM, Carroll MD, Kuczmarski RJ, et al. Overweight and obesity in the United States: Prevalence and trends, 1960–1994. *Int J Obes Relat Metab Disord* 1998;22:39–47.

2. Expert Panel on the Identification E, and Treatment of Overweight in Adults. Clinical guidelines on the identification, evaluation, and treatment of overweight and obesity in adults: The evidence report. National Institutes of Health. *Obes Res* 1998;6:51S–209S.

3. Pate RR, Pratt M, Blair SN, et al. Physical activity and public health. A recommendation from the Centers for Disease Control and Prevention and the American College of Sports Medicine. *JAMA* 1995;273:402–407.

4. NIH Consensus Development Panel on Physical Activity, and Cardiovascular Health. Physical activity and cardiovascular health. *JAMA* 1996;276:241–246.

5. Stefanick ML. Exercise and weight control. *Exerc Sport Sci Rev* 1993;21:363–396.

6. Ronnemaa T, Mattila K, Lehtonen A, et al. A controlled randomized study on the effect of long-term physical exercise on the metabolic control in type 2 diabetic patients. *Acta Med Scand* 1986;220:219–224.

7. Wood PD, Stefanick ML, Dreon DM, et al. Changes in plasma lipids and lipoproteins in overweight men during weight loss through dieting as compared with exercise. *N Engl J Med* 1988;319:1173–1179.

8. Fortmann SP, Haskell WL, Wood PD. Effects of weight loss on clinic and ambulatory blood pressure in normotensive men. *Am J Cardiol* 1988;62:89–93.

9. Frey-Hewitt B, Vranizan KM, Dreon DM, et al. The effect of weight loss by dieting or exercise on resting metabolic rate in overweight men. *Int J Obes* 1990;14:327–334.

10. Hammer RL, Barrier CA, Roundy ES, et al. Calorie-restricted low-fat diet and exercise in obese women. *Am J Clin Nutr* 1989;49:77–85.

11. Verity LS, Ismail AH. Effects of exercise on cardiovascular disease risk in women with NIDDM. *Diabetes Res Clin Pract* 1989;6:27–35.

12. Bertram SR, Venter I, Stewart RI. Weight loss in obese women: Exercise v. dietary education. *S Afr Med J* 1990;78:15–18.

13. King AC, Haskell WL, Taylor CB, et al. Group- vs home-based exercise training in healthy older men and women. A community-based clinical trial. *JAMA* 1991;266:1535–1542.

14. Hellenius ML, de Faire U, Berglund B, et al. Diet and exercise are equally effective in reducing risk for cardiovascular disease. Results of a randomized controlled study in men with slightly to moderately raised cardiovascular risk factors. *Atherosclerosis* 1993;103:81–91.

15. King AC, Haskell WL, Young DR, et al. Long-term effects of varying intensities and formats of physical activity on participation rates, fitness, and lipoproteins in men and women aged 50 to 65 years. *Circulation* 1995;91:2596–2604.

16. Katzel LI, Bleecker ER, Colman EG, et al. Effects of weight loss vs aerobic exercise training on risk factors for coronary disease in healthy, obese, middle-aged and older men. A randomized controlled trial. *JAMA* 1995;274:1915–1921.

17. Anderssen S, Holme I, Urdal P, et al. Diet and exercise intervention have favourable effects on blood pressure in mild hypertensives: The Oslo Diet and Exercise Study (ODES). *Blood Press* 1995;4:343–349.

18. Stefanick ML, Mackey S, Sheehan M, et al. Effects of diet and exercise in men and postmenopausal women with low levels of HDL cholesterol and high levels of LDL cholesterol. *N Engl J Med* 1998;339:12–20.

19. Ready AE, Drinkwater DT, Ducas J, et al. Walking program reduces elevated cholesterol in women postmenopause. *Can J Cardiol* 1995;11:905–912.
20. Huttunen JK, Lansimies E, Voutilainen E, et al. Effect of moderate physical exercise on serum lipoproteins. A controlled clinical trial with special reference to serum high-density lipoproteins. *Circulation* 1979;60:1220–1229.
21. Wood PD, Haskell WL, Blair SN, et al. Increased exercise level and plasma lipoprotein concentrations: A one-year, randomized, controlled study in sedentary, middle-aged men. *Metabolism.* 1983;32:31–39.
22. Duncan BB, Chambless LE, Schmidt MI, et al. Correlates of body fat distribution. Variation across categories of race, sex, and body mass in the atherosclerosis risk in communities study. The Atherosclerosis Risk in Communities (ARIC) Study Investigators. *Ann Epidemiol* 1995;5:192–200.
23. Pritchard JE, Nowson CA, Wark JD. A worksite program for overweight middle-aged men achieves lesser weight loss with exercise than with dietary change. *J Am Diet Assoc* 1997;97:37–42.
24. Sopko G, Leon AS, Jacobs DR Jr, et al. The effects of exercise and weight loss on plasma lipids in young obese men. *Metabolism* 1985;34:227–236.
25. Wing RR, Epstein LH, Paternostro-Bayles M, et al. Exercise in a behavioural weight control programme for obese patients with Type 2 (non-insulin-dependent) diabetes. *Diabetologia* 1988;31:902–909.
26. Wood PD, Stefanick ML, Williams PT, et al. The effects on plasma lipoproteins of a prudent weight-reducing diet, with or without exercise, in overweight men and women. *N Engl J Med* 1991;325:461–466.
27. Svendsen OL, Hassager C, Christiansen C. Effect of an energy-restrictive diet, with or without exercise, on lean tissue mass, resting metabolic rate, cardiovascular risk factors, and bone in overweight postmenopausal women. *Am J Med* 1993;95:131–140.
28. Blonk MC, Jacobs MA, Biesheuvel EH, et al. Influences on weight loss in type 2 diabetic patients: Little long-term benefit from group behaviour therapy and exercise training. *Diabet Med* 1994;11:449–457.
29. Marks BL, Ward A, Morris DH, et al. Fat-free mass is maintained in women following a moderate diet and exercise program. *Med Sci Sports Exerc* 1995;27:1243–1251.
30. Andersen RE, Wadden TA, Bartlett SJ, et al. Relation of weight loss to changes in serum lipids and lipoproteins in obese women. *Am J Clin Nutr* 1995;62:350–357.
31. Gordon NF, Scott CB, Levine BD. Comparison of single versus multiple lifestyle interventions: Are the antihypertensive effects of exercise training and diet-induced weight loss additive? *Am J Cardiol* 1997;79:763–767.
32. Wadden TA, Vogt RA, Foster GD, et al. Exercise and the maintenance of weight loss: 1-year follow-up of a controlled clinical trial. *J Consult Clin Psychol* 1998;66:429–433.
33. Wadden TA, Vogt RA, Andersen RE, et al. Exercise in the treatment of obesity: Effects of four interventions on body composition, resting energy expenditure, appetite, and mood. *J Consult Clin Psychol* 1997;65:269–277.
34. King AC, Tribble DL. The role of exercise in weight regulation in nonathletes. *Sports Med* 1991;11:331–349.
35. Hill JO, Schlundt DG, Sbrocco T, et al. Evaluation of an alternating-calorie diet with and without exercise in the treatment of obesity. *Am J Clin Nutr* 1989;50:248–254.

36. Donnelly JE, Pronk NP, Jacobsen DJ, et al. Effects of a very-low-calorie diet and physical-training regimens on body composition and resting metabolic rate in obese females. *Am J Clin Nutr* 1991;54:56–61.
37. Sweeney ME, Hill JO, Heller PA, et al. Severe vs moderate energy restriction with and without exercise in the treatment of obesity: Efficiency of weight loss. *Am J Clin Nutr* 1993;57:127–134.
38. Singh RB, Rastogi SS, Ghosh S, et al. The diet and moderate exercise trial (DAMET): Results after 24 weeks. *Acta Cardiol* 1992;47:543–557.
39. Dengel DR, Hagberg JM, Coon PJ, et al. Effects of weight loss by diet alone or combined with aerobic exercise on body composition in older obese men. *Metabolism* 1994;43:867–871.
40. Fox AA, Thompson JL, Butterfield GE, et al. Effects of diet and exercise on common cardiovascular disease risk factors in moderately obese older women. *Am J Clin Nutr* 1996;63:225–233.
41. Svendsen OL, Hassager C, Christiansen C. Six months' follow-up on exercise added to a short-term diet in overweight postmenopausal women: Effects on body composition, resting metabolic rate, cardiovascular risk factors and bone. *Int J Obes Relat Metab Disord* 1994;18:692–698.
42. Skender ML, Goodrick GK, Del Junco DJ, et al. Comparison of 2-year weight loss trends in behavioral treatments of obesity: Diet, exercise, and combination interventions. *J Am Diet Assoc* 1996;96:342–346.
43. Manning JM, Dooly-Manning CR, White K, et al. Effects of a resistive training program on lipoprotein–lipid levels in obese women. *Med Sci Sports Exerc* 1991;23:1222–1226.
44. Boyden TW, Pamenter RW, Going SB, et al. Resistance exercise training is associated with decreases in serum low-density lipoprotein cholesterol levels in premenopausal women. *Arch Intern Med* 1993;153:97–100.
45. Ross R, Rissanen J. Mobilization of visceral and subcutaneous adipose tissue in response to energy restriction and exercise. *Am J Clin Nutr* 1994;60:695–703.
46. Jakicic JM, Wing RR, Butler BA, et al. Prescribing exercise in multiple short bouts versus one continuous bout: Effects on adherence, cardiorespiratory fitness, and weight loss in overweight women. *Int J Obes Relat Metab Disord* 1995;19:893–901.
47. Perri MG, Martin AD, Leermakers EA, et al. Effects of group- versus home-based exercise in the treatment of obesity. *J Consult Clin Psychol* 1997;65:278–285.
48. Dunn AL, Marcus BH, Kampert JB, et al. Comparison of lifestyle and structured interventions to increase physical activity and cardiorespiratory fitness: A randomized trial. *JAMA* 1999;281:327–334.
49. Andersen RE, Wadden TA, Bartlett SJ, et al. Effects of lifestyle activity vs structured aerobic exercise in obese women: A randomized trial. *JAMA* 1999;281:335–340.

Chapter 17

Efficacy and Safety of Pharmacologic Interventions for the Overweight Patient

George A. Bray, MD

Introduction

Drug treatment for obesity has been tarnished by a number of disasters. Since the first drug was used in 1893, almost every drug treatment that has been tried in obese patients has generated undesirable outcomes that have resulted in their termination. Thus, caution must be used in accepting any new drugs for treatment of obesity, unless the safety profile would make it acceptable for almost everyone.

An additional serious negative aspect to the use of drug treatment for obesity is the negative halo spread by the addictive properties of amphetamine. Amphetamine stands for α-methyl-β-phenethylamine. It is an addictive β-phenethylamine that reduces food intake. The addictiveness of amphetamine probably is related to its effects on dopaminergic neurotransmission. On the other hand, its anorectic effects probably are caused by its modulation of noradrenergic neurotransmission. Because this β-phenethylamine is addictive, other β-phenethylamine derivatives were presumed to be addictive. Whether actually addictive or not, they were guilty by association. This has led to restrictions on the use of this entire class of drugs by the US Drug Enforcement Agency (DEA).

Drugs such as phentermine, diethylpropion, fenfluramine, sibutramine, and the antidepressant venlafaxine are all β-phenethylamines. Phentermine and diethylpropion are sympathomimetic amines, like amphetamine, but differ from amphetamine in having

From: Fletcher GF, Grundy SM, Hayman LL (eds). *Obesity: Impact on Cardiovascular Disease*. Armonk, NY: Futura Publishing Co., Inc.; © 1999.

little or no effect on dopamine release at the synapse. Abuse of either phentermine or diethylpropion is rare. On the other hand, fenfluramine has no effect on reuptake or release of either norepinephrine or dopamine in the brain, but increases serotonin release and partially inhibits serotonin reuptake. Sibutramine, likewise, has no evident abuse potential. Thus, derivatives of β-phenethylamine have a wide range of pharmacologic effects. However, if examined uncritically, they could all be lumped with amphetamine and carry its negative halo. It is misleading to use "amphetaminelike" in reference to appetite suppressant β-phenethylamine drugs except amphetamine and methamphetamine because of the negative linguistic images.

A third issue in drug treatment of obesity is the perception that because patients regain weight when drugs are stopped that the drugs are ineffective. Quite the contrary is true. Overweight is a chronic disease that has many causes. However, cure is rare, and treatment is thus aimed at palliation. As clinicians we do not expect to cure such diseases as hypertension or hypercholesterolemia with medications. Rather, we expect to palliate them. When the medications for any of these diseases are discontinued, we expect the disease to recur. This means that medications only work when used. The same arguments go for medications used to treat overweight. It is a chronic incurable disease for which drugs only work when used.

Recent reports of valvular heart disease associated with the use of fenfluramine, dexfenfluramine, and phentermine have provided the most recent problem for drug treatment of obesity. This is an example of the "law of unintended consequences." The report of valvulopathy in up to 35% of patients treated with the combination of fenfluramine and phentermine was totally unexpected. However, the finding will add caution to any future drugs that are marketed to treat obesity and will provide support for those who believe drug treatment of obesity is inappropriate.

Mechanisms of Drug Treatment for Obesity

Obesity results from an imbalance between energy intake and EE. Drugs can reduce food intake, alter metabolism, and/or increase EE. This approach will be used in discussing the available and potential drug leads for treatment of obesity.

Reduction of Food Intake

Noradrenergic Receptors

A number of monoamines and neuropeptides are known to modulate food intake. Both noradrenergic receptors and serotonergic receptors have served as the site for clinically useful drugs to decrease food intake[1-5] (Table 1). Activation of the α_1- and β_2-adrenoceptors decreases food intake. Stimulation of the α_2-adrenoceptor in experimental animals, on the other hand, increases food intake. Direct agonists and drugs that release neurotransmitter norepinephrine (NE) or block NE reuptake can activate one or more of these receptors depending on where the NE is released. Phenylpropanolamine is an α_1-agonist that decreases food intake by acting on α_1-adrenergic receptors in the paraventricular nucleus. The weight gain seen in patients treated for hypertension or prostatic hypertrophy with α_1-adrenergic antagonists indicates that the α_1-adrenoceptor is important clinically in regulation of body weight. Stimulation of the β_2-adrenoceptor by NE or agonists like terbutaline, clenbuterol, or salbutamol reduces food intake. The weight gain in patients treated with some β_2-adrenergic antagonists also indicates that this is a clinically important receptor for regulation of body weight.

Serotonergic Receptors

The serotonin receptor system consists of seven families of receptors. Stimulation of receptors in the hydroxytryptamine ($5HT_1$) and

Table 1

Monoamine Mechanisms That Reduce Food Intake

Neurotransmitter system	Mechanism of action	Examples
Noradrenergic	α_1-Agonist	Phenylpropanolamine
	β_2-Agonist	Terbutaline
	Stimulate NE release	Phentermine
	Block NE reuptake	Mazindol
Serotonergic	$5HT_{1B}$ or $5HT_{2C}$ Agonists	Cyproheptidine
	Stimulate 5HT release	Fenfluramine
	Block reuptake	Fluoxetine
Dopaminergic	D-1 Agonist	Bromocriptine
Histaminergic	H-1 Antagonist	Cimetidine

$5HT_2$ families have the major effects on feeding. Activation of the $5HT_{1A}$ receptor increases food intake but this acute effect is down-regulated rapidly and is not significant clinically in regulation of body weight. Activation of the $5HT_{2C}$ and possibly $5HT_{1B}$ receptor decreases food intake. Direct agonists (quipazine) or drugs that block serotonin reuptake (fluoxetine, sertraline, and fenfluramine) will reduce food intake by acting on these receptors or by providing the serotonin that modulates these receptors.

Altered Metabolism

Excess fat is the visible sign of obesity. Metabolic strategies have been directed to preabsorptive and postabsorptive mechanisms of modifying fat absorption or metabolism. Preabsorptive mechanisms that influence digestion and absorption of macronutrients have been utilized to develop orlistat, which inhibits intestinal digestion of fat and lowers body weight. The second strategy is to affect intermediary metabolism. Enhancing lipolysis, inhibiting lipogenesis, and affecting fat distribution between subcutaneous and visceral sites are strategies that can be developed.

Increased Energy Expenditure

Increased energy expenditure (EE) through exercise would be an ideal approach to treating obesity. Drugs that have the same physiological consequences as exercise would provide useful ways of treating obesity.

Drugs that Reduce Food Intake

Table 2 summarizes the effects of a number of drugs used to treat obesity.[1-5] They are discussed below in more detail.

Sympathomimetic Drugs Approved by the Food and Drug Administration to Treat Obesity

Pharmacology

The sympathomimetic drugs are grouped together because they can increase blood pressure and, in part, act like the NE. Drugs in this group work by a variety of mechanisms including the release of NE from synaptic granules (benzphetamine, phendimetrazine, phentermine, and diethylpropion), blockade of NE reuptake (mazindol), blockade of reuptake of both NE and 5HT (sibutramine), or direct action on adrenoceptors (phenylpropanolamine).

All of these drugs are absorbed orally and reach peak blood concentrations within a short time. The half-life in blood is short for all except the metabolites of sibutramine, which have a long half-life. Both metabolites of sibutramine are active, but this is not true of the other drugs in this group. Liver metabolism inactivates a large fraction of these drugs before excretion. Side effects include dry mouth, constipation, and insomnia. Food intake is suppressed either by delaying the onset of a meal or by producing early satiety. Both sibutramine and mazindol have been shown to increase thermogenesis experimentally.

Efficacy

The efficacy of an appetite-suppressing drug can be established by showing that in double-blind randomized clinical trials, it produces a significantly greater weight loss than a placebo drug[1] and that the weight loss is more than 5% below baseline weight. Clinical trials of sympathomimetic drugs done before 1975 generally were short term because it was widely believed that short-term treatment would "cure obesity."[5] This was unfounded optimism, but because the trials were of short duration, and often cross over in design, they provided little long-term data. In this discussion I will focus on longer term trials lasting over 24 weeks and on those trials in which there is an adequate control group.

Phentermine and Diethylpropion

A 36-week trial comparing continuous administration of phentermine with intermittent phentermine and placebo is shown in Figure 1.[6] Both continuous and intermittent phentermine therapy produced more weight loss than the placebo. In the drug-free periods the intermittently treated patients slowed their weight loss only to lose more rapidly when the drug was reinstituted. Phentermine and diethylpropion are schedule IV drugs indicating a regulatory classification as having the potential for abuse, although this appears to be very low. Phentermine and diethylpropion only are approved for a "few weeks," which is widely interpreted as up to 12 weeks. Weight loss with phentermine and diethylpropion persists for the duration of treatment

Table 2

Drugs That Reduce Food Intake

Drug group	FDA approval	Approved duration of treatment	DEA schedule	Trade names	Dosage form (mg)	Administration
Sympathomimetic drugs Norepinephrine releasers						
Methamphetamine	Yes (warning box)	Few weeks	II	Desoxyn	5, 10, 15	10 or 15 mg in morning
Amphetamine	Yes (warning box)	Few weeks	II	Dexedrine	5, 10, 15	5 mg two or three times daily Initial dose: 25 mg once daily Maximum dose: 25–50 mg three times daily
Benzphetamine	Yes	Few weeks	III	Didrex Standard release Bontril PDM Plegine X-Trozine	25–50	
Phendimetrazine	Yes	Few weeks	III	Slow release Bontril PDM Prelu-2 X-Trozine	35	35 mg before meals three times daily
					105	105 mg 30–60 min before morning meal
Diethylpropion	Yes	Few weeks	IV	Tenuate Tenuate Dospan	25	25 mg three times daily
					75	75 mg once daily

Norepinephrine reuptake inhibitor						
Phentermine	Yes	Few weeks	IV	Standard	37.5	37.5 mg/in morning
				Adipex-P	30	30 mg/d 2 h after breakfast
				Fastin	37.5	37.5 mg/d 9 in morning
				Obenix	30	30 mg/d 2 h after breakfast
				Oby-Cap	30	30 mg/d 2 h after breakfast
				Oby-Trim		
				Zantryl	30	30 mg/d 2 h after breakfast
				Slow release		15 mg/d before breakfast (30 mg
				Ionamin	15, 30	for less responsive patients)
Mazindol	Yes	Few weeks	IV	Sanorex	1, 2	Initial dose; 1 mg once daily Maximum dose: 1 mg three times daily with meals
				Mazanor	1	Initial dose; 1 mg/once daily Maximum dose: 1 mg three times daily with meals
Noradrenergic agonist						
Phenylpropanolamine	Yes	—	—	Dexatrim Accutrim	25, 75	25 mg three times daily
Serotonin-norepinephrine reuptake inhibitor						
Sibutramine	Yes	—	IV	Meridia Reductil	5, 10, 15	Initial dose, 10 mg/d Maximum dose 15 mg/d

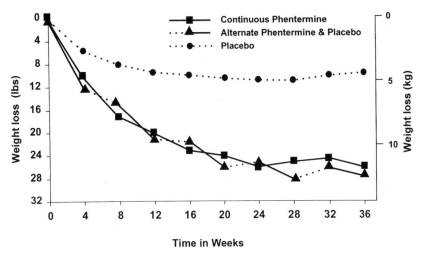

Time in Weeks

Figure 1. Comparison of weight loss with continuous and intermittent therapy with phentermine. Adapted with permission from Reference 6.

suggesting that tolerance does not develop to these drugs. If tolerance does develop, the drugs would be expected to lose their effectiveness or require increased amounts of drug for patients to maintain weight loss. This does not seem to occur.

Mazindol

No long-term double-blind placebo-controlled trials have been reported with mazindol. In 1-year-long open label trial, the weight loss was 9%, which is comparable with weight loss with other sympathomimetic drugs.

Sibutramine

In contrast to all of the other sympathomimetic drugs in Table 2, sibutramine has been evaluated extensively in several multicenter trials lasting 6 to 12 months. In a clinical trial lasting 8 weeks sibutramine was found to produce dose-dependent weight loss with doses of 5 and 20 mg/d. Three clinical trials are included in the package insert. They were conducted in men and women ages 18 to 65 with a body mass index (BMI) between 27 and 40 kg/m^2. In one trial enrolling 456 patients, 56% of those who stayed in the trial for 12 months lost at least 5% and 30% of the patients lost 10% of their initial body weight while taking the 10-mg dose. In a dose-ranging study of 1047 patients lasting

6 months, 67% achieved a 5% weight loss and 35% lost 10% or more. They show a dose-related reduction in body weight and body fat. Data from one site in a multicenter trial on over 1000 patients is shown in Figure 2.[7] There is a clear dose-response during treatment for 24 weeks and regain of weight when the drug was stopped indicating that the drug remained effective. Nearly 2/3 of the patients treated with sibutramine lost more than 5% of their body weight from baseline and nearly 1/3 lost more than 10%. The year-long trial showed that 10 and 15 mg produced significantly greater weight loss than placebo but that these doses were not different from one another. In a third trial, in patients who initially lost weight on a very low calorie diet before being randomized to sibutramine or placebo, sibutramine produced additional weight loss, whereas the placebo-treated patients regained weight. Lipids and uric acid were reduced across all trials in relation to the weight loss. The medication will be available in 5-, 10-, and 15-mg doses; 10 mg/d as a single daily dose is the recommended starting level with titration up or down based on response. Doses above 20 mg/d are not recommended. Of the patients who lost 4 lb in the first 4 weeks of treatment, 60% achieved a weight loss of more than 5%, compared with less than 10% of those who did not lose 4 lb in 4

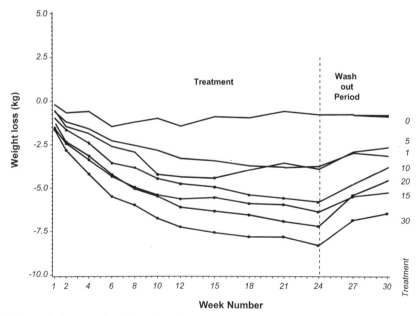

Figure 2. Dose-related weight loss with sibutramine. The regain in weight when the drug was discontinued indicates that it remained effective during treatment. Adapted with permission from Reference 7.

weeks. Combining data from the total of 11 studies on sibutramine showed a weight-related reduction in triglyceride, total cholesterol, and low-density lipoprotein (LDL) cholesterol and a weight-loss–related rise in high-density lipoprorein (HDL) cholesterol.

Safety

The side effect profile for sympathomimetic drugs is similar. They produce insomnia, dry mouth, asthenia, and constipation. The safety of older sympathomimetic appetite-suppressant drugs has been the subject of considerable controversy because dextroamphetamine is addictive. The sympathomimetic drugs phentermine, diethylpropion, and mazindol have very little abuse potential as assessed by the low rate of reinforcement when the drugs are available intravenously to test animals. In this same paradigm, neither phenylpropanolamine nor fenfluramine showed any reinforcing effects and no clinical data show any abuse potential for either of these drugs. Sibutramine, likewise, has no abuse potential in this paradigm, but it is nonetheless a schedule IV drug.

Sympathomimetic drugs can affect blood pressure. Phenylpropanolamine is an α_1-agonist and at doses of 75 mg or more it can increase blood pressure. Phenylpropanolamine has been associated with stroke and it should not be used above 75 mg/d. Phenylpropanolamine also has been reported in association with cardiomyopathy. In the placebo-controlled studies, systolic and diastolic blood pressure increased by 1 to 3 mm Hg and pulse increased by approximately 4 to 5 beats per minute. Caution should be used when combining sibutramine with other drugs that may increase blood pressure. Sibutramine should not be used in patients with a history of coronary artery disease, congestive heart failure, cardiac arrhythmias, or stroke. There should be a 2-week interval between termination of monoamine oxidase inhibitors (MAOIs) and beginning sibutramine and it should not be used with MAOIs or selective serotonin reuptake inhibitors (SSRIs). Because sibutramine is metabolized by the cytochrome P_{450} enzyme system (isozyme CYP3A4) it may interfere with metabolism of erythromycin and ketoconazole.

Sympathomimetic Drugs Not Approved by the Food and Drug Administration to Treat Obesity

There are several other sympathomimetic agents that either carry warning labels (amphetamine and methamphetamine) or have never been approved (fenproporex and chlobenzorex) by the US Food and Drug Administration (FDA) for treatment of obesity.

Nonsympathomimetic Drugs Not Approved by the Food and Drug Administration to Treat Obesity

Dexfenfluramine and Fenfluramine

Pharmacology

Fenfluramine and its dextroisomer, dexfenfluramine, are serotonergic drugs that are devoid of sympathomimetic activity but that are no longer licensed to treat obesity because of their association with valvular heart disease. Dexfenfluramine, which contains all of the appetite-suppressing properties of fenfluramine, releases serotonin from nerve endings and blocks its reuptake. The *d*-norfenfluramine metabolite of dexfenfluramine has a direct action on serotonin receptors, possibly the $5HT_{2C}$ type, to reduce food intake. These drugs are well absorbed orally but have a long half-life in the plasma.

Efficacy

Fenfluramine originally was licensed in 1972 for short-term use in the treatment of obesity. The International Dexfenfluramine (INDEX) Study was a 12-month long double-blind, placebo-controlled randomized clinical study of dexfenfluramine and was the cornerstone for its approval by the US FDA in April 1996.[8] The drug-treated patients lost significantly more weight than the placebo-treated patients, that is, 9% below baseline weight. The weight loss in the placebo-treated group also was noteworthy, being a 7.5% decrease from baseline. When the patients were stratified by the amount of weight lost, 64% of the drug-treated versus 43% of the placebo-treated patients lost more than 5% of their initial weight, and 40% of the dexfenfluramine-treated patients versus 21% of the placebo-treated patients lost more than 10%.

Safety

In addition to insomnia, dry mouth, asthenia, and loose stools, which are most prominent in the first 1 to 2 weeks of treatment and tend to subside, four serious problems have been associated with fenfluramine and dexfenfluramine. These include pulmonary hypertension, neuroanatomical changes, the serotonin syndrome, and an atypical valvular heart disease, which will be discussed after the discussion of combination therapy below.

Primary pulmonary hypertension is a rare complication associated with appetite-suppressant drugs.[9] Its spontaneous occurrence rate is 1 to 2 per million per year. Aminorex was the first β-phenethylamine to be associated with pulmonary hypertension. Initially, it was marketed in Europe in 1967 and withdrawn shortly afterward. Treatment with fenfluramine and other anorexigens for more than 3 months has been reported to increase the relative risk of developing pulmonary hypertension by 20- to 40-fold based on data from a retrospective case-controlled study.[9] This is comparable with the risk of anaphylaxis from penicillin.

The neuroanatomic changes attributed to dexfenfluramine are a depletion of serotonin levels in the brain in experimental animals. This has been reported after treatment with high doses of dexfenfluramine given parenterally. The depletion is long lived and blocked by serotonin reuptake inhibitors, which prevent dexfenfluramine from reaching serotonin storage vesicles. No functional impairments have been reported to accompany the depletion of serotonin other than reduced food intake.

The serotonin syndrome arises when too much serotonin is released. It usually occurs when two or more serotonergic drugs are used concomitantly. It consists of altered mental status such as confusion, hallucinations, agitation, or mania. It also produces dysfunction of the autonomic nervous system with sweating, hyperthermia, shivering, and diarrhea, as well as neuromuscular abnormalities including clonus, hyperreflexia, rigidity, and tremor. Treatment consists of withdrawal of the medications and supportive therapy.

Fluoxetine and Sertraline

Pharmacology

Fluoxetine and sertraline are highly specific inhibitors of serotonin reuptake into the nerve terminal. They are absorbed readily and have a long half-life in the blood. In experimental animals fluoxetine reduces food intake.

Efficacy

Both fluoxetine and sertraline have been approved by the FDA for treatment of depression but not for the treatment of obesity. In short-term clinical trials fluoxetine produced a dose-related decrease in body weight. In longer-term trials the maximum weight loss was seen after 20 to 30 weeks of treatment. This was followed by a return of body weight toward the baseline by 1 year.[10] In a trial with sertraline in patients who had lost weight using a very low calorie diet, the drug was no more effective than placebo in preventing weight gain.

In contrast to the limited potential for fluoxetine in long-term treatment of obesity, they may be of value in treating individuals with binge-eating disorder or to help prevent weight gain in individuals who have stopped smoking.

Safety

Both fluoxetine and sertraline are used widely to treat depression and have no major safety concerns.

Bromocriptine

Bromocriptine is a synthetic ergot alkaloid that acts directly on dopamine receptors. It is used most often for treating pituitary tumors. Experimental studies show that modulating prolactin will affect fat storage. Timed administration of bromocriptine has been reported to reduce body fat and improve diabetes. Confirmation is awaited.

Cimetidine

Cimetidine is an H-2 antagonist that is used widely in the treatment of peptic ulcer disease. A small clinical trial showed that patients treated with 200 mg three times a day lost significantly more weight than controls. More definitive data are awaited. The side effects from cimetidine are mild.

Combining Serotonergic and Noradrenergic Drugs

Efficacy

Drugs that act on either the noradrenergic or the serotonergic feeding system can reduce body weight. The possibility that combining drugs that act on the serotonergic system with drugs that act on the noradrenergic system, might produce more weight loss and/or have fewer side effects if submaximal doses of one drug from each group were combined was the rationale for a 4-year controlled trial of fenfluramine and phentermine.[11] The first double-blind, placebo-controlled portion of the trial is shown in Figure 3. During the baseline run-in, patients received an effective program of behavior therapy, diet, and exercise and they lost weight. When the patients were randomized with the drug-treated group, they lost 15.9% from baseline compared with the placebo-treated group, which lost only 4.9% from baseline. Some patients received long-term benefit by maintaining their weight at lower levels for up to 3 1/2 years during which time drug treatment was continued. This trial led to national enthusiasm for this drug combination. More than 18 million prescriptions were written in 1996 for this combination of drugs and an estimated 3–4 million people were treated with them.

Safety

Following this initial report, the use of the combination of phentermine and fenfluramine spread rapidly. In July 1997, 24 patients with

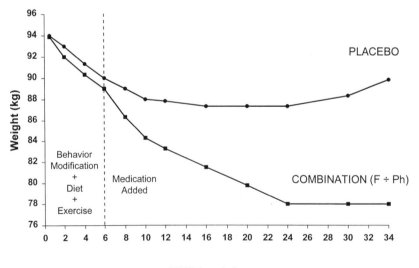

TIME (weeks)

Figure 3. Effect of combination treatment with fenfluramine and phentermine. During the 6-week run-in period both groups were treated with diet, exercise, and behavior modification. Patients were randomized using minimization techniques to assure a close match at the start of the double-blind period. During the double-blind period the placebo-treated patients lost almost no additional weight, whereas the drug-treated patients plateaued at a significantly lower weight. Adapted with permission from Reference 11.

an atypical valvular heart disease were reported to the medical profession.[12] In the three patients in whom histopathology of the heart valves was available, the valvular changes were identical to the changes seen in carcinoid syndrome. By the end of August 1997, the FDA had received reports of 291 patients, 92 of whom had valvular heart disease. Based on the concerns raised by this data both fenfluramine and dexfenfluramine were withdrawn from the market on September 15, 1997. An earlier report of cardiomyopathy developing during treatment with fenfluramine and mazindol went unnoticed but may represent an early example of the same problem.

The current recommendations are that all symptomatic patients treated with fenfluramine or dexfenfluramine alone or in combination with phentermine have an echocardiogram. Because careful clinical examination fails to detect a murmur in more than half of the patients with documented regurgitant lesions, it would be prudent to do an echocardiogram on any patient who might need prophylactic antibiotics as recommended by the American Heart Association.

Peptides that Reduce Food Intake and Are in Early Stages of Drug Development

Leptin

Leptin is a peptide produced exclusively in adipose tissue. Absence of leptin produces massive obesity in mice (ob/ob) and in humans. Treatment with the peptide decreases food intake in the ob/ob mouse. The diabetes mouse (db/db) and the fatty rat, which have genetic defects in the leptin receptor, also are obese but they do not respond to leptin. Leptin levels in the blood are highly correlated with body fat levels yet obesity persists, suggesting that there may be leptin resistance. Clinical trials currently are underway with leptin to see whether it can reduce food intake and body fat in overweight humans or diabetic humans.

Neuropeptide-Y

Neuropeptide-Y (NPY) is one of the most potent stimulators of food intake and appears to act through Y-5 and possibly Y-1 receptors. Antagonists to these receptors might block NPY and thus decrease feeding. Early trials of one antagonist to the NPY receptor are underway and more are expected soon.

Cholecystokinin

Cholecystokinin (CCK) reduces food intake in human beings and experimental animals. This effect does not require an intact hypothalamic feeding control system but does appear to require an intact vagus nerve. Peptide analogs have been developed and tested experimentally but clinical data have not been published yet. A second strategy to modify CCK activity is to reduce the degradation of CCK. This approach is likewise under evaluation.

Pancreatic Hormones

Glucagon Pancreatic glucagon produces a dose-related decrease in food intake. A fragment of glucagon (amino acids 6–29) called glucagonlike peptide-1 (GLP-1) reduced food intake when given either peripherally or into the brain.

Insulin

Circulating insulin levels are correlated directly with body fat and the level of insulin in the cerebrospinal fluid has been proposed as a feedback signal to reduce food intake. Infusion of insulin into the brain's ventricular system lowers body weight. A drug that reduces insulin secretion has been found to reduce body weight.

Amylin

Amylin is a pancreatic peptide released from the islet β-cell along with insulin. It, too, has been shown to decrease food intake and body weight in animals. In clinical trials it lowers glucose and has been used with success in type I diabetes. Clinical trials on weight loss are awaited.

Drugs that Alter Metabolism

Drugs Approved by the Food and Drug Administration

Orlistat (Xenical)

Pharmacology

Orlistat (formerly called tetrahydrolipostatin) is a potent selective inhibitor of pancreatic lipase and reduces intestinal digestion of fat.

The drug has a dose-dependent effect on fecal fat loss increasing it to approximately 30% on a diet that has 30% of energy as fat. Orlistat has little effect in subjects eating a low-fat diet as might be anticipated from the mechanism by which this drug works.

Efficacy

Five long-term clinical trials with orlistat lasting 1 to 2 years have been presented in abstract form. The results of one of the 2-year trials is shown in Figure 4.[13] The trial consisted of two parts. In the 1st year patients received a hypocaloric diet calculated to be 500 kcal/d below their requirements. During the 2nd year the diet was calculated to maintain weight. At the end of year 1 the placebo-treated patients lost 6.5% of their initial body weight and the drug-treated patients lost nearly 10%. Drug-treated patients regained less weight in year 2 than those receiving placebo. An analysis of quality of life in patients treated with orlistat showed improvements over the placebo group in spite of the concerns about gastrointestinal (GI) symptoms.

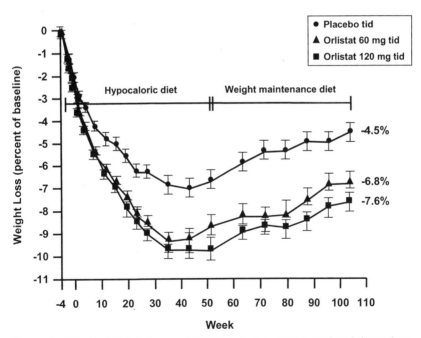

Figure 4. Effect of Orlistat on weight loss during year 1 and weight maintenance during year 2. Adapted with permission from Reference 13.

Safety

Orlistat is not absorbed to any significant degree and its side effects thus are related to the blockade of triglyceride digestion in the intestine. Fecal fat loss and related GI symptoms are common initially but subside as patients learn to use the drug. Some patients also need supplementation with fat-soluble vitamins, which can be lost in the stools. Absorption of other drugs does not seem to be affected significantly by orlistat.

Drugs Approved by the Food and Drug Administration for an Indication Other than Obesity

Androgens and Androgen Antagonists

Dehydroepiandrosterone

Dehydroepiandrosterone (DHEA) is a weak androgen that induces weight loss in several animal species. Clinical trials in humans have shown no effect.

Etiocholandione

Etiocholandione is a derivative of DHEA, which produced weight loss in one preliminary clinical trial. Additional trials are underway.

Testosterone

In men, testosterone and the anabolic steroid oxandrolone have been reported to reduce visceral fat. A trial of an antiandrogen and nandrolone in women did not show any effects on visceral fat.

Drugs that Increase Energy Expenditure

Drugs Approved by the Food and Drug Administration for an Indication Other than Obesity

Ephedrine/Caffeine

Pharmacology

Ephedrine is a sympathomimetic amine that is used to relax bronchial smooth muscle in patients with asthma. It also stimulates thermogenesis in human subjects. Caffeine is an xanthine that inhibits adenosine receptors and phosphodiesterase. In experimental animals the combination of ephedrine and caffeine reduce body weight probably through a stimulation of thermogenesis and a reduction in food intake.

Efficacy

One long-term placebo-controlled clinical trial with ephedrine, caffeine, or the combination has shown greater weight loss for the combination of ephedrine and caffeine than for either drug alone[14] (Figure 5). No other long-term data are available.

Safety

Although caffeine and ephedrine have a long record of clinical use separately, neither drug alone nor the combination is approved for treatment of obesity. Recent reports of problems associated with the use of ma huang, a natural source of ephedrine, raise concerns and it cannot be recommended until more data and FDA review have been done.

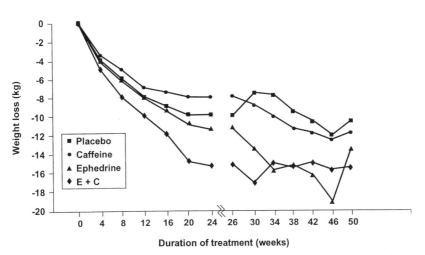

Figure 5. Effect of Ephedrine and caffeine on weight loss and weight maintenance for 1 year. Adapted with permission from Reference 14.

β_3-Adrenergic Receptor Agonists in Early Stages of Drug Development

The sympathetic nervous system has a tonic role in maintaining EE and blood pressure. Blockade of the thermogenic part of this system will reduce the thermic response to a meal. Norepinephrine, the neurotransmitter of the sympathetic nervous system also may decrease food intake by acting on β_2- or β_3-adrenergic receptors. Several synthetic β_3-agonists have been developed against rodent β_3-receptors, but the clinical responses have been disappointing. After cloning of the human β_3-receptor, a new round of compounds is being synthesized that will be tried in obese human subjects soon.

Patient Selection for Drug Treatment

Those patients who have a BMI above 30 are potential candidates for drug therapy. The presence of comorbidities such as dyslipidemia, hypertension, diabetes or impaired glucose tolerance, symptomatic osteoarthritis, or sleep apnea increases the rationale for treatment by shifting the BMI to 27–30 from 30 kg/m^2. The currently available sympathomimetic drugs can reduce body weight but only sibutramine is approved for long-term use. This drug should not be used in patients with stroke, congestive failure, or myocardial infarction. The likely approval of orlistat will further expand the therapeutic armamentarium of the physician.

Weight loss of 10%–15% can improve health risks. However, failure to lose weight or failure to improve comorbid conditions indicates either noncompliance with the drug or that the patient is not responding to the drug. Either setting requires reevaluation of therapy and addition of other medications or other modalities of treatment. As a guideline patients being treated with drugs should lose more than 2 kg (4 lb) in the 1st month and achieve more than a 5% weight loss by 6 months. As long as weight loss is more than 5% and/or the patient's comorbidities have responded, the drug may be continued. The data with phentermine suggests that intermittent use may be beneficial.

At least two groups of patients merit long-term drug therapy. The first are patients who are considered for surgical treatment of their obesity. Individuals with a BMI above 35 should first be treated with antiobesity drugs. If they respond with more than a 15% weight loss, drugs should be continued as long as they respond and their comorbidities improve. The second group of patients who deserve vigorous treatment are individuals with sleep apnea. A modest weight loss is often sufficient to alleviate their sleep apnea.

References

1. Bray GA, Atkinson RL, Inoue S. Pharmacologic treatment of obesity. *Obes Res* 1995;3:415S–632S.
2. Bray GA. Pharmacological treatment of obesity. In: Bray GA, Bouchard C, James WPT, eds. *Handbook of Obesity.* New York: Marcel Dekker; 1997:953–975.
3. Bray GA. Drug treatment of obesity. *Am J Clin Nutr* 1992;55:538S–544S.
4. Anonymous. Long-term pharmacotherapy in the management of obesity. National Task Force on the Prevention and Treatment of Obesity. *JAMA* 1996;276:1907–1915.
5. Bray GA. Use and abuse of appetite-suppressant drugs in the treatment of obesity. *Ann Intern Med* 1993;119:707–713.
6. Munro JF, MacCuish AC, Wilson EM, et al. Comparison of continuous and intermittent anorectic therapy in obesity. *Br Med J* 1968;1:352–356.
7. Bray GA, Ryan DH, Gordon D, et al. A double-blind randomized placebo-controlled trial of sibutramine. *Obes Res* 1996;4:263–270.
8. Guy-Grand B, Apfelbaum M, Crepaldi G, et al. International trial of long-term dexfenfluramine in obesity. *Lancet* 1989;2:1142–1145.
9. Abenhaim L, Moride Y, Brenot F, et al. Appetite-suppressant drugs and the risk of primary pulmonary hypertension. International Primary Pulmonary Hypertension Study Group. *N Engl J Med* 1996;335:609–616.
10. Darga LL, Carroll-Michals L, Botsford SJ, et al. Fluoxetine's effect on weight loss in obese subjects. *Am J Clin Nutr* 1991;54:321–325.
11. Weintraub M. Long-term weight control. The National Heart, Lung, and Blood Institute Funded Multimodal Intervention Study. *Clin Pharmacol Ther* 1992;51:581–585.
12. Connolly HM, Crary JL, McGoon MD, et al. Valvular heart disease associated with fenfluramine-phentermine. *N Engl J Med* 1997;337:581–588.
13. Sjostrom L, Rissanen A, Andersen T, et al. Randomised placebo-controlled trial of orlistat for weight loss and prevention of weight regain in obese patients. European Multicentre Orlistat Study Group. *Lancet* 1998;352:167–172.
14. Astrup A, Breum L, Toubro S, et al. The effect and safety of an ephedrine/caffeine compound compared to ephedrine, caffeine and placebo in obese subjects on an energy restricted diet. A double blind trial. *Int J Obes Relat Metab Disord* 1992;16:269–277.

Chapter 18

Behavioral Interventions

John P. Foreyt, PhD
and W. S. Carlos Poston, PhD

Summary

This chapter reviews the role of behavioral interventions in the treatment of obesity. Behavioral interventions include the systematic application of learning theories to modify behaviors that contribute to the development of obesity or its maintenance. Most behavioral interventions include the use of self-monitoring, stimulus control, cognitive restructuring, stress management, social support, contingency management, problem solving, physical activity, and relapse prevention. These interventions have been helpful in the achievement of short-term weight losses in obese individuals, but they have been less successful in long-term maintenance of lowered body weight. Because obesity is a chronic condition, unlikely to be cured, behavioral interventions need to focus on broader outcomes, including quality of life, improved psychological functioning, and lowered cardiovascular risk, in a continual care model of treatment rather than short-term, time-limited approaches.

Introduction

The goal of behavioral interventions is to help obese individuals improve their unhealthy dietary and sedentary habits.[1,2] A number of interventions based on learning theories have been developed to assist

---

This chapter was supported by National Institute of Diabetes and Digestive and Kidney Diseases grant DK43109 and a Minority Scientist Development Award from the American Heart Association and its Puerto Rican Affiliate.

From: Fletcher GF, Grundy SM, Hayman LL (eds). *Obesity: Impact on Cardiovascular Disease.* Armonk, NY: Futura Publishing Co., Inc.; © 1999.

patients in modifying their life habits. These interventions are based on the assumptions that by changing these unhealthy dietary and sedentary habits it is possible to lower body weight. We assume that these habits are modifiable and that their long-term change requires environmental restructuring.

Behavioral interventions include specific strategies for identifying and overcoming barriers to compliance with a healthy diet and increased physical activity. Most behavioral strategies are taught in weight-loss programs as a package that includes education about good nutrition and reasonable exercise. Within the overall package, the strategies are individualized, based on the specific needs of the obese patient.

No single strategy or combination of strategies have shown themselves to be superior. Therefore, several interventions typically are taught to an individual. All of the interventions are aimed at changing dietary patterns and physical activity permanently. The interventions usually are taught in group settings because of cost considerations and the support that groups can provide. However, the strategies also can be taught on an individual basis, either through self-help manuals or with a trained behavioral counselor.

Behavioral Interventions

Behavioral interventions typically include a number of specific strategies. These strategies include self-monitoring, stimulus control, cognitive restructuring, stress management, social support, contingency management, problem solving, physical activity, and relapse prevention.

Self-Monitoring

Self-monitoring includes the observing and recording of behavioral patterns, followed by feedback on the behaviors.[3] With obese patients, self-monitoring involves teaching the individual to record in a diary all food ingested. The diary can be a simple, inexpensive notebook. Recording ideally should be done as soon as possible after the food is ingested (even better before the food is eaten). Feedback can include looking up and recording the number of calories or fat grams that each food contained. The feedback should be done by the patient, and then positive changes should be reinforced at a meeting with the behavioral counselor. In addition to recording food ingested, other helpful behavioral patterns to record include time of day the food is eaten, mood state, location, and other individuals present. The behavioral counselor helps identify possible eating patterns that might need changing, such as eating when under stress or when bored.

Physical activity also can be recorded in the same diary. Minutes of exercise, along with time of day, should be noted. Weight on a bathroom scale should be measured on a regular schedule, but the question is how often. We find that the more frequently the patient weighs in, the better the results. Remember, when individuals are gaining weight, they tend to stay away from scales. Getting them back on a regular schedule of weighing, such as daily, can serve as a reminder to pay attention to eating and exercise patterns.

Obese patients typically will underreport their intake and overreport their physical activity. It is not unusual to find that individuals eat about one-third more calories than they report and exercise about one-half less than is recorded in the diary. It doesn't matter. The primary goal of self-monitoring is to serve as a reminder of their eating and exercise patterns. The results are clear; individuals who self-monitor do better than those who don't. Self-monitoring is one of the most helpful behavioral interventions for the management of eating and exercise. In our opinion, if the behavioral counselor chooses only one strategy to teach to obese individuals, it should be self-monitoring. Counselors should use all their training and skills to encourage their patients to use this important intervention.

Stimulus Control

Stimulus control involves identifying the environmental cues that are associated with unhealthy eating and sedentary patterns.[4] Modifying these cues, that is, controlling the stimuli, may help the obese patient to be more successful in managing weight control behaviors. We find that one of the most common problems reported to us by obese individuals is lack of time to exercise. Many individuals say that they are so busy during the day that by the time evening arrives they are just too exhausted to go for a brisk walk. Helping indviduals find time in their day, such as setting their alarm clock, which is on the other side of their bedroom, 30 minutes earlier and laying out their clothes and walking shoes before going to bed, may serve as reminders and encouragement to get up earlier and exercise before breakfast. We find that once patients get up earlier and exercise that many report that they feel good and some develop the habit.

Other common stimulus control strategies include the use of a shopping list, eliminating high-fat foods in the home, limiting the time and place of eating, and avoiding certain high-risk places, for example, the coffee machine with the donuts next to it at work. Depending on the barriers, the obese patient and behavioral counselor should individualize the stimulus control strategies.

Cognitive Restructuring

Cognitive restructuring involves helping obese individuals change their unrealistic goals and inaccurate beliefs about themselves.[5] For example, some patients believe that they can lose large amounts of weight. We recently worked with a patient who weighed 360 lb. When asked how much he expected to lose, he replied, "I just plan to get down to 170." Cognitive restructuring involves helping him modify his expectations. We said "Let's start with 30 lb and focus on the changes needed to achieve that goal." Over time, the patient did lose 30 lb and improved his cardiovascular risk factors and his psychological health. Although not a major cosmetic change, the patient's physical health and psychological attitude about himself improved significantly. He felt more in control of himself and his life. Cognitive restructuring involves helping patients focus on quality of life and improved health, not unrealistic cosmetic outcomes.

Stress Management

Stress triggers unhealthy eating patterns. It is one of the primary predictors of relapse from a healthy diet and frequently is associated with bouts of binging.[6] Stress management involves teaching obese individuals various strategies for identifying and counteracting stress and tension. Behavioral interventions include progressive relaxation, meditation, coping strategies such as physical activity, and diaphragmatic breathing. These interventions help patients reduce tension and sympathetic nervous system arousal and provide a distraction from the stressful situation. One patient told us that she attended a local dance at the community center. When she saw her favorite German chocolate cake on the dessert table, she almost lost control. However, before indulging, she went into a stall in the women's toilet and practiced the muscle-tensing and -relaxing exercises that we had taught her. She reported that she became so relaxed that when she returned to the dessert table she had no hunger for any food and danced the night away with her husband, never eating the cake or any other food. Stress management strategies can be very effective for helping individuals cope with high-risk situations.

Social Support

Individuals with strong support systems tend to do better in weight-loss programs than those trying to make changes on their own.[7] Family members, good friends, community programs, adult education classes, or other social activities can serve as support networks. It is not critical that the support system be weight related. We encourage our patients to get involved in volunteer work with others or take adult education classes at their local community college. Peer support is especially helpful because it helps obese individuals learn self-acceptance, build relationships with others, and handle stressful situations more effectively.

Contingency Management

Rewarding oneself for making healthy dietary and exercise behaviors can help reinforce those new habits.[5,6] It usually is helpful to reward specific behaviors that are being encouraged, such as minutes walked each day. Rewarding weight losses should be discouraged, because some individuals use unhealthy strategies, such as the use of diuretics, vomiting, or excessive exercise, to achieve their weight goals. It is helpful to reward changes in behaviors frequently with small rewards rather than infrequently. Small changes with small rewards make sense for most individuals.

Problem Solving

Problem solving includes the identification and correction of difficult, high-risk situations involving eating and exercise.[1,2,8] Generally, high-risk situations involve emotional issues and social events. Learning an effective approach to handling an anxious moment may involve examining possible solutions, choosing a possible solution, implementing the strategy, and evaluating the outcome. Being invited to a new, unknown restaurant may worry an individual who is trying to limit daily fat grams or calories. Calling the restaurant ahead of time and asking for suggestions can be an effective problem-solving approach to this common, high-risk event.

Physical Activity

A habit of regular physical activity is a strong predictor of long-term weight maintenance.[9] Although physical activity alone does not lead to significant weight losses, it does improve body image, psychological well-being, and feelings of control over eating behavior. Improvements in psychological functioning appear to help some individuals better cope with high-risk situations related to overeating. In one of our research studies, we found that obese individuals who were randomized into an exercise-only condition maintained their modest weight losses better than those randomized to diet-only and diet-exercise combination conditions. Small changes in physical activity daily seem to confer benefits exceeding the calories burned. The psychological benefits may be more powerful than the physiological benefits for maintenance of weight loss.

Relapse Prevention

Relapse prevention involves training obese individuals to cope with the inevitable lapses that occur during and following formal weight management programs.[1,4,6] Patients are taught that relapses are normal and need not be viewed as catastrophic. Relapse prevention strategies include teaching individuals to anticipate and recognize high-risk emotional and social situations. Negative emotions, including depression and anxiety, and common social events, including holidays, vacations, and traveling, frequently precipitate relapses. Behavioral counselors can teach patients a number of relapse prevention strategies, including visualization approaches, modeling, role-playing, and assertive techniques to help individuals cope with potential relapses.

Results of Behavioral Interventions

Behavioral interventions to help improve dietary and physical activity habits produce a gradual weight loss in obese individuals of approximately 10% of baseline weight in 6 months. Average losses are approximately 8.5 kg.[10] However, without continued care maintenance of the weight loss is unlikely. Acquisition of new habits is critical for long-term success. The majority of individuals return to their baseline weights without continued interventions. Only extended behavioral interventions have been able to show reasonable maintenance of intial weight losses.

Long-Term Maintenance

Physical activity appears to be the strongest predictor of weight maintenance.[11] We believe that the psychological benefits of exercise, including improved well-being, help patients better cope with high-risk situations and reduce the chances that they will relapse. Other predictors of long-term maintenance include self-monitoring of diet, exercise, and body weight, a good social support network, and a positive coping style, that is, the use of cognitive restructuring and stress management stategies. Because obesity is a chronic condition, unlikely to be cured, only a continual care model of treatment appears to be successful in helping individuals manage their modest weight losses.

Future Trends

The behavioral field has moved away from its reliance on body weight as the primary measure of success.[12] Today, there is greater emphasis on broader measures of improvement. These measures include beneficial changes in the individual's metabolic profile, such as improvements in lipids and lipoproteins, blood pressure, and glucose. Other outcomes include improved fitness, self-esteem, body image, quality of life, eating, self-efficacy, and functional capacity.

Rather than relying solely on restrictive dieting, which has shown limited long-term success, newer interventions are testing approaches that are aimed at helping obese individuals accept themselves by focusing on improving body image and resolving long-held issues related to food and exercise.[13–16] It is not clear yet how effective such approaches will be, but focusing on outcomes other than weight loss certainly may be beneficial to some individuals.

Increasing emphasis on encouraging physical activity rather than restrictive dieting seems to make sense for many obese patients.[14,16–18] Regular exercise leads to improvements in many medical comorbities, prevents weight regain, and increases psychological health.

The use of pharmacotherapy as an adjunct to lifestyle change appears to be increasingly popular.[19] With the approval of sibutramine and the pending approval of orlistat, the need for research aimed at determining the optimal combination of drug and lifestyle modification approaches is needed.

Summary

Behavioral interventions aimed at helping obese individuals adhere to a healthy diet and regular exercise program provide the most successful therapy for weight loss and weight maintenance.[20–22] The use of self-monitoring, stimulus control, cognitive restructuring, stress management, social support, contingency management, problem solving, physical activity, and relapse prevention help obese individuals lose about 10% of their baseline weight. Maintenance of those losses occurs in a subset of those patients as long as they continue to participate in active intervention. These modest losses are significant medically. In the future, behavioral interventions will continue to focus on broader outcomes, including improved quality of life, enhanced psychological functioning, and lowered cardiovascular risk factors, using a continual care model of intervention.

References

1. Foreyt JP, Poston WS II. The role of the behavioral counselor in obesity treatment. *J Am Diet Assoc* 1998;98:S27–S30.
2. Foreyt JP, Poston WS II. What is the role of cognitive-behavior therapy in patient management? *Obes Res* 1998;6:18S–22S.
3. Baker RC, Kirschenbaum DS. Self-monitoring may be necessary for successful weight control. *Beahvior Therapy* 1993;1993:377–394.
4. Foreyt JP, Goodrick GK. Factors common to successful therapy for the obese patient. *Med Sci Sports Exerc* 1991;23:292–297.
5. Foreyt JP, Goodrick GK. Evidence for success of behavior modification in weight loss and control. *Ann Intern Med* 1993;119:698–701.
6. Foreyt JP, Goodrick GK. Attributes of successful approaches to weight loss and control. *Appl Prev Psych* 1994;3:209–215.
7. Foreyt JP, Goodrick GK. Prediction in weight management outcome: Implications for practice. In: ALlison DB, Pi-Sunyer FX, eds. *Obesity Treatment*. New York: Plenum Press; 1995.
8. Goodrick GK, Poston WS II, Kimball KT, et al. Nondieting versus dieting treatment for overweight binge-eating women. *J Consult Clin Psychol* 1998; 66:363–368.
9. Grillo CM. The role of physical activity in weight loss and weight loss management. *Med Exer Nutr Health* 1995;4:60–76.
10. Institute of Medicine (IOM). *Weighing the Options: Criteria for Evaluating Weight Management Programs*. Washington, DC: National Academy Press; 1995.
11. Kayman S, Bruvold W, Stern JS. Maintenance and relapse after weight loss in women: Behavioral aspects. *Am J Clin Nutr* 1990;52:800–807.
12. Kirschenbaum DS, Fitzgibbon ML. Controversy about the treatment of obesity: Criticisms or challenges. *Behav Ther* 1995;26:43–68.
13. Perri MG, Fuller PR. Success and failure in the treatment of obesity: Where do we go from here. *Med Exer Nutr Health* 1995;4:255–282.
14. Perri MG, Martin AD, Leermakers EA, et al. Effects of group- versus home-based exercise in the treatment of obesity. *J Consult Clin Psychol* 1997;65:278–285.
15. Peri MG, Nezu AM, Viegener BJ. *Improving The Long-Term Management Of Obesity: Theory, Research, And Clinical Guidelines*. New York: Wiley; 1992.
16. Perri MG, Sears SF Jr, Clark JE. Strategies for improving maintenance of weight loss. Toward a continuous care model of obesity management. *Diabetes Care* 1993;16:200–209.

17. Safer DJ. Diet, behavior modification, and exercise: A review of obesity treatments from a long-term perspective. *South Med J* 1991;84:1470–1474.
18. Skender ML, Goodrick GK, Del Junco DJ, et al. Comparison of 2-year weight loss trends in behavioral treatments of obesity: Diet, exercise, and combination interventions. *J Am Diet Assoc* 1996;96:342–346.
19. Poston WS II, Foreyt JP, Borrell L, et al. Challenges in obesity management. *South Med J* 1998;91:710–720.
20. Stalonas PM, Perri MG, Kerzner AB. Do behavioral treatments of obesity last? A five-year follow-up investigation. *Addict Behav.* 1984;9:175–183.
21. Stunkard AJ. An overview of current treatments for obesity. In: Wadden TA, Van Itallie TB, eds. *Treatment of the Seriously Obese Patient.* New York: The Guilford Press; 1992:33–43.
22. Stunkard AJ. Current views on obesity. *Am J Med* 1996;100:230–236.

Chapter 19

Strategies to Enhance Compliance to Weight-Loss Treatment

Lora E. Burke, PhD, MPH, RN

Introduction

One of the most significant problems in the behavioral management of obesity is the failure of individuals to maintain the weight loss and behavioral changes achieved while in treatment.[1-3] In recent years behavioral treatment programs have been lengthened, which has produced an improvement in the initial weight loss.[4] However, maintenance of weight loss does not seem to have undergone the same improvement, and the larger initial losses are followed by larger weight regain.[4] In a recent review of studies (1990–1995), Wing[4] reported that participants maintained 60% of their initial weight loss 1 year after treatment. However, the weight loss at follow-up across the studies was no better than what was reported prior to 1990.[4] In 1989, Kramer et al[5] reported that individuals were returning to their baseline weight within 2–3 years after completion of treatment. These findings underscore the need to address the issue of weight-loss maintenance and to study alternative strategies that may lead to improved long-term outcome.

A review of the weight-loss maintenance literature underlines the dearth of studies focusing on this problem and accentuates the work of one particular investigator, Perri,[1,6,7] who has focused on strategies to improve long-term maintenance of weight loss. This chapter presents a review of the empirical literature of the last 15 years reporting on strategies to improve weight-loss maintenance. This chapter does not present an exhaustive review but rather one representative of the

From: Fletcher GF, Grundy SM, Hayman LL (eds). *Obesity: Impact on Cardiovascular Disease.* Armonk, NY: Futura Publishing Co., Inc.; © 1999.

Table 1

Strategies to Improve Weight-Loss Maintenance

Author/reference	Treatment and maintenance components		Treatment			Follow-up		
	Treatment	Maintenance	Duration (wk)	n	Weight loss (kg)	Duration (wk)	n	Weight loss (kg)
Perri et al 1984[7]	BT + relapse prevention	Contact	15	17	9.6 ± 7.2	52	17	10.3 ± 11.4[a]
	BT	Contact	15	15	8.7 ± 3.8	52	15	5.8 ± 4.2
	Non-BT	Contact	15	16	8.5 ± 4.5	52	16	6.2 ± 5.0[b]
	BT + relapse prevention	No contact	15	15	8.5 ± 7.3	52	15	2.9 ± 3.6
	BT	No contact	15	21	7.5 ± 3.8	52	21	6.3 ± 6.1
	Non-BT	No contact	15	15	8.2 ± 3.8	52	15	3.2 ± 4.8
King et al 1989[8]					Year 1			Year 2
	Diet	Contact	52	24	7.6 ± 3.9	104	20	+3.2 ± 2.9[b]
	Exercise	Contact	52	24	4.6 ± 3.8	104	21	+0.8 ± 3.1[a]
	Diet	No contact	52	20	6.4 ± 5.0	104	16	+2.6 ± 2.8[b]
	Exercise	No contact	52	22	5.5 ± 2.7	104	15	+3.9 ± 2.8[a]
Wing et al 1996[9]	BT	Weekly phone contact	24	26	12.8	78	22	9.31[a]
	BT	No contact	24	27	14.2	78	27	8.6[a]
Perri et al 1984[10]	BT	Booster sessions	14	26	5.6 ± 3.5	88	17	0.4 ± 3.6[a]
	BT	Multicomponent Program: buddy groups, mail/phone contacts	14	30	6.1 ± 3.3	88	26	4.6 ± 6.9[b]
Perri et al 1987[1]	BT	Peer self-help group	20	46	10.9	72	32	6.5[a]
	BT	Therapist contact	20	41	10.7	72	27	6.4[b]
		No contact	20		10.4	72	16	3.1[b]

Perri et al 1986[12]	BT + exercise	Multi-component	20	Data not available		72	18	+0.4[a]
	BT	Multi-component	20			72	17	+3.1[b]
	BT + exercise	No maintenance	20	—		72	16	+7.2[b]
	BT	No maintenance	20	—		72	16	+6.9[c]
Perri et al 1990[14]	BT	Relapse prevention training	20	8.9	29	52	29	7.3
	BT	Therapist contact	20	9.6	33	52	33	9.4
	BT	No maintenance	20	7.3	26	52	26	4.5
Perri et al 1988[15]	BT	Contacts (26 biweekly)	24	13.2 ± 5.4[a]	19	72	19	11.4 ± 12.1[a]
	BT	Contact + aerobic exercise	24	13.1 ± 4.8[a]	18	72	18	9.1 ± 6.4[a]
	BT	Contact + social influence	24	11.3 ± 3.1[a]	19	72	19	8.4 ± 7.5[a]
	BT	Contact + aerobic exercise + social influence	24	13.7 ± 5.9[a]	19	72	19	13.5 ± 15.2[a]
	BT	No maintenance	24	10.8 ± 7.6[b]	16	72	16	3.6 ± 6.2[b]
Perri et al 1989[16]	BT	Extended over 40 weeks	40	13.6 ± 9.0[a]	24	52	16	9.8 ± 8.2[a]
	BT	Given over 20 weeks	20	6.4 ± 5.9[b]	24	52	16	4.6 ± 5.2[b]
Wing et al 1996[9]	BT	Optional food provision	24	13.2	26	78	26	9.0[a]
	BT	Monthly sessions (control)	24	13.4	22	78	22	9.2[a]
Wing and Jeffery 1998[20]	Recruited alone	BT	16	7.0 ± 3.8	30	42	29	5.3 ± 6.8
	Recruited with friends	BT	16	8.6 ± 4.3	36	42	33	8.8 ± 6.6
	Recruited alone	Social support	16	6.9 ± 3.5	44	42	36	6.1 ± 4.7
	Recruited with friends	Social support	16	9.3 ± 4.0	39	42	38	8.7 ± 6.3

+ Weight gain instead of a loss.

[abc] Weight losses indicated with different letter superscript indicate significant difference between conditions; BT, behavioral therapy or treatment.

studies being conducted. Some of the strategies discussed are ongoing patient-therapist contact, peer support, inclusion of aerobic exercise, and extended treatment. Table 1 contains a summary of the studies, their strategies, and comparison of initial and long-term weight loss. A second table identifies those strategies that have been demonstrated as effective in improving long-term weight loss and refers the reader to the literature describing the study.

The epitome of compliance in the treatment of obesity is sustaining the dietary and behavior changes that created the initial weight loss and if maintained, would prevent weight regain. The title of this chapter emphasizes compliance. However, the term maintenance will be used when referring to long-term adherence or compliance to lifestyle and behavior changes.

Strategies to Improve Weight-Loss Maintenance

Post-Treatment Contact by Mail and Telephone

Ongoing contact with a health care provider allows the professional to provide reinforcement to the patient for continued adherence, directive problem solving should adherence become difficult, encouragement, motivational enhancement, and reminders to be vigilant about eating and exercise behavior.[6] Ongoing contact post-treatment was first tested in 1984 by Perri and colleagues[7] as a means to enhance weight-loss maintenance. The strategy used in their study consisted of continued self-monitoring of daily caloric intake and weight change on postcards and ongoing therapist contacts during the year following treatment. Participants mailed the postcards weekly to the therapist for the first 6 months following treatment and the therapists called the participants weekly during the first 3 months to provide additional guidance and support. The frequency of calls was reduced during the second 3-month period, at which point participant-therapist contacts were discontinued.[7]

The presence or absence of the post-treatment maintenance strategy was crossed with three treatment conditions: a nonbehavioral treatment, behavior therapy, and behavior therapy with relapse prevention training. The nonbehavioral treatment consisted of exchange diet plans, recommendations for exercise, and emphasis on the "underlying reasons" for overeating. Behavior therapy focused on the establishment of new eating and exercise habits that promote weight loss and included self-control techniques typically used in weight-reduction treatment, that is, self-monitoring and stimulus control. In the behavior therapy plus relapse prevention condition, participants received individualized training in the last 6 weeks of treatment that included training to recognize high-risk situations, in vivo practice in coping with the situations, and training in cognitive strategies to deal with the feelings associated with a slip or lapse.[7] As presented in Table 1, the post-treatment contacts improved weight-loss maintenance in two groups, the behavior therapy plus relapse prevention and the nonbehavioral therapy groups, but not the group receiving only behavior therapy. At the 12-month follow-up, the only group that maintained the weight loss was behavior therapy plus relapse prevention and continued contact.

King and colleagues[8] tested the use of an ongoing therapist contact as a maintenance strategy in a study of males using either energy restriction alone or exercise alone as a weight-reducing strategy (Table 1). At the end of the 1st year of treatment, approximately 87% of the participants agreed to participate in the 2nd-year study and were randomized to either a telephone-mail contact maintenance condition or to an assessment-only control condition. The major focus of the ongoing contact was preventing a return to behaviors unsupportive to weight-loss maintenance and included monthly mailings supplemented during the first 3 months and at months 6, 9, and 12 with a staff-initiated telephone contact that addressed participants' concerns or questions.

The weight regain that occurred in year 2 was different for the dieters and exercisers. The exercisers in the maintenance condition regained only 17.4% of their initial loss compared with 70.9% among the exercisers in the control condition, while the dieters in the maintenance condition regained 42.1% and the dieters in the control condition regained 40.6% of their initial loss. These findings suggest that the exercisers required the ongoing contact to prevent substantial regain.[8] The results of this study also suggest that exercise accompanied by contact may provide a stabilizing effect on weight post-treatment.

King used baccalaureate prepared staff for the ongoing contact and reported approximately 1 hour of staff time per participant in the 1-year follow-up.[8] Similarly, Wing and colleagues[9] utilized interviewers trained by a data center in their study testing the effectiveness of frequent phone calls from a staff member to improve weight-loss maintenance compared with a no-contact control condition (Table 1). Women who had lost at least 4.5 kg during the 6-month treatment phase were invited to participate in the maintenance study and were assigned randomly to one of the two conditions. All participants were provided goals for energy and fat intake, provided a year's supply of eating and exercise diaries, and were encouraged to use them. The control group received no further contact while the phone maintenance participants received a weekly call at a prearranged time for 1 year. The interviewer inquired if the participant was keeping a diary and, if so requested a report of energy and fat intakes and the amount of exercise being done. Counseling was not provided.

The weight-regain pattern was similar in the contact and control groups, but the mean weight regain in participants in the phone maintenance condition was 30% compared with 39% among those in the control condition; the difference was not statistically significant. It is possible that the sample of 53 was insufficient in size to draw conclusions from the effect size reported (0.30). Another possibility is that better results may have occurred had professional staff conducted the telephone contacts, possibly providing ongoing counseling and problem solving.[9] A drawback to this would be the added incurred expense. Ongoing contact through the telephone has been effective in additional studies when combined with other maintenance conditions, which will be discussed in the following section.

Booster Sessions

Use of this strategy provides periodic contact following treatment although its main purpose is to provide a review and reinforcement of previously learned behaviors to help ensure a persistence or habituation of the new habits. Perri[10] tested this strategy in comparison to a multicomponent maintenance program following a 14-week behavioral therapy program. Booster sessions were held every 2 weeks for 3 months and provided additional review and reinforcement of the strategies used during the initial treatment. The booster session strategy did not prevent weight regain beyond the 6-month mark and at the 21-month assessment there was nearly a full regain of initial weight loss[10] (Table 1). A possible explanation for the failure of booster sessions is that they provided a review and reinforcement of strategies implemented during treatment and may have provided insufficient support and guidance for the challenges faced during maintenance, or that additional behaviors needed to be learned during this phase. Furthermore, the sessions were limited in number.[6]

Multicomponent Maintenance Program

This program of strategies included continued self-monitoring of eating and exercise behavior, which was returned to the therapist through the mail, therapist initiated phone contacts, and participation in self-help groups. Building on their study of post-treatment contacts, Perri and colleagues[7] developed this multifaceted program and compared it with booster sessions. An additional component included instruction of participants in how to form self-help peer groups ("buddy groups") and to use problem-solving techniques when a fellow patient was challenged by difficulties in maintaining the weight loss. The self-help groups were encouraged to meet regularly throughout the 1-year follow-up period. Participants returned 43% of the weekly self-monitoring postcards and received 52% of the therapist phone calls. However, the self-help group met only 8.5 times during the year.

In comparing the multicomponent maintenance program to the booster strategy over the 21-month follow-up, there were no differences until the 9th month. Participants in the multicomponent group demonstrated significantly better maintenance at the 9-, 15-, and 21-month assessments and at 21-months had maintained 74% of their initial loss. However, the positive finding associated with this strategy needs to be balanced by the cost of weekly telephone calls placed by therapists during the first 3 months and then quarterly during the post-treatment year.[6,10]

Peer Support

Building on their earlier study examining the effectiveness of helping group participants form buddy groups, Perri and colleagues[1] examined therapist contact in comparison to peer support as a maintenance strategy. The strategy included instructing participants on how to form their own peer support groups and to utilize problem-solving techniques as described by D'Zurilla and Nezu.[11] Instruction was provided during the last 4 of the 20 treatment sessions and included providing reinforcement to peers, assisting with difficult situations through use of problem solving, and how to monitor peers' weight. Participants were provided a meeting place, a scale, and a schedule for 15 biweekly sessions during the maintenance period.[1] This strategy appeared to provide more structured support than the buddy groups of the multicomponent maintenance program.[7]

Therapist contact in this study included face-to-face contact in 15 biweekly sessions that included weigh-ins, progress review, and therapist-led problem solving to assist participants with maintenance of behavior change.[1] The behavior therapy–only condition had no therapist contact beyond the 20-week initial treatment, except for assessment during the post-treatment period.

The original sample was comprised of 109 males and females. Overall, attrition was 31%, which was distributed evenly across treatment conditions.[1] Table 1 presents the weight loss at end of treatment and at 18-month follow-up. At 1 year (7 months post-treatment end) the therapist contact group showed significantly better weight loss than the peer support or behavior therapy-only group. However, at 18 months all three groups showed significant weight regain, but the peer self-help and therapist contact groups experienced smaller regains.

Exercise

Perri's[12] multicomponent maintenance program was tested again in a 2 × 2 design study that tested the effectiveness of adding exercise to the treatment to increase initial weight loss and to improve maintenance by replicating use of the multicomponent maintenance program (Table 1). A sample of moderately obese adults was assigned randomly to one of four conditions: behavior therapy with or without aerobic exercise (walking and cycling) crossed with no post-treatment contact or the multicomponent program. The exercise component was structured with therapist-led demonstrations included in the weekly session. Participants in the nonaerobic exercise group were encouraged to increase their physical activity.

Participants in the exercise condition achieved better weight loss during treatment.[12] However, the groups receiving the multicomponent maintenance condition (with and without exercise) achieved significantly better weight loss than participants in the no-maintenance condition (Table 1). However, at the 18-month mark a significant weight increase was observed in the groups receiving the multicomponent maintenance intervention, with the regain being significantly smaller in the exercise group that received the maintenance program compared with the group that did not. This may be explained by the reported adherence to the treatment and maintenance program. Participants reported over 80% adherence to behavioral strategies and over 80% of the exercise group reported meeting or exceeding the prescribed regimen while nearly 90% of the no-exercise group adhered to the recommendation to increase physical activity. However, the self-reported adherence for both exercise programs fell. Moreover, over 40% of the exercise group reported no longer engaging in exercise at the 18-month follow-up, and the remainder of the group reported a 50% reduction in the time spent exercising. Adherence to the post-treatment maintenance program strategies was approximately 50%. The significant difference in the maintenance group appeared to be caused by the improved adherence to the behavioral strategies. However, during the final months of maintenance the improved weight loss seen in the early portion began to reverse itself, suggesting that the maintenance program was delaying rather than preventing this occurrence.

Relapse Prevention Training

A cognitive-behavioral model of relapse prevention was formulated by Marlatt and Gordon.[13] The model consists of specific strategies for use in minimizing or preventing a relapse following treatment for addictive behaviors. More specifically, these include four components: identification of high-risk situations, problem-solving training in how to deal with the situation, in vivo practice of the coping skills, and developing cognitive coping strategies for negotiating in the face of setbacks. Perri[10] tested this strategy in combination with ongoing contact in an earlier study. In another study, Perri[14] compared relapse prevention with frequent therapist contacts to determine which would be more effective as a maintenance strategy.

Following the standard 20-week behavior therapy treatment, participants were assigned randomly to one of the two maintenance conditions. The relapse prevention training included training and practice according to the four components described above and was conducted in 26 biweekly sessions during the year following treatment.[14] The therapist contact program was the same as described in the peer support study described previously and occurred over 26 biweekly meetings.[10]

Compared with the no-maintenance condition, both relapse prevention and therapist contact groups experienced better weight loss with no significant difference between them[14] (Table 1). These findings suggest that frequent therapist contact may be as effective as structured relapse prevention training and skill practice.[6] These findings differ from Perri's 1984 study that demonstrated improved weight loss in the combined relapse prevention training and therapist contact condition, but are similar in that therapist contact following behavior therapy was superior to relapse prevention following behavior therapy without maintenance.[10,15]

Social Influence

The social influence maintenance program was developed to enhance motivation and provide incentives for continued progress in weight loss and provide instructions on the provision of peer support through ongoing telephone contacts and peer group meetings. It also included active participation of participants in the preparation and presentation of lectures, as well as monetary contingencies for program adherence. Building on prior work, Perri[15] tested this strategy in combination with post-treatment strategies described previously, for example, therapist contact and aerobic exercise. The four treatment conditions are listed in Table 1 with the weight-loss results.

The attrition rate during the 20-week treatment phase was 23.6%, and 74% of the original sample of the 123 subjects who completed the 18-month evaluation. The four experimental conditions experienced improved weight-loss maintenance at the 12-month point compared with the behavior therapy–only condition, which demonstrated a regain of initial weight loss and sustained only 33% of their post-treatment loss at the final follow-up.[15] At 18-months, the four maintenance conditions were not significantly different and on average, maintained 82.7% of their mean post-treatment losses. In assessing self-reported adherence to the program strategies, participants in the behavior therapy plus contacts plus social influence condition reported significantly higher adherence at 12 months, but a significant decaying of adherence occurred by 18 months.[15]

Extended Treatment

The typical weight control program consists of 15–20 weekly sessions. This brief duration may be insufficient to allow adequate weight loss. Perri and colleagues[16] tested the effectiveness of extending the typical program to 40 weeks by introducing the topics in a more gradual manner.

The predominantly female sample of 48 had a 33% attrition rate over 72 weeks. In the period between 20- and 40-week follow-up, the extended treatment group lost a significant amount of additional weight while the standard treatment group regained. At 72 months, both groups had gained weight, but the extended group maintained a significantly greater net loss than the standard group. Examination of the weight loss that occurred between weeks 20 and 40 reveals that 62.5% of the extended group lost an additional 10 lb or more compared with only 6.3% of the standard group, demonstrating the benefit of the extended treatment.[16] However, the weight regain at 72 weeks shown in Table 1 suggests the extended treatment merely delayed the regain and did not affect the regain slope.

Optional Food Provision

Jeffery and colleagues[17] demonstrated the effectiveness of providing food for initial weight loss. Building on this work, Wing and colleagues[9] tested the effectiveness of food provision as a weight-loss maintenance strategy, with the rationale that this might reduce barriers or be used at a time of crisis when a lapse may be more likely. Subjects who completed a 6-month treatment program were eligible to participate; 57 subjects were enrolled and 48 completed the study. Subjects were randomized to either a control or the food provision group. Both groups met monthly for weigh-in and an interactive session on a health, behavior change, or nutrition topic. All participants were encouraged to self-monitor 1 week of each month and return the diary at the meeting. The treatment group was told they could obtain food boxes containing five breakfasts and five dinners 4 months out of the year and was encouraged to use these when anticipating difficult times, for example, the holiday season.

Forty-six percent of the food provision group took advantage of the food boxes, and these were participants who had lower weight losses during treatment. There was no difference between the two treatment conditions in weight loss during the 1-year maintenance program or in total loss over the 18-month study.[9] The researchers speculated that the food boxes were not utilized by a greater percentage of participants because they were required to pick up the boxes at weekly intervals, which should have eliminated the burden of going grocery shopping, but then added the burden of coming to the clinic. In reality, this may have added to the burden of shopping because all food needed could not be provided in the box, for example, milk and food only for the participant. Delivering food to the individual's home may have served as a better crisis intervention technique.[9]

Social Support

Overall, the literature on social support has shown a positive effect on efforts of long-term weight management.[18] Moreover, compared with the control group, adherence to exercise has improved when social support was created among strangers in a group.[19] However, most of the social support strategies have been employed during the active treatment phase, rather than during a follow-up period. Identifying this void, Wing and Jeffery[20] conducted a study that evaluated the effectiveness of a social support condition in the prevention of weight regain in a post-treatment 6-month maintenance study.

Individuals were recruited to join either alone or with three other people who could be friends, co-workers, or family members. A sample of 166 adults, balanced across genders, received a 4-month standard behavioral treatment program.[20] Participants were assigned randomly to one of four conditions: recruited alone and received either the standard treatment or the social support intervention, or recruited with friends and received either the standard treatment or the social support intervention. Those who enrolled alone and were assigned the social support condition were assigned to a team, and those who enrolled with friends and received the social support condition formed natural teams. Intragroup activities were conducted at each lesson and between lessons in the form of homework assignments for those in the social support condition. Following the 16-week treatment phase, intergroup competition was conducted during the 6-month maintenance phase through monetary contingency rewards for the team with the greatest proportion of its members retaining their initial weight loss.[20]

There was a significant difference between those who completed the study; for example, 95% of those who were recruited with friends and received the social support intervention completed the study compared with 75%–83% of those who were in the other three conditions.[20] Weight losses overall differed by the recruitment strategy. Participants who were recruited with friends experienced an overall weight loss of 8.7 kg compared with those who were recruited alone who experienced a 5.8-kg weight loss. There was a significant difference in maintenance of weight loss with those who had the greater initial weight loss having better maintenance. Those who were recruited with friends and received the intervention retained 66% of their weight loss, in contrast to those who were recruited alone and received only the standard behavioral treatment retained 24% of their loss.

Discussion

The 11 studies reviewed in this chapter demonstrated varying responses to the strategies that were evaluated in varying combinations. Some of these results are more promising than others. Ongoing contact between therapist and participant provided the most consistent results of improved maintenance. Interestingly, the only study that did not show a significant difference in the ongoing contact group was reported by Wing and colleagues[9] and implemented weekly phone calls for a 1-year maintenance program. In contrast, Perri and colleagues[7,10] as well as King[8] utilized a less intensive schedule of weekly phone calls during the first 3 months followed by calls at 3-month intervals. Each of the investigators utilized a different level of staff to conduct the phone calls. Perri[7] noted that the favorable results were tempered by the cost of a therapist conducting the phone calls over a year. Wing[9] speculated that the use of a therapist for the weekly phone calls may have resulted in an improved outcome. Although

King and colleagues[8] noted that weight maintenance among exercisers was easier to maintain than dietary strategies, it is worth noting that a baccalaureate level staff person conducted the contacts in that study in approximately 1 hour per participant over the year. These findings suggest that possibly less frequent contact with higher level staff may result in favorable weight maintenance.

Another strategy that demonstrated consistent improved outcome was the addition of exercise to standard treatment. However, Perri[12] reported reduced adherence to the exercise regimen at 18 months and a trend toward reversal of weight loss, indicating that long-term maintenance needs to be in place to reinforce continued exercise. Other approaches to the implementation of exercise have been studied in active treatment programs and demonstrated improved adherence to exercise. Pavlou[21] used exercise as an adjunctive modality in an 8-week clinical weight-loss program and crossed exercise/no-exercise conditions with four diet programs. Follow-up measures at 18 months post-treatment revealed follow-up weight loss in the four exercise-treated groups of 12 kg compared with the nonexercise-treated participants who regained 92% of their weight loss. Moreover, those who exercised more frequently fared better in weight-loss maintenance, reinforcing the role of exercise in long-term success.[21] Jakicic et al[22] reported that the use of short bouts of 10 minutes of exercise four times a day resulted in greater total exercise time compared with the standard 40-minute bout of exercise. Another promising approach is the home-based exercise program which, when compared with group-based exercise, demonstrated improved adherence and great weight loss.[23] These latter strategies warrant further investigation in studies that incorporate a maintenance phase.

Relapse prevention training was tested in two studies by Perri[10,14] and demonstrated somewhat unexpected results. In one study[10] relapse prevention only was effective if combined with the therapist contact condition, and in the second study did not yield an improvement over therapist contact.[14] These findings suggest that therapist-led problem solving through ongoing contacts is more effective and probably less time-consuming than the comprehensive training provided participants in these treatment maintenance conditions.

The social support intervention reported by Wing and Jeffery[20] was a provocative study that highlighted some points to be considered in our current approach to treatment. First, recruitment of participants with their friends into a weight-reduction program seemed to reduce the dropout rate and increased the weight maintenance rate. The lowest rate of attendance and of weight maintenance was observed in those who enrolled in the study alone and received the standard behavioral weight control program, which typically is the standard way in which weight reduction is conducted. The researchers suggested that this approach needs to be reconsidered or strategies for providing social support need to be added to standard behavioral programs.

Other strategies tested may have made a difference in the short term but did not provide any sustained change in behavior, for example, the extended treatment program.[16] Others such as peer self-help[1] or relapse prevention[10,14] did not have as positive an effect as therapist contact or a multicomponent maintenance program was observed to have.[10,12] However, these may need to be studied further in larger samples or different populations.

The strategies that demonstrated beneficial effects on long-term weight-loss maintenance, for example, ongoing contact with the provider through mail and/or telephone, inclusion of aerobic exercise, and provision of social support, need to be incorporated into future and ongoing programs. Other strategies that also provided improved results, such as a multicomponent maintenance program, which included self-help groups, or social influence programs in combination with ongoing contact, need to be included when possible, particularly in long-term treatment programs. These strategies are displayed in Table 2. Review articles on adherence to dietary treatment are available for additional reading.[24–26]

Summary and Conclusions

The studies reviewed in this chapter represent the current state of maintenance strategies for preventing weight regain. Implementation

---

Table 2

Strategies Demonstrated to Improve Weight-Loss Maintenance

Successful strategies	Investigators/studies in which improved maintenance demonstrated (reference)
Ongoing contact	Perri et al 1984;[7] King et al 1989[8]
Peer self-help group	Perri et al 1987[1]
Social influence	Perri et al 1988[15]
(active participant participation)	
Social support	Wing and Jeffery 1998[20]
Relapse prevention/skill training	Perri et al 1994,[7] 1990[14]
Multicomponent maintenance	Perri et al 1984,[10] 1986[12]
(buddy system, client-therapist contact by mail/phone)	
Aerobic exercise	Perri et al 1986[12]

of the nine strategies in differing combinations yielded varied results, some not always favorable. Taken collectively, the results underscore the point that participants eventually will abandon the behavioral techniques they learned during active treatment. Furthermore, it emphasizes the need for additional strategies to promote long-term adherence to the behavioral and dietary changes that are necessary for successful weight-loss maintenance. Ongoing contact was used successfully in several of the studies reported here. The telephone is but one mode available for continued contact. Future research needs to examine alternative communication modalities and evaluate their use in this treatment arena.

Taken one step further, the results of the studies reviewed suggest that obesity, not unlike hyperlipidemia and hypertension, is a chronic condition requiring both life-long supervision by a health care provider and active self-management by the patient. However, before management and supervision can be provided it is important that physicians, nurses, and other members of the health care team be knowledgeable in how to treat and manage this important risk factor and how to reinforce long-term maintenance of weight loss. One approach to addressing this issue could be educating and training health care professionals in a manner similar to that established by the National Cholesterol Education Program.[27] This educational program provides a model on which we could base our approach to reducing obesity in a manner similar to how hypercholesterolemia was addressed in the 1980s. Moreover, it would provide an additional opportunity for numerous professionals to help ensure long-term maintenance of achieved weight loss.

Acknowledgments: The author acknowledges Rena R. Wing, PhD, who critiqued an earlier draft of this chapter.

References

1. Perri MG, McAdoo WG, McAllister DA, et al. Effects of peer support and therapist contact on long-term weight loss. *J Consult Clin Psychol* 1987;55: 615–617.
2. Perri MG, Sears SF Jr, Clark JE. Strategies for improving maintenance of weight loss. Toward a continuous care model of obesity management. *Diabetes Care* 1993;16:200–209.
3. Foreyt JP, Goodrick GK. Evidence for success of behavior modification in weight loss and control. *Ann Intern Med* 1993;119:698–701.
4. Wing RR. Behavioral approaches to the treatment of obesity. In: Bray G, Bourchard C, James PT, eds. *Handbook of Obesity*. New York: Marcel Dekker; 1997.
5. Kramer FM, Jeffery RW, Forster JL, et al. Long-term follow-up of behavioral treatment for obesity: Patterns of weight regain among men and women. *Int J Obes* 1989;13:123–136.

6. Perri MG. Improving maintenance of weight loss following treatment by diet and lifestyle modification. In: Wadden TA, Van Itallie TB, eds. *Treatment of the Seriously Obese Patient*. New York: Guilford Press; 1992:456–477.
7. Perri MG, Shapiro RM, Ludwig WW, et al. Maintenance strategies for the treatment of obesity: An evaluation of relapse prevention training and posttreatment contact by mail and telephone. *J Consult Clin Psychol* 1984; 52:404–413.
8. King AC, Frey-Hewitt B, Dreon DM, et al. Diet vs exercise in weight maintenance. The effects of minimal intervention strategies on long-term outcomes in men. *Arch Intern Med* 1989;149:2741–2746.
9. Wing RR, Jeffery RW, Hellerstedt WL, et al. Effect of frequent phone contacts and optional food provision on maintenance of weight loss. *Ann Behav Med* 1996;18:172–176.
10. Perri MG, McAdoo WG, Spevak PA, et al. Effect of a multicomponent maintenance program on long-term weight loss. *J Consult Clin Psychol* 1984;52:480–481.
11. D'Zurilla TJ, Nezu AM. Social problem solving in adults. In: Kendall PC, ed. *Advances in Cognitive-Behavioral Research and Therapy*. New York: Academic Press, 1982:202–274.
12. Perri MG, McAdoo WG, McAllister DA, et al. Enhancing the efficacy of behavior therapy for obesity: Effects of aerobic exercise and a multicomponent maintenance program. *J Consult Clin Psychol* 1986;54:670–675.
13. Marlatt GA, Gordon JR. Implications for the maintenance of behavior change. In: Davidson PO, Davidson SM, eds. *Behavioral Medicine: Changing Health Lifestyles*. New York: Brunner/Mazel, 1980:410–452.
14. Perri MG, McKelvey WF, Schein RL, et al. Relapse prevention training versus frequent therapist contacts as weight loss maintenance strategies. Annual Meeting of the Association for Advancement of Behavior Therapy, San Francisco, Calif; 1990.
15. Perri MG, McAllister DA, Gange JJ, et al. Effects of four maintenance programs on the long-term management of obesity. *J Consult Clin Psychol* 1988;56:529–534.
16. Perri MG, Nezu AM, Patti ET, et al. Effect of length of treatment on weight loss. *J Consult Clin Psychol* 1989;57:450–452.
17. Jeffery RW, Wing RR, Thorson C, et al. Strengthening behavioral interventions for weight loss: A randomized trial of food provision and monetary incentives. *J Consult Clin Psychol* 1993;61:1038–1045.
18. Black DR, Gleser LJ, Kooyers KJ. A meta-analytic evaluation of couples weight-loss programs. *Health Psychol* 1990;9:330–347.
19. King AC, Fredericksen LW. Low cost strategies for increasing exercise behavior: Relapse prevention and social support. *Behav Modif* 1984;8:13–21.
20. Wing RR, Jeffery RW. Benefits of recruiting participants with friends and increasing social support for weight loss and maintenance. *J Consult Clin Psychol* 1999;67:142–138.
21. Pavlou KN, Krey S, Steffee WP. Exercise as an adjunct to weight loss and maintenance in moderately obese subjects. *Am J Clin Nutr* 1989;49:1115–1123.
22. Jakicic JM, Wing RR, Butler BA, et al. Prescribing exercise in multiple short bouts versus one continuous bout: Effects on adherence, cardiorespiratory fitness, and weight loss in overweight women. *Int J Obes Relat Metab Disord* 1995;19:893–901.

23. Perri MG, Martin AD, Leermakers EA, et al. Effects of group- versus home-based exercise in the treatment of obesity. *J Consult Clin Psychol* 1997;65:278–285.
24. Brownell KD, Cohen LR. Adherence to dietary regimens. 1: An overview of research. *Behav Med* 1995;20:149–154.
25. Brownell KD, Cohen LR. Adherence to dietary regimens. 2: Components of effective interventions. *Behav Med* 1995;20:155–164.
26. Burke LE, Dunbar-Jacob JM, Hill MN. Compliance with cardiovascular disease prevention strategies: A review of the research. *Ann Behav Med* 1997;19:239–263.
27. National Cholesterol Education Program. Second report of the expert panel on detection, evaluation, and treatment of high blood cholesterol in adults. NIH Publication 93–3095; 1993.

Chapter 20

Quality of Life and Obesity

Marguerite R. Kinney, RN, DNSc, FAAN

Although quality of life traditionally has been a matter of clinical concern, it has in recent years achieved respectability as a focus of research and evaluation and in many clinical trials it is an expected outcome measure.[1] Current conceptualization of quality of life includes patients' perceptions in the following areas: physical and occupational functioning, psychological functioning, social interaction and role activities, overall life satisfaction, and perceptions of health status.[2] It is important to note that for quality of life to be measured in a particular study, all of these dimensions should be included. If fewer dimensions are included, as may at times be appropriate, then the restriction should be acknowledged and defended. As noted by Schipper and colleagues[1] only limited conclusions can be drawn about quality of life when examining fewer than the complete set of fundamental dimensions.

Quality of Life Research and Obesity

Although quality of life has been studied extensively in a number of chronic conditions including cancer, heart disease, arthritis, and others, the literature is somewhat limited in obesity even though authors frequently comment that impaired quality of life accompanies obesity. Atkinson[3] proposed that standards for the successful treatment of obesity be enlarged beyond the classic standard of weight loss to include other measures of body size (percent of excess body weight, body mass index, and body fat mass), improvement in complications associated with obesity, and maintenance of the weight loss. In his discussion of complications associated with obesity, Atkinson included psychosocial problems along with diabetes mellitus, hypertension, sleep apnea, and others. He noted that obese persons experience

From: Fletcher GF, Grundy SM, Hayman LL (eds). *Obesity: Impact on Cardiovascular Disease.* Armonk, NY: Futura Publishing Co., Inc.; © 1999.

a lower quality of life than nonobese persons and recommended research aimed at assessing the success of weight reduction in improving quality of life for obese persons.

The actual quality of life-related goals of a study vary considerably and may include the following: (1) establishing detailed quality of life data on a particular population, (2) assessing patterns of a quality of life dimension over time, (3) assessing the effects of treatment on overall quality of life or on specific dimensions of quality of life in more detail, (4) assessing the dimensions and moderators of quality of life most amenable to interventions, and (5) using quality of life as baseline data to predict morbidity and mortality.[2]

Challenges in Quality of Life Research

Because quality of life is a subjective assessment and represents an individual's perception of the dimensions of quality of life, there are a number of challenges to those wishing to include quality of life as a measure of success of treatment. These challenges include conceptualization, design, measurement, and interpretation of data. In an excellent discussion of the contributions of conceptual models, Cleary[4] observes that progress in quality of life research has been hampered by the absence of conceptual or theoretical models. He proposes that investigators focus on (1) including the full range of variables in studies of quality of life, (2) specifying proposed links between variables, (3) investigating relationships between quality of life dimensions and traditional measures of health status, and (4) empirical testing of proposed models.

Cleary and Wilson[5] have proposed a model for conceptualizing the relationships between clinical variables and measures of quality of life including potential intervening variables that mediate the effects of treatment on quality of life (Figure 1). The model includes five measures of health thought of as existing on a continuum of increasing biological, social, and psychological complexity. Characteristics of the individual and of the environment play an important role at several points in the model. Nonmedical factors that may influence an individual's overall perception of quality of life also are included in the model. A model such as this one can be useful in addressing the conceptual or theoretical challenges in quality of life research.

A second challenge in quality of life research has to do with measurement. Good measurement is necessary for studying and understanding any phenomenon and quality of life is no exception. Unfortunately, many published studies of quality of life reported in the literature have used inadequate measures and have failed to capture the full impact of disease and its treatment on the lives of patients

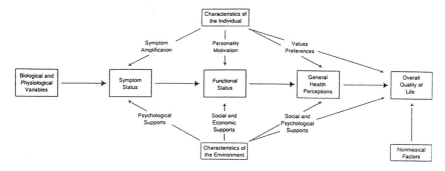

Figure 1. Relationships among measures of patient outcome in a health-related quality of life conceptual model. Reprinted with permission from reference 5.

and their families.[6] Evaluation of candidate instruments includes examination of the following properties: (1) coverage of each objective and subjective component important to those in a given patient population (such as the obese), (2) reliability, (3) validity, (4) responsiveness (ie, a measure of the association between the change in the observed score and the change in the true value of the construct), and (5) sensitivity (ie, the ability of the measurement to reflect true changes or differences in quality of life).[7]

Schipper and Levitt[8] have suggested that the following basic properties and characteristics of instruments should be considered when selecting a tool for measuring quality of life:

- takes into account the patient's diagnosis and focuses on distinguishing functional states within disease groups (eg, moderately obese and morbidly obese);
- is oriented functionally and addresses the concerns of day-to-day living that represent a multidimensional conceptualization of quality of life;
- is designed for self-administration;
- includes questions of general applicability, ease and consistency of interpretation, and the questions are limited in number so that patients will answer them in repeated administrations of the instrument;
- is repeatable so that scores can be tracked over time to capture trends both within individuals and between groups of patients;
- is sensitive across the range of clinical practice to distinguish between patients with varying severity of illness and between intensity of therapy; and
- has demonstrated adequate validity and reliability.

Osoba and colleagues[9] propose an algorithm to assist in the selection of the most appropriate measure for assessing quality of life in a given situation. The first step is to identify the purpose for including quality of life in the assessment and whether the data will be used for description, for making comparisons, or for purposes of stratification. The second step is to determine which method of measurement is most appropriate for the determined purpose (ie, structured, unstructured, or semistructured interview or questionnaire). If a questionnaire is to be employed, Osoba and colleagues offer a list of questions to be asked about proposed questionnaires when using the algorithm. The questions are (1) who developed the questionnaire? (2) what is its scope? (3) who will administer it? (4) what is the question timeframe and response structure? (5) what dimensions are included? (6) what is the questionnaire's reliability? (7) are the results likely to be valid? and (8) will the questionnaire yield a dimension score or an aggregate score? The third step in the algorithm is to determine whether the scope of the assessment will be general (all dimensions of quality of life) or specific (restricted dimensions) followed by an assessment of the psychometric properties of candidate instruments. The next step is an evaluation of the feasibility of assessing quality of life in the particular situation and the final step is to determine if the results are likely to be meaningful, that is, statistically significant and clinically relevant.

A third challenge relates to design of the study. Testa and Simonson[7] describe the three study designs most commonly used in quality of life evaluations: (1) cross sectional or nonrandomized longitudinal designs to describe predictors of quality of life, (2) randomized controlled trials (in which measures must reflect the nature of the disease being studied), and (3) cost-effectiveness and cost-benefit analysis to estimate the incremental costs of a program or treatment compared with its incremental effects on health. Wellisch[10] suggests a hierarchy of research strategies in which the most optimal approach is the prospective design where the same group of patients is studied sequentially and the least rigorous strategy is the cross-sectional design in which patients are assessed at variable times after treatment. The former design yields a coherent picture of quality of life as a pattern begins to emerge but is expensive and time-consuming and is likely to experience subject attrition. The latter design is relatively inexpensive and maximizes the number of subjects enrolled but is plagued by history effects and other threats to validity that limit comparability of patient responses.

Finally, there are challenges in quantifying and explaining important or meaningful differences in measurements of quality of life. Sullivan and colleagues[11] suggest several criteria for assessing clinical change in quality of life: (1) physicians' or patients' overall judgment of improvement or deterioration; (2) a combination, requiring agreement between independent assessments by the patient and physician; and (3) a significant change in specific clinical variables over time. Lydick and Epstein[12] note that the clinical significance of statistically significant changes in quality of life often is difficult to interpret. They provide an excellent discussion of distribution-based interpretations (such as effect size) and anchor-based interpretations (such as population norms). The relevant anchor or amount of change judged clinically significant will differ with different populations and it may be necessary to establish clinical significance in different patient groups (such as moderately obese and morbidly obese). Cleary[4] adds to the discussion of clinical significance the patient's perception of change or a "just noticeable difference" where patients are asked to evaluate the size or importance of a change in quality of life scores.

Studies of Quality of Life in Obesity

Measures of quality of life generally are categorized as generic or disease specific.[6] Generic instruments are comprehensive in their coverage of the dimensions of quality of life and, thus, are applicable in many groups. In addition, findings can be compared across groups. This category includes profiles and utility measures. In contrast, disease-specific instruments are designed specifically for use in a particular patient group (eg, obese patients) or for assessing a particular function (eg, activities of daily living or symptoms). These instruments have the advantage of helping in the understanding of the impact of a disease and its treatment on dimensions of quality of life but have the disadvantage of limited comparison of interventions across patient groups. In the fairly sparse literature addressing quality of life and obesity, both generic (such as the SF-36 or the Sickness Impact Profile) and disease-specific instruments [such as the Impact of Weight on Quality of Life (IWQOL) or the Obesity-related Problem (OP) Scale]) have been used.

The IWQOL questionnaire was developed and is being tested by Kolotkin and colleagues[13] at Duke University's Diet and Fitness Center. Aims of their work include developing a questionnaire that reliably and validly will measure the extent to which weight affects quality of life, determine the aspects of quality of life most affected by weight, and measure improvements in quality of life associated with treatment. In the development of the IWQOL questionnaire, morbidly obese patients enrolled in a university-based weight-loss program were asked in clinical interviews and group discussions to describe the effects of being overweight in their everyday life. From these responses, 74 items were created and divided into eight scales: health, social/interpersonal, work, mobility, self-esteem, sexual life, activities of daily living, and comfort with food. A five-point Likert-type scale is used for scoring individual items. Except for the comfort with food scale, the higher the score, the poorer the quality of life in that area.

Preliminary reports support the clinical utility of the IWQOL questionnaire for assessing problems of living associated with weight and for measuring treatment outcomes. Findings reported to date indicate that scores worsen as size increases, women experience a greater impact than men, and the impact of weight on quality of life lessens with age. It is important to recognize that the sample studied to date typically is white, upper-middle class to upper-class, morbidly obese individuals treated in a unique treatment environment. Work is ongoing to study comparison groups such as minority groups, obese persons who are not in treatment, persons with obesity who are enrolled in a community weight control program instead of a university health center–sponsored program, individuals who are not obese, and individuals with eating disorders to achieve broader clinical and research applicability and increased generalization of the IWQOL.

The Swedish Obese Subjects (SOS)[14] Study has both a registry component and an intervention component. The main objective of the registry study is to define health-related quality of life characteristics in the severely obese and to identify predictors of these characteristics. The intervention study addresses quality of life after surgical treatment for obesity. Both generic and disease-specific measures are used in this study. Generic instruments include the General Health Rating Index (Swedish version), the Mood Adjective Check List (short form), the Hospital Anxiety and Depression Scale (Swedish version), and the Sickness Impact Profile (Swedish version). An eight-item disease-specific instrument, the Obesity-related Problem (OP) Scale, was modified from a cancer survivor's questionnaire. Items are scaled on a range of 0–3 in terms of how much they are bothered by their obesity and ask about such things as going to a restaurant, trying on and buying clothes, intimate relations with a partner, going to community activities, etc. Finally, body image is measured with a male or female series of drawings from lean to massively obese using a scale of 1–9 to indicate the drawing subjects feel best applies to them.

Findings to date include that both men and women who are severely obese report poorer current health, a less positive mood state, and more social dysfunction than the general population. Anxiety and depression scores were higher in women than in men. Comparisons with nonobese individuals suggest that differences between the severely obese and the nonobese populations may be underestimated.

The Technology Assessment Group in San Francisco[15] is testing a self-administered health-related quality of life instrument and an interviewer-administered health state preference instrument targeting the moderately obese. The health-related quality of life instrument contains 55 items with approximately two-thirds of the questionnaire consisting of the following existing, widely used measures: Center for Epidemiologic Studies Scale for Depression, the Fleming Self-Rating Scale, and the distress scale from the Medical Outcomes Study (wording modified to be weight specific). The remainder of the questionnaire contains original measures addressing issues relevant to obese individuals, such as work loss and productivity, and physical and social activities.

The Health State Preference (HSP) interview takes about 15 minutes and asks subjects to provide preference scores for their current health state, as well as three other hypothetical health states. Preliminary data support reliability and validity of both assessments, suggest that the questionnaire is responsive to changes in weight, and suggest that the instrument is able to detect many differences between normal weight and obese individuals. Further, the HSP values were quite low for the obese population indicating that obese individuals evaluate their current health state as undesirable.

In a focus group of eight moderately obese individuals enrolled in a weight-reduction program, we asked subjects to respond to the question "How does your weight affect your everyday life?" Participants' responses could be categorized into the following four groups: physical functioning, psychological functioning, social and role activities, and economic and/or vocational states. In the physical functioning category, respondents noted problems with energy and exercise, esophageal reflux, and pain. As noted by Fontaine and colleagues,[16] obese patients report a significant amount of pain, and the pain is perceived to have a debilitating effect on normal daily activities. In the psychological functioning category, respondents described a cycle of pain, depression, and weight gain as well as problems with self-image and self-esteem. Some of the participants said they hated to look at themselves, which is consistent with the writings of Louderback.[17] In his book titled *Fat Power: Whatever You Weigh is Right,* Louderback emphasizes that American society's message to the obese is fat is ugly (an aesthetic crime), fat is immoral (indulgent), fat is sick, and fat is unhealthy. Compensation for these messages led participants to buy larger clothes than necessary to hide their imperfections. In the category of social functioning and role activities, some participants described avoiding people and withdrawal from social activities. Others noted limitations in entertainment and travel opportunities because of narrow seats in theaters and on airplanes. In the final category of economic and/or vocational status, one young woman described the negative effect of her weight on parenting her young child as she chose to remain at home as much as possible. Others commented on the expense associated with buying larger clothing and diet foods.

Research Recommendation

A number of recommendations can be made for further research in quality of life and obesity and include the following.

1. Refine theoretical/conceptual models. As noted by Stewart,[18] conceptual/theoretical frameworks could help to clarify the distinction between what is quality of life and what contributes to quality of life as well as clarify terms such as health status, functional status, and quality of life, which often are used interchangeably.
2. Assess impact of moderate obesity on quality of life. As reported by Mathias and colleagues,[15] an important gap in the literature is research addressing those issues that are most relevant and important to moderately obese individuals.
3. Compare outcomes of different treatments. The work to date focuses primarily on surgical treatment for obesity. Further research is needed to compare the effects of different treatments (eg, dieting, exercise) on short- and long-term changes in quality of life dimensions.
4. Include pain as a variable because it has been found to be a prevalent problem in this population.
5. Attend to potential effects of culture on the impact of weight on quality of life. Brownell and Wadden[19] observe that culture shapes our perceptions of ideal body weight and configuration and that the aesthetic ideal in the United States has grown consistently leaner over several decades. As noted by Hutchinson,[20] it is important to recognize that an individual's perception of quality of life is conditioned by cultural norms and quality of life may have different dimensions among different groups of obese individuals.[21] Thus, it is important to learn the value an ethnic group places on quality of life dimensions. In addition, ethnic groups differ in the manner in which they respond to physical abnormalities and disabilities. Thus, obesity may not always be viewed as a negative attribute.

6. Focus on children and adolescents as the work here is very limited.
7. Because obesity is lived through interpretation, expectation, meaning, past experiences, and future intentions, we use novel data-gathering techniques such as narratives or stories to learn about quality of life in obese individuals. As described by Gordon and Paci,[22] narratives can be used to (1) improve theoretical understanding, as a means for understanding what is quality of life in the obese, how it is lived, and how it is evaluated; (2) generate quality of life outcomes that are closer to actual experience; (3) describe and evaluate the quality of life of particular individuals, groups, and subgroups; (4) identify and evaluate how narrative influences quality of life and reaction to therapy; (5) understand and interpret individual and group contexts of quality of life evaluations; and (6) contribute to the evaluation of medical technologies in clinical trials and clinical decisions for individuals.

References

1. Schipper H, Clinch JJ, Olweny LM. Quality of life studies: Definitions and conceptual issues. In: Spilker B, ed. *Quality of life and Pharmacoeconomics in Clinical Trials.* 2nd ed. Philadelphia, Pa: Lippencott-Raven; 1996:11–23.
2. Naughton MJ, Shumaker SA, Anderson RT, et al. Aspects of health related quality of life measurement: Tests and scales. In: Spilker B, ed. *Quality of Life and Pharmacoeconomics in Clinical Trials.* 2nd ed. Philadelphia, PA: Lippencott-Raven; 1996:117–131.
3. Atkinson RL. Proposed standards for judging the success of the treatment of obesity. *Ann Intern Med* 1993;119:677–680.
4. Cleary PD, Greenfield S, Mulley AG, et al. Variations in length of stay and outcomes for six medical and surgical conditions in Massachusetts and California. *JAMA* 1991;266:73–79.
5. Wilson IB, Cleary PD. Linking clinical variables with health-related quality of life. A conceptual model of patient outcomes. *JAMA* 1995;273:59–65.
6. Mayou R, Bryant B. Quality of life in cardiovascular disease. *Br Heart J* 1993;69:460–466.
7. Testa MA, Simonson DC. Assesment of quality-of-life outcomes. *N Engl J Med* 1996;334:835–840.
8. Schipper H, Levitt M. Measuring quality of life: Risks and benefits. *Cancer Treat Rep* 1985;69:1115–1125.
9. Osoba D, Aaronson NK, Till JE. Practical guide for selecting quality-of-life measures in clinical trials and practice. In: Osoba D, ed. *Effect of Cancer on Quality of Life.* Boca Raton, Fla: CRC Press; 1991:89–104.
10. Wellisch DK. Methodology in behavioral and psychosocial cancer research. Work, social, recreation, family, and physical status. *Cancer* 1984; 53:2290–2302.

11. Sullivan MBE, Sullivan LGM, Kral JG. Quality of life assessment in obesity: Physical, psychological, and social function. *Gastroenterol Clin North Am* 1987;16:433–442.
12. Lydick EG, Epstein RS. Clinical significance of quality of life data. In: Spilker B, ed. *Quality of Life and Pharmacoeconomics in Clinical Trials*. 2nd ed. Philadelphia, Pa: Lippencott-Raven; 1996:461–465.
13. Kolotkin RL, Head S, Hamilton M, et al. Assessing impact of weight on quality of life. *Obes Res* 1995;3:49–56.
14. Sullivan M, Karlsson J, Sjostrom L, et al. Swedish obese subjects (SOS): An intervention study of obesity. Baseline evaluation of health and psychosocial functioning in the first 1743 subjects examined. *Int J Obes Relat Metab Disord* 1993;17:503–512.
15. Mathias SD, Williamson CL, Colwell HH, et al. Assessing health-related quality-of-life and health state preference in persons with obesity: A validation study. *Qual Life Res* 1997;6:311–622.
16. Fontaine KR, Cheskin LJ, Barofsky I. Health-related quality of life in obese persons seeking treatment. *J Fam Pract* 1996;43:265–270.
17. Louderback L. *Fat Power: Whatever You Weigh Is Right*. New York: Hawthorn Books; 1970.
18. Stewart A. Conceptual and methodologic issues in defining quality of life: State of the art. *Prog Cardiovasc Nurs* 1992;7:3–11.
19. Brownell KD, Wadden TA. Etiology and treatment of obesity: Understanding a serious, prevalent, and refractory disorder. *J Consult Clin Psychol* 1992;60:505–517.
20. Hutchinson JF. Quality of life in ethnic groups. In: Spilker B, ed. *Quality of Life and Pharmacoeconomics in Clinical Trials*. 2nd ed. Philadelphia, Pa: Lippencott-Raven; 1996:587–593.
21. Salio-Lahteenkorva S, Strunkard A, Rissanen A. Psychosocial factors and quality of life in obesity. *Int J Obes* 1995;19:1S–5S.
22. Gordon DR, Paci E. Narrative and quality of life. In: Spilker B, ed. *Quality of Life and Pharmacoeconomics in Clinical Trials*. 2nd ed. Philadelphia: Lippencott-Raven; 1996:387–395.

Chapter 21

Economic Impact of Obesity and its Cardiovascular Sequelae in Managed Care Settings

Kathy McManus, MS, RD

Introduction

Obesity is a major risk factor for a number of chronic diseases, including cardiovascular disease (CVD) and diabetes mellitus. Obesity and overweight also exacerbate many chronic conditions (eg, dyslipidemia and hypertension).[1–3]

Over one-third of US adults are overweight and the prevalence of overweight people has increased steadily over the past 20 years.[4] The prevalence of people who are overweight and obese in the United States ranks among the highest in the world.[5] National surveys in the United States have shown a marked increase in the prevalence of obesity over time. Between 1960 and 1980, there only was a slight increase in overweight people. However, between 1980 and 1994 a striking increase in the prevalence of people who are overweight occurred.[5] This increase was seen for all age groups, for both men and women, and for non-Hispanic whites, non-Hispanic blacks, and Mexican Americans. The magnitude of the increase was similar for all these groups. The US experience shows that a populationwide increase in the prevalence of overweight people may occur relatively quickly after a long period during which the prevalence of overweight people is fairly stable.

To date, the United States, the Netherlands, France, Sweden, and Australia have reported the estimated economic impact of obesity.

In the United States, a number of studies have examined the economic costs associated with obesity. Gorsky et al[6] used an

From: Fletcher GF, Grundy SM, Hayman LL (eds). *Obesity: Impact on Cardiovascular Disease*. Armonk, NY: Futura Publishing Co., Inc.; © 1999.

incidence-based model and determined the direct costs of a hypothetical cohort of 10 000 women, aged 40, followed over 25 years. Compared with the reference women who had a body mass index (BMI) < 25 kg/m^2, the economic impact of the moderately overweight women (BMI, 25–28.9 kg/m^2) was an additional $22 million. The health care costs for the obese women (BMI > 29 kg/m^2) were $53 million.[6] Extrapolating the costs to the US population, the authors estimated that the 25-year cost of obesity for women aged 40–64 years was approximately $16.1 billion or $4132 per individual for a woman with a BMI > 25 kg/m^2. The authors conclude that each woman who maintains a BMI of ≥ 25 kg/m^2 while she is between 40 and 65 years of age will accrue $4132 in excess costs for health care and medication, discounted at 3%.[6] These excess costs range from an average of $2229 for moderately overweight women to an average of $5325 for severely overweight women.[6] Successful weight-reduction programs that cost less than these amounts (in present dollars, during the same 25-year period) could be effective in reducing the total costs associated with overweight people.

Wolf and Colditz examined the cost associated with weight gain and obesity using different definitions of overweight (BMI, 25–29.9 kg/m^2).[7] Using a prevalence-based approach to the cost of illness, the authors estimated the economic costs in 1993 dollars associated with illnesses of different strata of BMI and varying increments of weight gain. They observed total direct costs of $5.89 billion attributed to a body weight that is considered healthy (BMI, 23–24.9 kg/m^2).[7] However, the direct costs continue to rise with increasing BMIs, reflecting the increased risk of disease even at a moderate BMI of 25 kg/m^2. When the direct costs by disease were examined, the authors concluded that the health risks of non–insulin-dependent diabetes mellitus (NIDDM) associated with body weight rose steadily with increasing BMI and have a significant economic effect at a BMI > 30 kg/m^2.[7] The economic effect of body weight for coronary heart disease (CHD) is significant at a BMI > 25 kg/m^2.[7] Wolf and Colditz conclude that total direct cost of illness attributable to body weight becomes economically significant at a BMI ≥ 25 kg/m^2.[7] They observed increased economic costs associated with adult weight gains as little as 5 kg, though the costs appear greatest at weight gains of 11–20 kg.[7]

Colditz reported the direct and indirect costs of obesity in 1986[8] and 1990[9] dollars for cardiovascular-related conditions, including non–insulin-dependent diabetes, CHD, and hypertension. More recently, Colditz and Wolf[10] have updated the estimates to 1995 dollars using more recent published estimates of the costs of several diseases. The authors used a prevalence-based approach to the cost of illness to estimate the economic costs in 1995 dollars attributed to obesity for

NIDDM; coronary disease; hypertension; gallbladder disease; breast, endometrial, and colon cancer; and osteoarthritis. Additionally and independently, excess physician visits, work-lost days, restricted activity, and bed days attributed to obesity were analyzed cross-sectionally using the 1988 and 1994 National Health Interview Survey (NHIS). For the purposes of this chapter, the economic impact of obesity will focus on the costs associated with diabetes mellitus, CVD, and hypertension.

In the most recent update of economic impact of obesity, Wolf and Colditz[10] categorized the burden of disease into two parts, direct medical costs and indirect morbidity and mortality costs. Direct costs were the costs of preventive, diagnosis, and treatment services related to the disease (eg, hospital and nursing home care, physician visits, and medications). The authors' current estimate does not include the cost of weight-loss programs or the cost people spend on over-the-counter weight-loss aids. Nor does the cost estimate include nonmedical estimates of obesity caused by transportation, food, and lodging when visiting the physician or hospital or caregiver time. Indirect costs were the value of lost output because of cessation or reduction of productivity caused by morbidity and mortality. Morbidity costs are the wages lost by people who are unable to work because of illness and disability. Mortality costs are the value of future earnings (translated into the current monetary value) lost by people who die prematurely.

To estimate the proportion of disease in a population that could have been prevented by eliminating obesity, the authors calculated the population attributable risk percent (PAR%), which was the maximum proportion of disease (eg, NIDDM and CHD) in the population that was attributable to a specific exposure (eg, obesity).[10] The PAR% was based on the incidence of disease in the exposed (ie, obese) as compared with the nonexposed group (ie, nonobese) using a method that controls for potential confounding factors (eg, age, smoking, dietary intake, and physical activity).[10] Obesity was defined as a BMI ≥ 29 kg/m^2. The PAR% was calculated using $P(RR - 1)/1 + P(RR - 1)$ where P was the prevalence of obesity in the study population and RR was the relative risk for contracting the disease comparing the obese with the lean subjects.[10] The PAR% was estimated using data from two large epidemiological studies, the Nurses Health Study and the Health Professionals Follow-Up Study, to assure for consistency in study methodology and definitions of obesity.

For NIDDM, the incidence increased with rising BMI.[11] The authors cite a recent report indicating 63.5% of the cases of NIDDM were diagnosed among women with BMI ≥ 29 kg/m^2.[12] Among these cases, 96.4% of NIDDM was attributable to obesity.[12] Thus 61% (0.635 ×

0.964) of the costs of NIDDM was attributable to obesity, $32.4 billion direct and $30.74 billion indirect in 1995 dollars.[10]

For CHD, Wolf and Colditz[13] estimated that 24% of CHD was diagnosed among women with BMI $\geq$ 29 kg/m^2 and that among the obese, 72% of CHD was attributed to obesity. Therefore, 17% (0.24 $\times$ 0.72) of the $40.4 billion direct cost of CHD was attributed to obesity; this amounted to $6.99 billion in 1995.[10] There is no updated direct cost estimate for CHD. The estimate for CHD is independent of stroke.

For hypertension, the authors cite data that estimate obese individuals have approximately 5–6 times greater risk of developing hypertension as compared with lean people.[14] The authors calculated 23% of the cases of hypertension were diagnosed with BMI $\geq$ 29 kg/m^2. Among the cases, 74% of hypertension was attributed to obesity.[15] Thus, 17% (0.23 $\times$ 0.74) of the costs of hypertension was attributable to obesity, with a direct health care cost attributable of $3.23 billion in 1995 dollars.[10]

Wolf and Colditz[10] concluded that the economic impact of obesity in the United States was approximately $99.2 billion in 1995. This included both direct and indirect costs of obesity for NIDDM, CHD, and hypertension in addition to gallbladder disease, osteoarthritis, and cancers. The direct medical costs of disease attributed to obesity was approximately $51.6 billion while the indirect costs (excluding CHD and hypertension) was $47.46 billion.[10] The direct costs associated with obesity represent 5.7% of the US health expenditure in 1995.[10] Approximately 63% of the direct costs associated with obesity are from NIDDM, 14% from CHD, and 6% from hypertension.[10]

Using the 1988 NHIS, Wolf and Colditz[10] also estimated the costs associated with productivity lost as a result of obesity and associated diseases. The annual number of work days lost was estimated by stratifying the population by age, gender, and the presence of obesity. In 1988, there was a total of 52 591 480 work days lost as a result of obesity-related disease, which amounted to indirect costs of approximately US $4 billion.[10] The authors noted that this amount slightly underestimated the actual indirect costs, because work days lost by individuals older than 64 were not included.

Obesity is not only a major economic drain in the United States, but Australia and a number of countries in Europe have reported economic costs associated with obesity. In European countries, obesity, defined as a BMI > 30 kg/m^2, is a common disorder prevalent in more than 10% of the adult male population and more than 15% in women.[16] The prevalence among women varies more than among men, and a particularly high prevalence has been found in women from Mediterranean countries and in women from eastern European countries.[16] If the definition of overweight is made somewhat broader (eg, BMI > 25 kg/m^2) at least one-half of adult Europeans can be considered overweight.[16] There also is evidence that the prevalence of obesity has been increasing over the last 15 years by 10%–40% in most countries.[17]

It seems that, in most countries, obesity is increasing in prevalence, although preliminary data from Denmark show that in the period of 1960–1980, the prevalence increased in men and decreased in women.[5] Subgroup analyses by sex, age, and educational level with regard to time trends yield different results in different countries. In some studies, the increase in the prevalence of obesity is most pronounced in young adults, whereas in others it is more pronounced in older subjects.[5] Usually, there is a greater increase in the prevalence of obesity in those with relatively low educational levels compared with those with higher education.

In The Netherlands, Jacob Seidell examined the age-adjusted odds ratios for being a user of diuretics and drugs for treatment of cardiovascular disorders in obese and overweight subjects in comparison with nonoverweight subjects. In examining the direct costs of obesity the same formula used by Wolf and Colditz for PAR, PAR = P(RR − 1)/(P(RR − 1) + 1), was used by Seidell.

HIS conducted from 1981 to 1989 that included 28 000 men and 30 000 women aged 20–65 years was the basis for the data. The direct cost associated with overweight and obesity included consultations with general practitioners, medical specialists, hospital admissions, and medications. These costs amounted to 1 billion Dutch guilders, which is equivalent to 4% of the total costs of health care (3% for overweight and 1% for obesity).[18] These data show that a significant proportion of health care costs can be attributed to excess weight. For comparison, the authors note all forms of cancer contribute to only 4.6% of health care costs in The Netherlands. Because of the high prevalence of people who are overweight, the contribution of people having BMIs between 25 and 30 kg/m^2 actually is larger than that of obesity (BMI > 30 kg/m^2).[18]

In France, Lévy et al[19] analyzed the economic impact of obesity using a prevalence-based approach identifying the costs incurred during a given year (1992) by obese subjects. Direct costs included personal health care, hospital care, physician's services, drugs, etc. The direct costs reflected the value of resources that could be allocated for alternative use if obesity was absent from the population. The direct medical costs represented the personal health care, hospital care, physician's services, and drugs. Indirect costs were the value of lost output as a result of cessation or reduction of productivity caused by morbidity and mortality. The definition of indirect costs is debated, especially in countries with a high level of unemployment. The measurement of the impact of morbidity and mortality on the total value of production is difficult because production is not affected simply by changes in the supply of labor. Nevertheless, Lévy et al[19] calculated "production losses" that appeared as a maximum figure, the minimum being put together by financial allocations from the Health Insurance System to those who are not attending work for obesity-related medical reasons.

In this study, only the diseases with well-established epidemiological relationships with obesity and that generated tangible monetary costs were considered. The list included NIDDM, hyperlipidemia, hypertension, CHD, stroke, venous thromboembolism, osteoarthritis of the knee, gallbladder disease, and cancer (colorectal, breast, and genitourinary tract).

Sources for the data were evaluated through a variety of means including ambulatory data from a survey called IMS Doreme, which reports annually on the number of consultations, visits, prescriptions of drugs, and laboratory investigations in France.[19] General practitioner services were factored by relevant average fees. Another panel provided information on drug prescriptions value in terms of producer prices. Hospital costs were derived from hospital morbidity data classified by the principal diagnosis (International Classification of Diseases, ICD9-CM). Sources were a survey conducted by the French Department of Health on the number and duration of stays for each disease for 1 year. The distribution of those stays between different categories of hospitals (public, private, and university) and between different disciplines were used.

Indirect costs were measured using data from the medical control department of electricity and gas on 150 000 wage earners.[19] On the basis of the mean daily wages for an active person the cost of total days lost in relation with all obesity-associated diseases was calculated. All costs are valued at their real prices, including the nonreimbursed part from the health insurance. All costs were expressed in 1992 French francs (US $1 = Fr5).

The direct costs of obesity (BMI $\geq$ 27kg/m^2) were Fr11.89 billion, which corresponded approximately to 2% of the expenses of the French care system.[19] Hypertension represented 33% of the total amount and cancer 2.5% of the direct costs of obesity.[19] Indirect costs represented Fr0.6 billion.[19]

In Sweden, Sjöström and colleagues[20] have reported on an ongoing nationwide intervention study of obesity, the Swedish Obese Subjects (SOS). The project consists of one Registry Study and one Intervention Study; 200 patients will be included in each group with a 10-year follow-up time. The SOS patients weigh 100–200 kg with an average of 120 kg; 90% of the males and 80% of the females have at least one cardiovascular risk factor.

Independent of age and gender, the annual number of sick-leave days is twice as high among the obese SOS patients as in the general Swedish population.[20] Similarly, the frequency of disability pensions approximately is doubled in obese subjects as compared with the general Swedish population.

In a situation with 100% employment, the authors estimate absence from work caused by obesity would be equivalent to a cost of 6 billion crowns during 1 year in Sweden or US $1 million per 10 000 inhabitants.[20] Six billion crowns corresponds to 7% of the total indirect costs of sick leave and disability pensions during 1 year.[20] However, the authors note Sweden does not have full employment but closer to 10% unemployment. Therefore, the net costs of obesity currently are lower than 6 billion crowns in the Swedish society.

The Australian Institute of Health and Welfare estimated that in 1989, 13 229 potential years of life were lost before age 65 (and 29 845 years were lost before age 75) as a result of death caused by obesity (BMI > 30 kg/m^2).[21] Segal et al[21] examined the direct health care costs resulting from obesity in Australia using a formal assessment of the cost of diet-related disease. The authors reported on comprehensive data on health care utilization and total health care costs and attribution of costs to disease as well as the epidemiology of disease. The authors used the same relative risks for selective diseases used by Colditz.[8]

The authors reported health service costs resulting from obesity from 1989 to 1990 in Australia were estimated at $A395 million.[21] Segal et al[21] noted that this amount was an underestimate, because approximately 15% of total health expenditure was not captured in the categories costed by the model and hospital expenditure did not include outpatients. Obesity accounted for 2% of total recurrent health expenditure in the disease categories investigated and amounts to $A25 per individual.

This summary of US, European, and Australian health economists has given us a fairly comprehensive picture of the economic costs of obesity. In 1994, Americans spent over $36 billion annually on weight-reduction products, which include both diet foods and drinks and other services.[22] Low-calorie soda and health clubs accounted for almost 70% or $25 billion of the Weight Control Field. Diet meals and appetite suppressants accounted for 14% or $5 billion, while exercise equipment accounted for 11% or $4 billion. Commercial weight-loss programs generated $2 billion a year in revenue and medically supervised weight-loss programs generated $600 million in revenue.

The staggering cost of obesity coupled with this expenditure of money by the US consumer would seem to emphasize the necessity to examine the advantages of early intervention to prevent disabilities and limit additional costs, which are a prime interest of managed care plans.

To assess the availability and costs of nutrition, weight loss, and exercise programs that may impact the incidence and treatment of obesity, a short survey was mailed to 16 Health Maintenance Organi-

---

Table 1.

Survey of Weight Reduction/Exercise Programs at HMOs

HMO: _____

DATE: _____

ADDRESS: _____

Please check any of the following weight reduction or exercise programs offered by your plan to members:

	YES	NO
● Nutrition counseling with a registered dietitian.	☐	☐
● Contract or commercial weight-loss programs, such as:		
Weight Watchers	☐	☐
Jenny Craig	☐	☐
Other: _____	☐	☐
Our Plan contributes to the initiation fee for the program.	☐	☐
If YES, what is the monetary contribution/ member? $_____		
Our Plan offers the program at a reduced cost.	☐	☐
If YES, what is the monetary contribution/ member? $_____		
● Exercise programs, such as:		
YWCA/YMCA:	☐	☐
Local gym:	☐	☐
Facilities at hospital/HMO site:	☐	☐
Other: _____	☐	☐
Our Plan contributes to the initiation fee for the program.	☐	☐
If YES, what is the monetary contribution/ member? $_____		
Our Plan offers membership at a reduced cost.	☐	☐
If YES, what is the monetary contribution/ member? $_____		
Other comments welcomed: _____		

Thank you for your cooperation. Please return in the stamped envelope. Information regarding your specific HMO will not be shared. Data identifying numbers and monies will be reported in general numbers only. Any questions, feel free to call at (617) 732-7494.

Please send me a copy of the summary   Yes ☐   No ☐

Kathy McManus, MS, RD

zations (HMOs) and Preferred Provider Organizations (PPOs) in Massachusetts (Table 1); 50% of the HMOs returned the survey with the following results: all eight (100%) of the HMOs/PPOs, offered nutrition counseling with a registered dietitian; one (13%) contracted with a commercial weight-loss program, while two plans (20%) supported members with their own "in-house" weight-loss programs. Thirty-eight percent offer a small contribution to either the initiation fee of the program or a contribution to reduce the cost of the program. The rates varied by plan from a 10% reduction in the initiation fee to a lump sum of $50 off the entire program. Seven of the plans (88%) offered exercise programs to their members, including the YWCA/YMCA, local gyms or fitness centers, or facilities at the HMO/PPO site. Eighty percent of the plans that offered exercise programs contributed money toward the initiation fee and/or reduction in membership costs. Again, this contribution varied widely depending on the plan, with some offering a $50 discount off the initiation fee while others offered members a 20% discount on the annual membership.

From this preliminary data, it appears that a number of HMOs and PPOs are offering small monetary contributions to encourage members to participate in nutrition and exercise programs. However, additional study is necessary to examine the efficacy and cost-effectiveness of these programs.

In light of the increasing prevalence and economic burden of overweight and obesity, it is clear that cost-effective programs are necessary. A number of goals should be considered to prevent unnecessary disease burden and the related health care costs. These include a two-prong approach, which addresses both prevention and treatment.

The prevention part of the approach includes the following:

- nutrition education in primary schools with integration into the general curriculum targeted at teachers and students,
- emphasis on individual physical education,
- community-based programs that encourage prevention through local-level initiatives for all ages and populations,
- encouragement and support for community groups that advocate healthy lifestyles through a variety of sites (eg, supermarkets, churches, and malls),
- physical activity programs that are easily accessible and are readily available to the public,
- systems to enhance early identification of high-risk individuals.

The treatment part of the approach includes the following:

- establishment of comprehensive, multidisciplinary, cost-effective programs that provide high-quality care while monitoring and reducing the cost of care;
- patient-centered service initiatives that will focus on and support long-term weight management and minimize attrition rates;
- development of national and state databases to track and measure outcome measures, which include long-term weight loss, improvement in obesity related comorbidities, and improvement in health practices;
- actively engaging in both clinical and basic research to enhance and support our knowledge of obesity.

In summary, the economic burden of obesity is a major contributor to health care costs. Our current health care system offers limited monetary support for the prevention and treatment of obesity. It appears that prevention and treatment of obesity can have a significant impact on health and potentially can reduce costs by saving a large portion of the health care dollar.

References

1. Pi-Sunyer FX. Medical hazards of obesity. *Ann Intern Med* 1993;119: 655–660.
2. Van Itallie TB. Obesity: Adverse effects on health and longevity. *Am J Clin Nutr* 1979;32:2723–2733.
3. Mann GV. The influence of obesity on health (first of two parts). *N Engl J Med* 1974;291:178–185.
4. Kuczmarski RJ, Flegal KM, Campbell SM, et al. Increasing prevalence of overweight among US adults. The National Health and Nutrition Examination Surveys, 1960 to 1991 [see comments]. *JAMA* 1994;272:205–211.
5. Seidell JC, Flegal KM. Assessing obesity: Classification and epidemiology. *Br Med Bull* 1997;53:238–252.
6. Gorsky RD, Pamuk E, Williamson DF, et al. The 25-year health care costs of women who remain overweight after 40 years of age. *Am J Prev Med* 1996;12:388–394.
7. Wolf AM, Colditz GA. Social and economic effects of body weight in the United States. *Am J Clin Nutr* 1996;63:466S–469S.
8. Colditz GA. Economic costs of obesity. *Am J Clin Nutr* 1992;55:503S–507S.
9. Wolf AM, Colditz GA. The cost of obesity: The US perspective. *Pharmacol Economics* 1994;5:34–37.
10. Wolf AM, Colditz GA. Current estimates of the economic cost of obesity in the United States [see comments]. *Obes Res* 1998;6:97–106.

11. Colditz GA, Willett WC, Rotnitzky A, et al. Weight gain as a risk factor for clinical diabetes mellitus in women [see comments]. *Ann Intern Med* 1995; 122:481–486.
12. Roy NF, Wills S, Thamer M, et al. *Direct and Indirect Costs of Diabetes in the US in 1992*. Alexandria, Va: American Diabetes Association; 1992.
13. Willett WC, Manson JE, Stampfer MJ, et al. Weight, weight change, and coronary heart disease in women. Risk within the "normal" weight range [see comments]. *JAMA* 1995;273:461–465.
14. Stamler R, Stamler J, Riedlinger WF, et al. Weight and blood pressure. Findings in hypertension screening of 1 million Americans. *JAMA* 1978; 240:1607–1610.
15. Witteman JC, Willett WC, Stampfer MJ, et al. A prospective study of nutritional factors and hypertension among US women. *Circulation* 1989; 80:1320–1327.
16. Seidell JC. Obesity in Europe: Prevalence and consequences for use of medical care. *Pharmacol Economics* 1994;5:38–44.
17. Seidell JC. Obesity in Europe. Scaling an epidemic. *Int J Obes Relat Metab Disord* 1995;19:S1–S4.
18. Seidell JC. The impact of obesity on health status: Some implications for health care costs. *Int J Obes Relat Metab Disord* 1995;19:S13–S16.
19. Levy E, Levy P, Le Pen C, et al. The economic cost of obesity: The French situation. *Int J Obes Relat Metab Disord* 1995;19:788–792.
20. Sjostrom L, Narbro K, Sjostrom D. Costs and benefits when treating obesity. *Int J Obes Relat Metab Disord* 1995;19:S9–S12.
21. Segal L, Carter R. The cost of obesity: An Australian perspective. *Pharmacol Economics* 1994;5:45–52.
22. Palmer J. Hey, Fatso. *Barron's* 1996;1996:25–29.

Summary

This book has addressed in depth the monumental problem of obesity and its impact on cardiovascular disease. The prevalence of obesity in childhood has been highlighted in context with genetic and environmental factors that influence the overweight state.

Specific sequela of obesity are discussed with emphasis on abdominal obesity and the metabolic syndrome. In addition the variable effects of obesity on blood lipids are included with discussions of hormonal interactions.

The important role of physical activity in long-term weight loss is well studied and these data are presented. It is clear that both exercise and diet provoke better long-term control of body weight.

Both compliance and behavioral modification are crucial in the process of losing weight. Impacts on quality of life relative to obesity must include psychological, social, and perception of health dimensions.

It is clear that if the current trend continues to the year 2020, 100% of Americans will be overweight. Health care costs, that is, lost wages, morbidity, and mortality, increase with body mass indices greater than 25. Therefore it is likely that long-term maintenance of weight loss will involve a public policy change.

Obesity must therefore be considered a major public health problem that is escalating rapidly to a pandemic level in the civilized world. There is emerging data to support both genetic and environmental influences for obesity and drugs and being developed to aid in its control. However, reduction of caloric intake and proper physical activity will always be the essential behavioral strategies needed to combat this enormous problem and its numerous medical sequela.

Gerald F. Fletcher, MD

From: Fletcher GF, Grundy SM, Hayman LL (eds). *Obesity: Impact on Cardiovascular Disease.* Armonk, NY: Futura Publishing Co., Inc.; © 1999.

Index

Page numbers followed by "t" indicate
tables.

367